Lecture Notes in Artificial Intelligence   3430

Edited by J. G. Carbonell and J. Siekmann

Subseries of Lecture Notes in Computer Science

W0114810

Shusaku Tsumoto   Takahira Yamaguchi
Masayuki Numao   Hiroshi Motoda (Eds.)

Active Mining

Second International Workshop, AM 2003
Maebashi, Japan, October 28, 2003
Revised Selected Papers

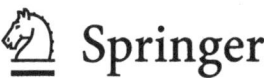 Springer

Series Editors

Jaime G. Carbonell, Carnegie Mellon University, Pittsburgh, PA, USA
Jörg Siekmann, University of Saarland, Saarbrücken, Germany

Volume Editors

Shusaku Tsumoto
Shimane University, School of Medicine
Department of Medical Informatics
89-1 Enya-cho, Izumo, Shimane 693-8501, Japan
E-mail: tsumoto@computer.org

Takahira Yamaguchi
Keio University, Faculty of Science and Technology
Department of Administration Engineering
3-14-1 Hiyoshi, Kohoku-ku, Yokohama, Kanagawa 223-8522, Japan
E-mail: yamaguti@ae.keio.ac.jp

Masayuki Numao
Osaka University, The Institute of Scientific and Industrial Research
Division of Intelligent Systems Science, Dept. of Architecture for Intelligence
8-1 Mihogaoka, Ibaraki, Osaka 567-0047, Japan
E-mail: numao@ai.sanken.osaka-u.ac.jp

Hiroshi Motoda
Osaka University, The Institute of Scientific and Industrial Research
Division of Intelligent Systems Science, Dept. of Advance Reasoning
8-1 Mihogaoka, Ibaraki, Osaka 567-0047, Japan
E-mail: motoda@ar.sanken.osaka-u.ac.jp

Library of Congress Control Number: 2005926624

CR Subject Classification (1998): H.2.8, I.2, F.2.2, J.3

ISSN   0302-9743
ISBN-10   3-540-26157-5 Springer Berlin Heidelberg New York
ISBN-13   978-3-540-26157-5 Springer Berlin Heidelberg New York

Springer is a part of Springer Science+Business Media

springeronline.com

© Springer-Verlag Berlin Heidelberg 2005
Printed in Germany

Typesetting: Camera-ready by author, data conversion by Scientific Publishing Services, Chennai, India
Printed on acid-free paper   SPIN: 11423270   06/3142   5 4 3 2 1 0

Foreword

This volume contains the papers selected for presentation at the 2nd International Workshop on Active Mining (AM 2003) which was organized in conjunction with the 14th International Symposium on Methodologies for Intelligent Systems (ISMIS 2003), held in Maebashi City, Japan, 28–31 October, 2003. The workshop was organized by the Maebashi Institute of Technology in cooperation with the Japanese Society for Artificial Intelligence. It was sponsored by the Maebashi Institute of Technology, the Maebashi Convention Bureau, the Maebashi City Government, the Gunma Prefecture Government, JSAI SIGKBS (Japanese Artificial Intelligence Society, Special Interest Group on Knowledge-Based Systems), a Grant-in-Aid for Scientific Research on Priority Areas (No. 759) "Implementation of Active Mining in the Era of Information Flood," US AFOSR/AOARD, the Web Intelligence Consortium (Japan), the Gunma Information Service Industry Association, and Ryomo Systems Co., Ltd.

ISMIS is a conference series that was started in 1986 in Knoxville, Tennessee. Since then it has been held in Charlotte (North Carolina), Knoxville (Tennessee), Turin (Italy), Trondheim (Norway), Warsaw (Poland), Zakopane (Poland), and Lyon (France).

The objective of this workshop was to gather researchers as well as practitioners who are working on various research fields of active mining, share hard-learned experiences, and shed light on the future development of active mining. This workshop addressed many aspects of active mining, ranging from theories, methodologies, and algorithms to their applications. We believe that it also produced a contemporary overview of modern solutions and it created a synergy among different branches but with a similar goal—facilitating data collection, processing, and knowledge discovery via active mining.

We express our appreciation to the sponsors of the symposium and to all who submitted papers for presentation and publication in the proceedings. Our sincere thanks especially go to the Organizing Committee of AM 2003: Shusaku Tsumoto, Hiroshi Motoda, Masayuki Numao, and Takahira Yamaguchi. Also, our thanks are due to Alfred Hofmann of Springer for his continuous support.

March 2005   Ning Zhong, Zbigniew W. Raś
                                                   ISMIS'03 Symposium Chairs

Preface

This volume contains the papers based on the tutorials of ISMIS 2003 and the papers selected from the regular papers presented at the 2nd International Workshop on Active Mining (AM 2003) held as part of ISMIS 2003, held at Maebashi, Gunma, October 28, 2003. (URL: http://www.med.shimane-u.ac.jp/med_info/am2003)

There were 38 paper submissions from Japan, US, Korea, China and Vietnam for AM 2003. Papers went through a rigorous reviewing process. Each paper was reviewed by at least three Program Committee members. When all the reviews of a paper were in conflict, another PC member was asked to review this paper again. Finally, 20 submissions were selected by the Program Committee members for presentation.

The PC members who attended this workshop reviewed all the papers and the presentations during the workshops and decided that 12 of them could be accepted with minor revisions, and 8 of them could be accepted with major revisions for the publication in the postproceedings. The authors were asked to submit the revised versions of their papers and, again, the PC members reviewed them for about four months. Through this process, we accepted 16 out of 20 papers. Thus, of 38 papers submitted, 16 were accepted for this postproceedings, corresponding to an acceptance ratio of only 42.1%.

AM 2003 provided a forum for exchanging ideas among many researchers in various areas of decision support, data mining, machine learning and information retrieval and served as a stimulus for mutual understanding and cooperation.

The papers contributed to this volume reflect advances in active mining as well as complementary research efforts in the following areas:

- Discovery of new information sources
- Active collection of information
- Tools for information collection
- Information filtering
- Information retrieval, collection, and integration on the WWW for data mining
- Data mining processes
- Inspection and validation of mined pieces of knowledge
- Description languages for discovery evaluation and accountability
- Interactive mining design and deployment of customer response models in CRM
- Adaptive modeling in data mining
- Selection, transformation, and construction of features
- Selection and construction of instances
- Exception/deviation discovery visualization
- Spatial data mining

- Text mining
- Graph mining
- Success/failure stories in data mining and lessons learned
- Data mining for evidence-based medicine
- Distributed data mining
- Data mining for knowledge management
- Active learning
- Meta learning
- Active sampling
- Usability of mined pieces of knowledge
- User interface for data mining

We wish to express our gratitude to Profs. Zbigniew W. Raś and Ning Zhong, who accepted our proposal on this workshop and helped us to publish the postproceedings. Without their sincere help, we could not have published this volume.

We wish to express our thanks to all the PC members, who reviewed the papers at least twice, for the workshop and the postproceedings. Without their contributions, we could not have selected high-quality papers with high confidence.

We also want to thank all the authors who submitted valuable papers to AM 2003 and all the workshop attendees.

This time, all the submissions and reviews were made through the CyberChair system (URL: http://www.cyberchair.org/). We wish to thank the Cyber-Chair system development team. Without this system, we could not have edited this volume in such a speedy way.

We also extend our special thanks to Dr. Shoji Hirano, who launched the CyberChair system for AM 2003 and contributed to editing this volume.

Finally, we wish to express our thanks to Alfred Hofmann at Springer for his support and cooperation.

March 2005

Shusaku Tsumoto
Takahira Yamaguchi
Masayuki Numao
Hiroshi Motoda

AM 2003 Conference Committee

Organizing Committee

Hiroshi Motoda (Osaka University, Japan)
Masayuki Numao (Osaka University, Japan)
Takahira Yamaguchi (Keio University, Japan)
Shusaku Tsumoto (Shimane University, Japan)

Program Committee

Hiroki Arimura (Hokkaido University, Japan)
Stephen D. Bay (Stanford University, USA)
Wesley Chu (UCLA, USA)
Saso Dzeroski (Jozef Stefan Institute, Slovenia)
Shoji Hirano (Shimane University, Japan)
Tu Bao Ho (JAIST, Japan)
Robert H.P. Engels (CognIT, Norway)
Ryutaro Ichise (NII, Japan)
Akihiro Inokuchi (IBM Japan, Japan)
Hiroyuki Kawano (Nanzan University, Japan)
Yasuhiko Kitamura (Kwansei Gakuin University, Japan)
Marzena Kryszkiewicz (Warsaw University of Technology, Poland)
T.Y. Lin (San Jose State University, USA)
Bing Liu (University of Illinois at Chicago, USA)
Huan Liu (Arizona State University, USA)
Tsuyoshi Murata (NII, Japan)
Masayuki Numao (Osaka University, Japan)
Miho Ohsaki (Doshisha University, Japan)
Takashi Onoda (CRIPEI, Japan)
Luc de Raedt (University of Freiburg, Germany)
Zbigniew Raś (University of North Carolina, USA)
Henryk Rybinski (Warsaw University of Technology)
Masashi Shimbo (NAIST, Japan)
Einoshin Suzuki (Yokohama National University, Japan)
Masahiro Terabe (MRI, Japan)
Ljupico Todorovski (Jozef Stefan Institute, Slovenia)
Seiji Yamada (NII, Japan)
Yiyu Yao (University of Regina, Canada)
Kenichi Yoshida (University of Tsukuba, Japan)
Tetsuya Yoshida (Hokkaido University, Japan)
Stefan Wrobel (University of Magdeburg, Germany)
Ning Zhong (Maebashi Institute of Techonology, Japan)

Table of Contents

Overview

Active Mining Project: Overview
Shusaku Tsumoto, Takahira Yamaguchi, Masayuki Numao,
Hiroshi Motoda   1

Tutorial Papers

Computational and Statistical Methods in Bioinformatics
Tatsuya Akutsu   11

Indexing and Mining Audiovisual Data
Pierre Morizet-Mahoudeaux, Bruno Bachimont   34

Active Information Collection

Relevance Feedback Document Retrieval Using Support Vector
Machines
Takashi Onoda, Hiroshi Murata, Seiji Yamada   59

Micro View and Macro View Approaches to Discovered Rule Filtering
Yasuhiko Kitamura, Akira Iida, Keunsik Park   74

Mining Chemical Compound Structure Data Using Inductive Logic
Programming
Cholwich Nattee, Sukree Sinthupinyo, Masayuki Numao,
Takashi Okada   92

First-Order Rule Mining by Using Graphs Created from Temporal
Medical Data
Ryutaro Ichise, Masayuki Numao   112

Active Data Mining

Extracting Diagnostic Knowledge from Hepatitis Dataset by Decision
Tree Graph-Based Induction
Warodom Geamsakul, Tetsuya Yoshida, Kouzou Ohara,
Hiroshi Motoda, Takashi Washio, Hideto Yokoi,
Katsuhiko Takabayashi   126

Data Mining Oriented CRM Systems Based on MUSASHI: C-MUSASHI
Katsutoshi Yada, Yukinobu Hamuro, Naoki Katoh, Takashi Washio,
Issey Fusamoto, Daisuke Fujishima, Takaya Ikeda 152

Investigation of Rule Interestingness in Medical Data Mining
Miho Ohsaki, Shinya Kitaguchi, Hideto Yokoi, Takahira Yamaguchi .. 174

Experimental Evaluation of Time-Series Decision Tree
Yuu Yamada, Einoshin Suzuki, Hideto Yokoi,
Katsuhiko Takabayashi 190

Spiral Multi-aspect Hepatitis Data Mining
Muneaki Ohshima, Tomohiro Okuno, Yasuo Fujita, Ning Zhong,
Juzhen Dong, Hideto Yokoi 210

Sentence Role Identification in Medline Abstracts: Training Classifier
with Structured Abstracts
Masashi Shimbo, Takahiro Yamasaki, Yuji Matsumoto 236

$CHASE_2$ – Rule Based Chase Algorithm for Information Systems of
Type λ
Agnieszka Dardzińska, Zbigniew W. Raś 255

Active User Reaction

Empirical Comparison of Clustering Methods for Long Time-Series
Databases
Shoji Hirano, Shusaku Tsumoto 268

Spiral Mining Using Attributes from 3D Molecular Structures
Takashi Okada, Masumi Yamakawa, Hirotaka Niitsuma 287

Classification of Pharmacological Activity of Drugs Using Support
Vector Machine
Yoshimasa Takahashi, Katsumi Nishikoori, Satoshi Fujishima 303

Cooperative Scenario Mining from Blood Test Data of Hepatitis B and C
Yukio Ohsawa, Hajime Fujie, Akio Saiura, Naoaki Okazaki,
Naohiro Matsumura 312

Integrated Mining for Cancer Incidence Factors from Healthcare Data
Xiaolong Zhang, Tetsuo Narita 336

Author Index 349

Active Mining Project: Overview

Shusaku Tsumoto[1], Takahira Yamaguchi[2],
Masayuki Numao[3], and Hiroshi Motoda[3]

[1]Department of Medical Informatics, Faculty of Medicine, Shimane University,
89-1 Enya-cho, Izumo 693-8501, Japan
tsumoto@computer.org
http://www.med.shimane-u.ac.jp/med_info/tsumoto
[2] Faculty of Science and Technology, Keio University
yamaguti@ae.keio.ac.jp
http://www.yamaguti.comp.ae.keio.ac.jp/
[3] The Institute of Scientific and Industrial Research, Osaka University
numao@ai.sanken.osaka-u.ac.jp
motoda@ar.sanken.osaka-u.ac.jp

Abstract. Active mining is a new direction in the knowledge discovery
process for real-world applications handling various kinds of data with
actual user need. Our ability to collect data, be it in business, government, science, and perhaps personal, has been increasing at a dramatic
rate, which we call "information flood". However, our ability to analyze
and understand massive data lags far behind our ability to collect them.
The value of data is no longer in "how much of it we have". Rather, the
value is in how quickly and effectively can the data be reduced, explored,
manipulated and managed. For this purpose, Knowledge Discovery and
Data mining (KDD) emerges as a technique that extracts implicit, previously unknown, and potentially useful information (or patterns) from
data. However, recent extensive studies and real world applications show
that the following requirements are indispensable to overcome information flood: (1) identifying and collecting the relevant data from a huge
information search space (active information collection), (2) mining useful knowledge from different forms of massive data efficiently and effectively (user-centered active data mining), and (3) promptly reacting to
situation changes and giving necessary feedback to both data collection
and mining steps (active user reaction). Active mining is proposed as
a solution to these requirements, which collectively achieves the various
mining need. By "collectively achieving" we mean that the total effect
outperforms the simple add-sum effect that each individual effort can
bring.

1   What Is Active Mining?

Data Mining is a fundamental tool for network-based society, which enables us
to discover useful knowledge hidden in a large scale of data. However, under the
environment in which our ability to collect data is increasing at a dramatic rate,

S. Tsumoto et al. (Eds.): AM 2003, LNAI 3430, pp. 1–10, 2005.

called "information flood", we can observe the following three serious problems to be solved: (1) identification and collection of the relevant data from a huge information search space, (2) mining useful knowledge from different forms of massive data efficiently and effectively, and (3) promptly reacting to situation changes and giving necessary feedback to both data collection and mining steps. Due to these problems, all the organizations cannot be efficient without a sophisticated framework for data analysis cycle dealing with data collection, data analysis and user reaction.

Active mining is proposed as a solution to these requirements, which collectively achieves the various mining need. By "collectively achieving" we mean that the total effect outperforms the simple add-sum effect that each individual effort can bring. Especially, a active mining framework proposes a "spiral model" of knowledge discovery rather than Fayyad's KDD process [1] and focuses on the feedback from domain experts in the cycle of data analysis (data mining).

In order to validate this framework, we have focused on common medical and chemical datasets and developed techniques to realize this spiral model. As a result, we have discovered knowledge unexpected to domain experts, whose results are included in this postproceedings.

2   Objectives of Active Mining Project

Corresponding to the above three major problems, we have set up the following three subgoals: (1) active information collection, where relevant data and information are autonomously identified and collected from a huge information space. (2) user-centered active data mining, where users flexibly mine useful knowledge from different forms of massive data, such as temporal medical data or chemical structure data. (3) active user reaction, where sophisticated presentation of mining results evokes experts' active feedback to data mining.

The main goal of this project is not only to achieve these subgoals, but also to develop the environment of strong collaborations with these subareas(Fig. 1).

Medical and Chemical Datasets are selected for application of active mining spiral model. Especially, all the project members except for chemical domain experts challenges medical data mining (hepatitis data) and validated this proposed model, which integrated the above three subprocess.

The practice of the spiral model has obtained interesting discovered results with evidence from hospital data, including knowledge about estimation of the degree of liver fibrosis from laboratory data, classification of temporal patterns. These results enables us to give a new non-invasive method evaluating liver function in place of invasive liver biopsy. This process can be viewed as a new approach of data-engineering methodologies to Evidence-Based Medicine (EBM), which is paid attention as a guideline to medicine in 21st century.

Concerning chemical domain, we investigate the possibility of acquiring a new risk report of newly developed chemical agents from datasets on the correspondence between bioactivities and partial chemical structure of chemicals.

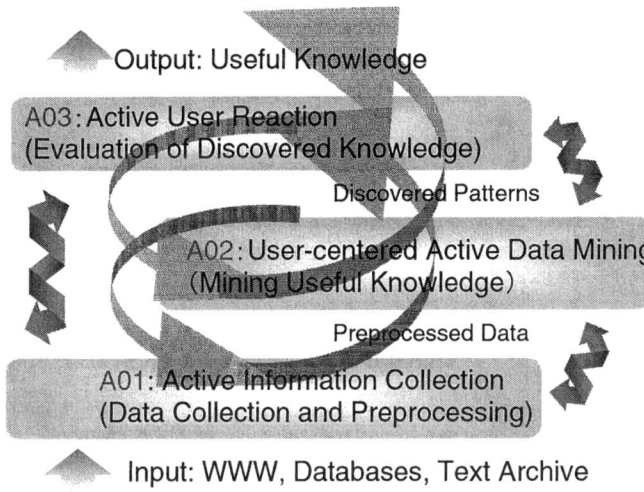

Fig. 1. Active Mining Project(Spiral Model)

3 Organization of Active Mining Project

This project was accepted as a national project in the Grant-in-Aid for Scientific Research on Priority Areas (No.759) "Implementation of Active Mining in the Era of Information Flood" by the Ministry of Education, Science, Culture, Sports, Science and Technology of Japan from September 2001 to March 2005.

The project leader was Hiroshi Motoda, who organized three teams corresponding to the above three goals: active information collection, user-centered active data mining, and active user reaction. Each team consists of three, four and three research groups, respectively. The organization of each team and group are given as follows.

1. A01 Team: Active Information Collection (Leader: Masayuki Numao)
    (a) A01-02: Seiji Yamada: Acquiring Meta Information Resource in the World Wide Web
    (b) A01-03: Yasuhiko Kitamura: Active Information Gathering from Distributed Dynamic Information Sources
    (c) A01-04: Masayuki Numao: Data gathering and automated preprocessing by a multiple learning method
2. A02 Team: User-centered Active Data Mining (Leader: Takahira Yamaguchi)
    (a) A02-05: Hiroshi Motoda: Active Mining for Structured Data
    (b) A02-06: Takahira Yamaguchi: Active Mining based on Meta Learning Scheme
    (c) A02-07: Einoshin Suzuki: Spiral Active-Mining based on Exception Discovery

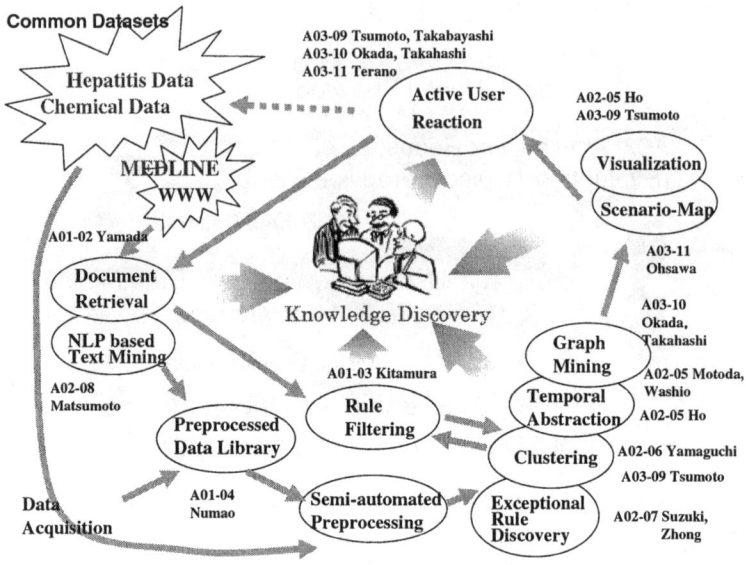

Fig. 2. Collaboration Map of Research Groups

   (d) A02-08: Yuji Matsumoto: Goal-oriented Knowledge Extraction from Sci-
        entific Text
3. A03 Team: Active User Reaction (Leader: Shusaku Tsumoto)
   (a) A03-09: Shusaku Tsumoto: Development of the Active Mining System
        in Medicine based on Rough Sets
   (b) A03-10: Takashi Okada: Discovery of Risk Molecules from Chemicals by
        Active Mining
   (c) A03-11: Yukio Ohsawa: Evaluation and Selection of Knowledge based on
        Human System Interactions

As discussed in Section 2, the main goal of this project is not only to achieve
these subgoals, but also to develop the environment of strong collaborations with
these subareas. To achieve the latter goal, we organized more than 40 face to
face meetings and workshops with domain experts every several months, where
all the project members grasp the progress of other research groups and discuss
their technical problems together. Furthermore, domain experts who donated
the datasets evaluated the results presented in the meeting. Fig. 2 illustrates
these collaborations between each research group.

In parallel with those common medical and chemical data analysis, many
studies related with active mining were reported and useful discussions were
made during the meetings. Therefore, mining common medical and chemical
datasets play a central role not only in practicing a spiral model of knowledge
discovery but also in collaboration with domain experts and each research group.
Furthermore, Internet strengthened such collaborations, complementing the interval between face to face meetings. In total, each research group focused on

each research goal, but could experience the total process of active mining due
to these meetings.

4   Main Results: Summary

This active mining have produced the following interesting elemental technologies to achieve the above research goal.

1. Active Information Collection
   - (a) Automated Learning of Meta Information Resources
   - (b) Relevance Feedback Document Retrieval
   - (c) Efficient Information Gathering from Distributed Information Sources
   - (d) Micro View and Macro View Approaches to Discovered Rule Filtering
   - (e) Automated Acquisition of Preprocessing Procedures
2. Usr-centered Active Data Mining
   - (a) Decision Tree Graph-Based Induction
   - (b) Temporal Abstraction
   - (c) Data Mining oriented CRM system
   - (d) Comprehensive Approach to Rule Interestingness Measures
   - (e) Rule Mining based on Meta-Learning Scheme
   - (f) Decision Tree Learning for Time-series Data
   - (g) Peculiarity Rule Mining
   - (h) Spiral Multi-aspect Data Mining
   - (i) Clustering of Long Temporal Sequences (Multi-Scale Matching)
3. Active User Reaction
   - (a) Visualization of Rule Similarities
   - (b) Visualization of Clustering
   - (c) Detection of Homogeneity/Inhomogeneity of Temporal Sequences
   - (d) Cascade Model
   - (e) Analysis of Topological Fragment Spectra (Support Vector Machine)
   - (f) Double Helical Model of Chance Discovery
   - (g) Key-graph based User Reaction (Human System Interaction)
   - (h) Scenario Mapping

5   In This Volume

This volume gives selection of the best papers presented at the Second International Workshop on Active Mining (AM2003), which includes papers from
research groups in Active Mining Project, but also from other data miners. This
section categorizes the papers from the project into three subgoals and summarizes those papers and contributions to our research goals.

5.1   Active Information Collection

Relevance Feedback Document Retrieval Using Support Vector Machines [2]. The
following data mining problems from the document retrieval were investigated:
From a large data set of documents, we need to find documents that relate

to human interest as few iterations of human testing or checking as possible. In each iteration a comparatively small batch of documents is evaluated for relating to the human interest. They apply active learning techniques based on Support Vector Machine for evaluating successive batches, which is called relevance feedback. The proposed approach has been very useful for document retrieval with relevance feedback experimentally.

Micro View and Macro View Approaches to Discovered Rule Filtering [3]. The authors try to develop a discovered rule filtering method to filter rules discovered by a data mining system to be novel and reasonable ones by using information retrieval technique. In this method, they rank discovered rules according to the results of information retrieval from an information source on the Internet. The paper shows two approaches toward discovered rule filtering; the micro view approach and the macro view approach. The micro view approach tries to retrieve and show documents directly related to discovered rules. On the other hand, the macro view approach tries to show the trend of research activities related to discovered rules by using the results of information retrieval. They discuss advantages and disadvantages of the micro view approach and feasibility of the macro view approach by using an example of clinical data mining and MEDLINE document retrieval.

5.2   User-Centered Active Data Mining

Extracting Diagnostic Knowledge from Hepatitis Dataset by Decision Tree Graph-Based Induction [4]. The authors have proposed a method called Decision Tree Graph- Based Induction (DT-GBI), which constructs a classifier (decision tree) for graph-structured data while simultaneously constructing attributes for classification. Graph-Based Induction (GBI) is utilized in DT-GBI for efficiently extracting typical patterns from graph-structured data by stepwise pair expansion (pairwise chunking). Attributes, i.e., substructures useful for classification task, are constructed by GBI on the fly while constructing a decision tree in DT-GBI.

Data Mining Oriented CRM Systems Based on MUSASHI: C-MUSASHI [5]. MUSASHI is a set of commands which enables us to efficiently execute various types of data manipulations in a flexible manner, mainly aiming at data processing of huge amount of data required for data mining. Data format which MUSASHI can deal with is either an XML table written in XML or plain text file with table structure. In this paper we shall present a business application system of MUSASHI, called C-MUSASHI, dedicated to CRM oriented systems. Integrating a large amount of customer purchase histories in XML databases with the marketing tools and data mining technology based on MUSASHI, C-MUSASHI offers various basic tools for customer analysis and store management based on which data mining oriented CRM systems can be developed at extremely low cost.We apply C-MUSASHI to supermarkets and drugstores in Japan to discover useful knowledge for their market- ing strategy and present possibility to construct useful CRM systems at extremely low cost by introducing MUSASHI.

Investigation of Rule Interestingness in Medical Data Mining [6]. This research experimentally investigates the performance of conventional rule interestingness measures and discusses their usefulness for supporting KDD through human-system interaction in medical domain. We compared the evaluation results by a medical expert and those by selected sixteen kinds of interestingness measures for the rules discovered in a dataset on hepatitis. χ^2 measure, recall, and accuracy demonstrated the highest performance, and specificity and prevalence did the lowest. The interestingness measures showed a complementary relationship for each other. These results indicated that some interestingness measures have the possibility to predict really interesting rules at a certain level and that the combinational use of interestingness measures will be useful.

Experimental Evaluation of Time-Series Decision Tree [7]. The authors give experimental evaluation of our time-series decision tree induction method under various conditions. Their time-series tree has a value (i.e. a time sequence) of a time-series attribute in its internal node, and splits examples based on dissimilarity between a pair of time sequences. The method selects, for a split test, a time sequence which exists in data by exhaustive search based on class and shape information. It has been empirically observed that the method induces accurate and comprehensive decision trees in time-series classification, which has gaining increasing attention due to its importance in various real-world applications. The evaluation has revealed several important findings including interaction between a split test and its measure of goodness.

Spiral Multi-Aspect Hepatitis Data Mining [8]. When therapy using IFN (interferon) medication for chronic hepatitis patients, various conceptual knowledge/rules will benefit for giving a treatment. The paper describes our work on cooperatively using various data mining agents including the GDT-RS inductive learning system for discovering decision rules, the LOI (learning with ordered information) for discovering ordering rules and important features, as well as the POM (peculiarity oriented mining) for finding peculiarity data/rules, in a spiral discovery process with multi-phase such as pre-processing, rule mining, and post-processing, for multi-aspect analysis of the hepatitis data and meta learning. Their methodology and experimental results show that the perspective of medical doctors will be changed from a single type of experimental data analysis towards a holistic view, by using our *multi-aspect mining* approach.

Sentence Role Identification in Medline Abstracts: Training Classifier with Structured Abstracts [9]. The abstract of a scientific paper typically consists of sentences describing the background of study, its objective, experimental method and results, and conclusions. The authors discuss the task of identifying which of these "structural roles" each sentence in abstracts plays, with a particular focus on its application in building a literature retrieval system. By annotating sentences in an abstract collection with role labels, we can build a literature retrieval system in which users can specify the roles of the sentences in which query terms should be sought. They argue that this facility enables more goal-oriented search, and also makes it easier to narrow down search results when adding extra query terms does not work.

5.3   Active User Reaction

Empirical Comparison of Clustering Methods for Long Time-Series Databases [10]. This paper reports empirical comparison of both time-series comparison methods and clustering methods. First, the authors examined basic characteristics of two sequence comparison methods, multiscale matching (MSM) and dynamic time warping (DTW), using a simple sine wave and its variants. Next, they examined the characteristics of various combinations of sequence comparison methods and clustering methods in terms of interpretability of generating clusters, using a time-series medical database. The results demonstrated that (1) shape representation parameters in MSM could capture the structural feature of time series; (2) However, the dissimilarity induced by MSM lacks linearity compared with DTW. It was also demonstrated that (1) combination of DTW and complete-linkage-AHC constantly produced interpretable results, (2) combination of DTW and RC would be used to find core sequences of the clusters.

Spiral Mining Using Attributes from 3D Molecular Structures [11]. Active responses from analysts play an essential role in obtaining insights into structure activity relationships (SAR) from drug data. Experts often think of hypotheses, and they want to reflect these ideas in the attribute generation and selection process. The authors analyzed the SAR of dopamine agonists and antagonists using the cascade model. The presence or absence of linear fragments in molecules constitutes the core attribute in the mining. In this paper, the authors generated attributes indicating the presence of hydrogen bonds from 3D coordinates of molecules. Various improvements in the fragment expressions are also introduced following the suggestions of chemists. Attribute selection from the generated fragments is another key step in mining. Close interactions between chemists and system developers have enabled spiral mining, in which the analysis results are incorporated into the development of new functions in the mining system. All these factors are necessary for success in SAR mining.

Classification of Pharmacological Activity of Drugs Using Support Vector Machine [12]. The authors investigated an applicability of Support Vector Machine (SVM) to classify of pharmacological activities of drugs. The numerical description of each drug's chemical structure was based on the Topological Fragment Spectra (TFS) proposed by the authors. 1,227 Dopamine antagonists that interact with different types of receptors (D1, D2, D3 and D4) were used for training SVM. For a prediction set of 137 drugs not included in the training set, the obtained SVM classified 123 (89.8 %) drugs into their own activity classes correctly. The comparison between using SVM and artificial neural network will also be discussed.

Mining Chemical Compound Structure Data Using Inductive Logic Programming [13]. The authors apply Inductive Logic Programming (ILP) for classifying chemical compounds. ILP provides comprehensibility to learning results and capability to handle more complex data consisting of their relations. Nevertheless, the bottleneck for learning first-order theory is enormous hypothesis search space which causes inefficient performance by the existing learning approaches compared to the propositional approaches. The authors introduces an improved ILP approach capable of handling more efficiently a kind of data called multiple-part data, i.e., one instance of data consists of several parts as well as relations among parts. The approach tries to find hypothesis describing class of each training example by using both individual and relational characteristics of its part which is similar to finding common substructures among the complex relational instances.

Cooperative Scenario Mining from Blood Test Data of Hepatitis B and C [14]. Chance discovery, to discover events significant for making a decision, can be regarded as the emergence of a scenario with extracting events at the turning points of valuable scenarios, by means of communications exchanging scenarios in the mind of participants. The authors apply a method of chance discovery to the data of diagnosis of hepatitis patients, for obtaining scenarios of how the most essential symptoms appear in the patients of hepatitis of type B and C. In the process of discovery, the results are evaluated to be novel and potentially useful for treatment, under the mixture of objective facts and the subjective focus of the hepatologists' concerns. Hints of the relation between f iron metabolism and hepatitis cure, the effective condition for using interferon, etc. has got visualized.

Acknowledgment

This work was supported by the Grant-in-Aid for Scientific Research on Priority Areas (No.759) "Implementation of Active Mining in the Era of Information Flood" by the Ministry of Education, Science, Culture, Sports, Science and Technology of Japan.

References

1. Fayyad, U., Piatetsky-Shapiro, G., Smyth, P.: The kdd process for extracting useful knowledge from volumes of data. CACM **29** (1996) 27–34
2. Onoda, T., Murata, H., Yamada, S.: Relevance feedback document retrieval using support vector machines. In Tsumoto, S., Yamaguchi, T., Numao, M., Motoda, H., eds.: Active Mining. Volume 3430 of Lecture Notes in Artificial Intelligence, Berlin, Springer (2005) 59–73
3. Kitamura, Y., Iida, A., Park, K.: Micro view and macro view approaches to discovered rule filtering. In Tsumoto, S., Yamaguchi, T., Numao, M., Motoda, H., eds.: Active Mining. Volume 3430 of Lecture Notes in Artificial Intelligence, Berlin, Springer (2005) 74–91
4. Geamsakul, W., Yoshida, T., Ohara, K., Motoda, H., Washio, T., Yokoi, H., Katsuhiko, T.: Extracting diagnostic knowledge from hepatitis dataset by decision tree graph-based induction. In Tsumoto, S., Yamaguchi, T., Numao, M., Motoda, H., eds.: Active Mining. Volume 3430 of Lecture Notes in Artificial Intelligence, Berlin, Springer (2005) 128–154

5. Yada, K., Hamuro, Y., Katoh, N., Washio, T., Fusamoto, I., Fujishima, D., Ikeda, T.: Data mining oriented crm systems based on musashi: C-musashi. In Tsumoto, S., Yamaguchi, T., Numao, M., Motoda, H., eds.: Active Mining. Volume 3430 of Lecture Notes in Artificial Intelligence, Berlin, Springer (2005) 155–176
6. Ohsaki, M., Kitaguchi, S., Yokoi, H., Yamaguchi, T.: Investigation of rule interestingness in medical data mining. In Tsumoto, S., Yamaguchi, T., Numao, M., Motoda, H., eds.: Active Mining. Volume 3430 of Lecture Notes in Artificial Intelligence, Berlin, Springer (2005) 177–193
7. Yamada, Y., Suzuki, E., Yokoi, H., Takabayashi, K.: Experimental evaluation of time-series decision tree. In Tsumoto, S., Yamaguchi, T., Numao, M., Motoda, H., eds.: Active Mining. Volume 3430 of Lecture Notes in Artificial Intelligence, Berlin, Springer (2005) 194–214
8. Ohshima, M., Okuno, T., Fujita, Y., Zhong, N., Dong, J., Yokoi, H.: Spiral multi-aspect hepatitis data mining. In Tsumoto, S., Yamaguchi, T., Numao, M., Motoda, H., eds.: Active Mining. Volume 3430 of Lecture Notes in Artificial Intelligence, Berlin, Springer (2005) 215–241
9. Shimbo, M., Yamasaki, T., Matsumoto, Y.: Sentence role identification in medline abstracts: Training classifier with structured abstracts. In Tsumoto, S., Yamaguchi, T., Numao, M., Motoda, H., eds.: Active Mining. Volume 3430 of Lecture Notes in Artificial Intelligence, Berlin, Springer (2005) 242–261
10. Hirano, S., Tsumoto, S.: Empirical comparison of clustering methods for long time-series databases. In Tsumoto, S., Yamaguchi, T., Numao, M., Motoda, H., eds.: Active Mining. Volume 3430 of Lecture Notes in Artificial Intelligence, Berlin, Springer (2005) 275–294
11. Okada, T., Yamakawa, M., Niitsuma, H.: Spiral mining using attributes from 3d molecular structures. In Tsumoto, S., Yamaguchi, T., Numao, M., Motoda, H., eds.: Active Mining. Volume 3430 of Lecture Notes in Artificial Intelligence, Berlin, Springer (2005) 295–310
12. Takahashi, Y., Nishikoori, K., Fujishima, S.: Classification of pharmacological activity of drugs using support vector machine. In Tsumoto, S., Yamaguchi, T., Numao, M., Motoda, H., eds.: Active Mining. Volume 3430 of Lecture Notes in Artificial Intelligence, Berlin, Springer (2005) 311–320
13. Nattee, C., Sinthupinyo, S., Numao, M., Okada, T.: Mining chemical compound structure data using inductive logic programming. In Tsumoto, S., Yamaguchi, T., Numao, M., Motoda, H., eds.: Active Mining. Volume 3430 of Lecture Notes in Artificial Intelligence, Berlin, Springer (2005) 92–113
14. Ohsawa, Y., Fujie, H., Saiura, A., Okazaki, N., Matsumura, N.: Cooperative scenario mining from blood test data of hepatitis b and c. In Tsumoto, S., Yamaguchi, T., Numao, M., Motoda, H., eds.: Active Mining. Volume 3430 of Lecture Notes in Artificial Intelligence, Berlin, Springer (2005) 321–344

Computational and Statistical Methods in Bioinformatics

Tatsuya Akutsu[*]

Bioinformatics Center, Institute for Chemical Research, Kyoto University,
Uji-city, Kyoto 611-0011, Japan
takutsu@kuicr.kyoto-u.ac.jp

Abstract. Many computational and statistical methods have been developed and applied in bioinformatics. Recently, new approaches based on support vector machines have been developed. Support vector machines provide a way of combining computational methods and statistical methods. After overviewing fundamental computational and statistical methods in bioinformatics, this paper surveys how these methods are used with support vector machines in order to analyze biological sequence data. This paper also overviews a method to handle chemical structures using support vector machines.

1 Introduction

Due to progress of high throughput experimental technology, complete genome sequences of many organisms have been determined. However, it is unclear how organisms are controlled by genome sequences. Therefore, it is important to decipher meanings of genomes and genes. Though many experimental technologies have been developed for that purpose, it is also important to develop information technologies for analyzing genomic sequence data and related data (e.g., protein structures, gene expression patterns) because huge amount of data are being produced. One of major goals of *bioinformatics* (and almost equivalently, *computational biology*) is to develop methods and software tools for supporting such analysis.

In this paper, we overview computational and statistical methods developed in bioinformatics. Since bioinformatics has become a very wide area, it is difficult to make comprehensive survey. Thus, we focus on a recent and important topic: *kernel methods in bioinformatics*. Though kernel methods can be used in several ways, the most studied way is with the *support vector machine* (SVM) [5, 6], where SVM is a kind of machine learning algorithms and is based on statistical learning theory. SVMs provide a good way to combine computational methods with statistical methods. We shows how computational and statistical methods are combined using SVMs in bioinformatics. It is worthy to note that we do not intend to give comprehensive survey on SVMs in bioinformatics. Instead,

---

[*] This paper is based on a tutorial at ISMIS 2003 conference.

S. Tsumoto et al. (Eds.): AM 2003, LNAI 3430, pp. 11–33, 2005.

we focus on SVMs for analyzing biological sequence data and chemical structure data, and try to explain these in a self-contained manner so that readers not familiar with bioinformatics (but familiar with computer science) can understand the ideas and methods without reading other papers or books.

Organization of this paper is as follows. First, we overview sequence alignment, which is used to compare and search similar biological sequences. Sequence alignment is one of the most fundamental and important computational methods in bioinformatics. Next, we overview computational methods for discovery of common patterns from sequences with common properties. Then, we overview the *Hidden Markov Model* (HMM) and its applications to bioinformatics, where HMM is a statistical model for generating sequences. Though HMMs were originally developed in other fields such as statistics and speech recognition, these have been successfully applied to bioinformatics since early 1990's. Then, we overview the main topic of this paper: recent development of kernel methods in bioinformatics. In particular, we focus on kernel functions for measuring similarities between biological sequences because designing good kernel functions is a key issue for applying SVMs to analysis of biological sequences. We also overview the marginalized graph kernel, which can be used for comparing chemical structures. It should be noted that chemical structures are also important in organisms and understanding of interaction between chemical structures and proteins of one of key issues in bioinformatics. Finally, we conclude with other applications of kernel methods in bioinformatics.

2   Sequence Alignment

Sequence alignment is a fundamental and important problem in bioinformatics and is used to compare two or multiple sequences [7, 26, 31]. Sequence alignment is classified into two categories: *pairwise sequence alignment* and *multiple sequence alignment*.

First, we briefly review pairwise sequence alignment. Let $\mathcal{A}$ be the set of nucleic acids or the set of amino acids (i.e., $|\mathcal{A}| = 4$ or $|\mathcal{A}| = 20$). For each sequence s over $\mathcal{A}$, $|s|$ denotes the length of s and $s[i]$ denotes the i-th letter of s (i.e., $s = s[1]s[2]\ldots s[n]$ if $|s| = n$). Then, a *global alignment* between sequences s and t is obtained by inserting gap symbols (denoted by '-') into or at either end of s and t such that the resulting sequences s' and t' are of the length l, where it is not allowed for each $i \leq l$ that both $s'[i]$ and $t'[i]$ are gap symbols.

Score matrix $f(a, b)$ is a function from $\mathcal{A}' \times \mathcal{A}'$ to the set of reals, where $\mathcal{A}' = \mathcal{A} \cup \{-\}$. We reasonably assume $f(a, b) = f(b, a)$ and $f(a, -) = f(-, b) = -d$ ($d > 0$) for all $a, b \in \mathcal{A}$, $f(-, -) = 0$ and $f(a, a) > 0$ for all $a \in \mathcal{A}$. Then, the score of alignment (s', t') is defined by

$$score(s', t') = \sum_{i=1}^{l} f(s'[i], t'[i]).$$

A *local alignment* between s and t is an alignment between $\hat{s}$ and $\hat{t}$, where $\hat{s}$ and $\hat{t}$ are substrings of s and t, respectively. An *optimal alignment* (resp. an *optimal local alignment*) is an alignment (resp. a local alignment) having the largest score. For example, consider sequences ACAGTGTCCT, GTTAGTC-TAAC Then, the followings are examples of global alignments.

M1	M2	M3
-ACAGTGTCCT	-ACAGTGTC-CT	--ACAGT-G-TC--CT-
GTTAGTCTAAC	GTTAGTCTAAC-	GT-TA-GTCT-AAC---

If we define $f(x,x) = 1$ and $f(x,-) = f(-,x) = -1$ for $x \in \mathcal{A}$, $f(x,y) = -1$ for $x \neq y$, and $f(-,-) = 0$, the score of both M1 and M2 is -3, and the score of M3 is -15. In this case, both M1 and M2 are optimal alignments.

The followings are examples of local alignments for the same input sequences.

M4	M5	M6	M7
AGT	AGTGT	AGT-GT--C	ACAGTGT---
AGT	AGTCT	AGTC-TAAC	--AGTCTAAC

If we use the same score function as above, the scores of M4, M5, M6 and M7 are 3, 3, 1 and -2, respectively. In this case, both M4 and M5 are optimal local alignments.

It is well known that an optimal alignment for two sequences can be computed in $O(mn)$ time using a simple *dynamic programming* algorithm [7], where $m = |s|$ and $n = |t|$. The following procedure is the core part of the algorithm:

$$F[i][0] = i \cdot -d, \qquad F[0][j] = j \cdot -d,$$
$$F[i][j] = \max(\ F[i-1][j] - d,\ F[i][j-1] - d,\ F[i-1][j-1] + f(s[i],t[j])\ ),$$

where $F[i][j]$ corresponds to the optimal score between $s[1\ldots i]$ and $t[1\ldots j]$, where $s[i\ldots j]$ denotes $s[i]s[i+1]\ldots s[j]$. An optimal alignment can be obtained from this matrix by using the *traceback* technique [7]. In order to compute the score of an optimal local alignment, it is enough to modify the above procedure into

$$F[i][0] = 0, \qquad F[0][j] = 0,$$
$$F[i][j] = \max(\ 0,\quad F[i-1][j] - d,\ F[i][j-1] - d,\ F[i-1][j-1] + f(s[i],t[j])\ ),$$

and to find $\max_{i,j} F[i][j]$. An optimal local alignment can also be obtained from this matrix. The algorithm for computing local alignment is also known as the Smith-Waterman algorithm.

In the above, we assumed that gap penalty per symbol is constant. However, several schemes have been proposed for gap penalty. Among them, *afine gap cost* is most widely used [7, 26]. It gives high penalty $(-d)$ for the first gap symbol in each consecutive gap region and low penalty $(-e)$ for each of the remaining gap symbols. For example, the score of alignment M7 is

$$-d - e + f(A,A) + f(G,G) + f(T,T) + f(G,C) + f(T,T) - d - 2e,$$

where $-d - e$ is assigned to the first gap region and $-d - 2e$ is assigned to the second gap region. Both global and local alignments can be computed in

$O(mn)$ time using dynamic programming procedures even if this afine gap cost is employed [7]. The Smith-Waterman algorithm with afine gap cost is most widely used for comparing two sequences.

The above dynamic programming algorithms are fast enough to compare two sequences. But, in the case of *homology search* (search for similar sequences), pairwise alignment between the query sequence and all sequences in the database should be performed. Since more than several hundreds thousands of sequences are usually stored in the database, simple application of pairwise alignment would take a lot of time. Therefore, several heuristic methods have been proposed for fast homology search, among which FASTA and BLAST are widely used [26]. Most of heuristic methods employ the following strategy: candidate sequences having fragments (short length substrings) which are the same as (or very similar to) a fragment of the query sequence are first searched and then pairwise alignments are computed using these fragments as anchors. Using these methods, homology search against several hundreds thousands sequences can be done in several seconds.

Next, we briefly review multiple sequence alignment. In this case, more than two sequences are given. Let $s_1, s_2, \ldots, s_h$ be input sequences. As in pairwise alignment, an alignment for $s_1, s_2, \ldots, s_h$ is obtained by inserting gap symbols into or at either end of s_i such that the resulting sequences $s'_1, s'_2, \ldots, s'_h$ are of the same length l. For example, consider three sequences AGCCAGTG, GCCGTGG, AGAGAGG, Then, the followings are examples of alignments.

M8	M9	M10
AGCCAGTG-	AGCCAGT-G	AGCCAGT-G-
-GCC-GTGG	-GCC-GTGG	-GCC-GT-GG
AG--AGAGG	AG--AGAGG	-AGA-G-AGG

Though there are various scoring schemes for multiple alignment, *SP-score* (Sum-of-Pairs score) is simple and widely used. SP-score is defined by

$$score(s'_1, \cdots, s'_h) = \sum_{1 \le p < q \le h} \sum_{i=1}^{l} f(s'_p[i], s'_q[i]).$$

Using the score function defined before, the score of both M8 and M9 is 3, and the score of M10 is -5. In this case, both M8 and M9 are optimal alignments.

The dynamic programming technique for pairwise alignment can be extended for multiple alignment. But, it is not practical because it takes $O(2^h \cdot n^h)$ time [7], where n is the maximum length of input sequences. Indeed, multiple alignment is known to be NP-hard if h is a part of an input (i.e., h is not fixed) [36]. Thus, a variety of heuristic methods have been applied to multiple alignment, which include simulated annealing, evolutionary computation, iterative improvement, branch-and-bound search, and stochastic methods [7, 29].

Among them, *progressive strategy* is widely used [7, 34]. In this strategy, we need alignment between two profiles, where a profile corresponds to a result of alignment. Alignment between profiles can be computed in a similar way as in

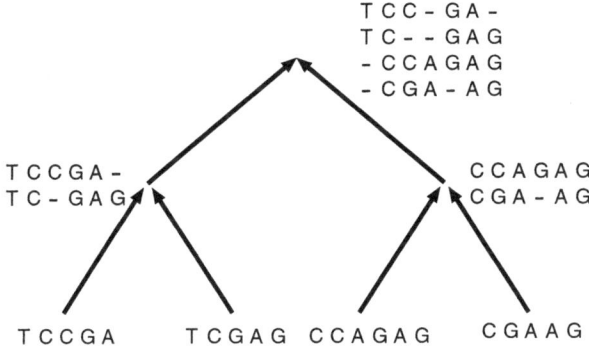

Fig. 1. Progressive alignment

pairwise alignment. An outline of the progressive strategy used in CLUSTAL-W [34] (the most widely used software for multiple sequence alignment) is as follows (see also Fig. 1):

(i) Construct a distance matrix for all pairs of sequences by pairwise sequence alignment, followed by conversion of alignment scores into distances using an appropriate method.
(ii) Construct a rooted tree whose leaves correspond to input sequences, using a method for phylogenetic tree construction.
(iii) Progressively perform sequence-sequence, sequence-profile and profile-profile alignment at nodes in order of decreasing similarity.

Though we have assumed that score functions were given, derivation of score functions is also important. Score functions are usually derived by taking log-ratios of frequencies [11]. However, some other methods have been proposed for optimizing score functions [12, 14].

3   Discovery of Common Patterns from Sequences

Discovering common string patterns from multiple sequences is important in bioinformatics because sequences with a common function have a common sequence pattern in many cases. Such a pattern is called a *motif* (precisely, a sequence motif) [4, 18]. Though there are various ways of defining motif patterns, these can be classified into *deterministic patterns* and *probabilistic patterns* [4].

Deterministic patterns are usually described using syntax like regular expressions. For example, "A-x(3,5)-[CT]" is a pattern matching any sequence containing a substring starting with A, followed by between three and five arbitrary symbols, followed by C or T. Though discovery of deterministic patterns is computational hard (NP-hard) in general, various machine learning techniques have been applied [4].

profile

	w(x,1)	w(x,2)	w(x,3)
A	2.2	2.8	-2.1
C	3.2	-2.5	-1.7
G	-1.5	0.2	3.5
T	0.5	3.3	3.1

threshold: $\theta = 9.0$

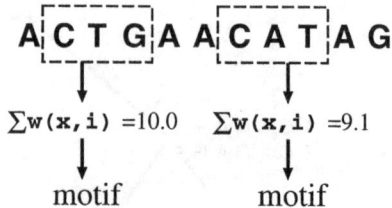

Fig. 2. Motif detection using profile

Probabilistic patterns are represented using statistical models. For example, *profiles* (also called as *weight matrices*, or *position specific score matrices*) and HMMs are widely used [7]. Here, we introduce profiles. A profile is a function $w(x, j)$ from $\mathcal{A} \times [1 \ldots L]$ to $\mathcal{R}$, where L denotes the length of subsequences corresponding to a motif, and $[1 \ldots L]$ denotes the set of integers between 1 and L. It should be noted in this case that the length of motif regions (i.e., subsequence corresponding to a motif) must be the same and gaps are not allowed in the motif regions. A profile can be represented by a two-dimensional matrix of size $L \cdot |\mathcal{A}|$. A subsequence $s[i \ldots i+L-1]$ of s is regarded as a motif if $\sum_{j=1,\ldots,L} w(s[i+j-1], j)$ is greater than a threshold θ.

Various methods have been proposed in order to derive a profile from sequences $s_1, s_2, \ldots, s_h$ having a common function. For example, algorithms based on the EM (*Expectation Maximization*) method [1] and Gibbs sampling [18] have been widely used.

4   Hidden Markov Model

The hidden Markov model was originally developed in the areas of statistics and speech recognition. In early 1990's, HMMs were applied to analysis of DNA/protein sequences. After that, HMMs and variants were applied to solving various problems in bioinformatics. Here, we briefly review HMM and its application to bioinformatics. Readers interested in more details may refer to [7].

An HMM is defined by quadruplet $(\mathcal{A}, Q, A.E)$, where $\mathcal{A}$ is an alphabet (a set of symbols), $Q = \{q_0, \ldots, q_m\}$ is a set of states, $A = (a_{kl})$ is an $(m+1) \times (m+1)$ matrix of state transition probabilities, and $E = (e_k(b))$ is an $(m+1) \times |\mathcal{A}|$ matrix of emission probabilities. Precisely, a_{kl} denotes the transition probability from state q_k to q_l, and $e_k(b)$ denotes the probability that a symbol b is emitted at state q_k. Θ denotes the collection of parameters of an HMM (i.e., $\Theta = (A, E)$), where we assume that $\mathcal{A}$ and Q are fixed.

A *path* $\pi = \pi[1] \ldots \pi[n]$ is a sequence of (indices of) states. The probability that both π and a sequence $s = s[1] \ldots s[n]$ over $\mathcal{A}$ are generated under Θ is defined by

$$P(s, \pi | \Theta) = \prod_{i=1}^{n} a_{\pi[i-1]\pi[i]} e_{\pi[i]}(s[i]),$$

where $\pi[0] = 0$ is introduced as a fictitious state, a_{0k} denotes the probability that the initial state is q_k, and $a_{k0} = 0$ for all k.

There are three important algorithms for utilizing HMMs: *Viterbi algorithm*, *Forward/Backward algorithm* and *Baum-Welch algorithm*. The Viterbi algorithm computes the most plausible path for a given sequence. Precisely, it computes $\pi^*(s)$ defined by

$$\pi^*(s) = \arg\max_{\pi} P(s, \pi | \Theta)$$

when sequence s is given. This path can be computed using dynamic programming as in pairwise sequence alignment. Let $c_k(i)$ be the probability of the most probable path for prefix $s[1 \ldots i]$ of s that ends with state q_k. The following is the core part of the Viterbi algorithm:

$$c_k(i) = e_k(s[i]) \cdot \max_{q_l \in Q}\{c_l(i-1) \cdot a_{lk}\}.$$

It is not difficult to see that the Viterbi algorithm works in $O(nm^2)$ time. Once $c_k(i)$'s are computed, $\pi^*(s)$ can be obtained using the traceback technique as in sequence alignment.

The Forward algorithm computes the probability that a given sequence is generated. It computes

$$P(s|\Theta) = \sum_{\pi} P(s, \pi | \Theta)$$

when sequence s is given. This probability can also be computed using dynamic programming. Let $f_k(i)$ be the probability of emitting prefix $s[1 \ldots i]$ of s and reaching the state q_k. Then, the following is the core part of the Forward algorithm:

$$f_k(i) = e_k(s[i]) \cdot \sum_{q_l \in Q} f_l(i-1) \cdot a_{lk}.$$

It should be noted that the only difference between the Forward algorithm and the Viterbi algorithm is that 'max' in the Viterbi algorithm is replaced with 'Σ' in the Forward algorithm.

Here, we define the backward probability $b_k(i)$ as the probability of being at state q_k and emitting the suffix $s[i+1 \ldots n]$ of s. Then, the following is the core part of the Backward algorithm:

$$b_k(i) = \sum_{q_l \in Q} e_l(s[i+1]) \cdot b_l(i+1) \cdot a_{kl}.$$

Using $f_k(i)$ and $b_k(i)$, we can compute the probability that an HMM takes state q_k at i-th step (i.e., just after emitting $s[i]$) is given by

$$P(q_{\pi[i]} = q_k | s) = \frac{P(s, q_{\pi[i]} = q_k)}{P(s)} = \frac{f_k(i) \cdot b_k(i)}{\sum_{q_k \in Q} f_k(|s|)}.$$

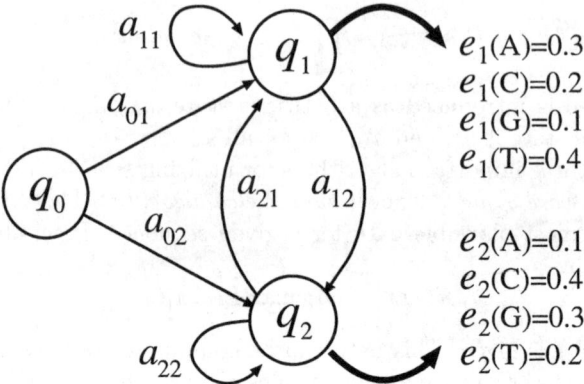

Fig. 3. Example of HMM

This $P(q_{\pi[i]} = q_k|s)$ is to be used in computing the marginalized count kernel (see Section 5.5).

Fig. 3 shows an example of HMM. Suppose that $a_{kl} = 0.5$ for all k, l ($l \neq 0$). Then, for sequence $s =$ATCGCT, we have $\pi^*(s) = 0112221$ and $P(s, \pi^*|\Theta) = 0.5^6 \cdot 0.4^4 \cdot 0.3^2$.

We assumed in both algorithms that Θ was fixed. However, it is sometimes required to train HMMs from sample data. The Baum-Welch algorithm is used to estimate Θ when a set of sequences is given. Suppose that a set of h sequences $\{s_1, \ldots, s_h\}$ is given. The likelihood of observing these h sequences is defined to be $\prod_{j=1}^{h} P(s_j|\Theta)$ for each Θ. Then, it is reasonable to estimate Θ by using the maximum likelihood method. That is, the goal is to find an optimal set of parameters Θ^* defined by

$$\Theta^* = \arg\max_{\Theta} \prod_{j=1}^{h} P(s_j|\Theta).$$

However, it is computationally difficult to find an optimal set of parameters. Therefore, various heuristic methods have been proposed for finding a locally optimal set of parameters. Among them, the Baum-Welch algorithm is most widely used. It is a kind of EM algorithms and computes a locally optimal set of parameters using the following iterative improvement procedure.

Suppose that we have an initial set of parameters Θ for a_{kl} and $e_k(b)$. Let A_{kl} be the number of transitions from state q_k to state q_l and $E_k(b)$ be the number of times that b is emitted from state q_k when a set of sequences $\{s_1, \ldots, s_h\}$ is given. Then, A_{kl} and $E_k(b)$ can be computed as

$$A_{kl} = \sum_{j=1}^{h} \frac{1}{P(s_j|\Theta)} \sum_{i} f_k^j(i) \cdot a_{kl} \cdot e_l(s_j[i+1]) \cdot b_l^j(i+1),$$

$$E_k(b) = \sum_{j=1}^{h} \frac{1}{P(s_j|\Theta)} \sum_{i|s_j[i]=b} f_k^j(i) b_k^j(i),$$

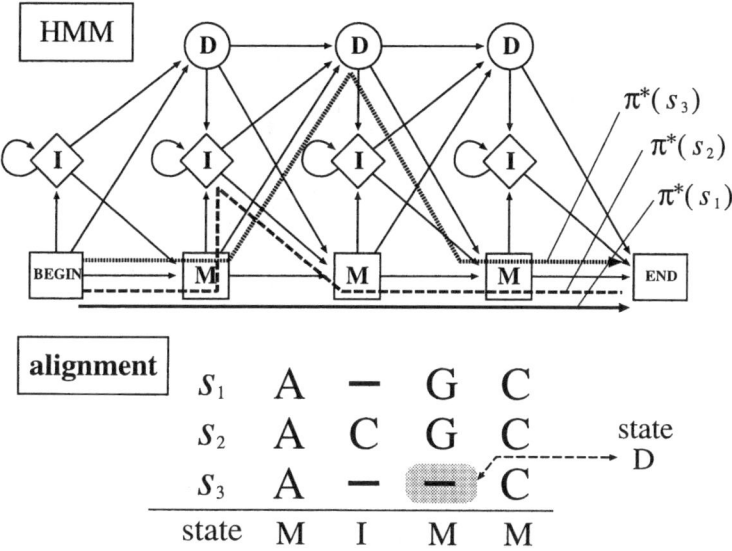

Fig. 4. Computation of multiple alignment using profile HMM

where $f_k^j(i)$ and $b_k^j(i)$ denote $f_k(i)$ and $b_k(i)$ for sequence s_j respectively. Then, we can obtain a new set of parameters $\hat{a}_{kl}$ and $\hat{e}_k(b)$ by

$$\hat{a}_{kl} = \frac{A_{kl}}{\sum_{q_{l'} \in Q} A_{kl'}}, \quad \hat{e}_k(b) = \frac{E_k(b)}{\sum_{b' \in \mathcal{A}} E_k(b')}.$$

It is proved that this iterative procedure does not decrease the likelihood [7].

HMMs are applied to bioinformatics in various ways. One common way is the use of *profile HMMs*. Recall that a profile is a function $w(x, j)$ from $\mathcal{A} \times [1 \ldots L]$ to $\mathcal{R}$, where L denotes the length of a motif region. Given a sequence s, the score for s was defined by $\sum_{j=1,\ldots,L} w(s[j], j)$. Though profiles are useful to detect short motifs, these are not so useful to detect long motifs or remote homologs (sequences having weak similarities) because insertions or deletions are not allowed. A profile HMM is considered to be an extension of a profile such that insertions and deletions are allowed.

A profile HMM has a special architecture as shown in Fig. 4. The states are classified into three types: *match states, insertion states* and *deletion states*. A match state corresponds to one position in a profile. A symbol b is emitted from a match state q_i according to probability $e_i(b)$. A symbol b is emitted with probability $P(b)$ from any insertion state q_i, where $P(b)$ is the background frequency of occurrence of the symbol b. No symbol is emitted from any deletion state. Using a profile HMM, we can also obtain multiple alignment of sequences by combining $\pi^*(s_j)$ for all input sequences s_j. Though alignments obtained by profile HMMs are not necessarily optimal, these are meaningful from a biological viewpoint [7].

Using profile HMMs, we can classify sequences. Though there are various criteria for sequence classification, one of well-known criteria is classification

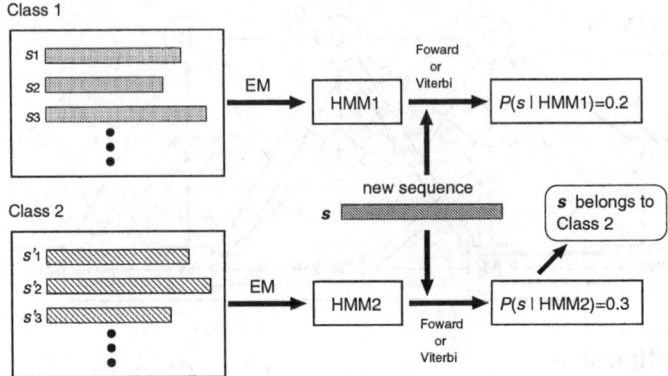

Fig. 5. Classification of protein sequences using profile HMMs. In this case, a new sequence s is predicted to belong to Class 2 because the score for HMM2 is greater than that for HMM1

based on similarities among three-dimensional structures of proteins that are coded by amino acid sequences. Usually experimental determination of protein structures are much more difficult than experimental determination of amino acid sequences. Therefore, extensive studies have been done for *protein structure prediction* (i.e., inference of three-dimensional structures) from amino acid sequences [22, 25]. One approach for protein structure prediction is *remote homology* detection, which is a problem of finding weak similarities between protein sequences. This approach is useful because it is recognized that similar sequences have similar structures in most cases.

There already exist databases, which classify known protein structures in terms of structural similarity. The most famous one is the SCOP database [28]. In the SCOP database, protein structures are classified in a hierarchical way. Proteins are first classified into classes, then are classified into folds, then into superfamilies, and finally into families. Once this database is constructed, we can consider the following problem: given a sequence whose structure is unknown, infer to which superfamily (resp. fold) the sequence belongs. This problem is called *superfamily recognition* (resp. *fold recognition*). Since recognition of classes is not so informative and recognition of families can be done well by using the Smith-Waterman algorithm, most of existing studies have been focusing on superfamily recognition and fold recognition. Since sequences in a superfamily are considered to have some homology, superfamily recognition is considered as a remote homology detection problem.

We can apply profile HMMs to classification of protein sequences (e.g., superfamily recognition). Let $C_1, \ldots, C_N$ be the classes. For each of C_i, we construct an HMM H_i and train H_i by using the Baum-Welch algorithm and the sequences in class C_i. Then, given a new sequence s, we compute the score $P(s|H_i)$ for each H_i, where $P(s|H_i)$ denotes the probability that s is generated from H_i. Then, we infer that s belongs to class C_i for which $P(s|H_i)$ is the highest (see Fig. 5).

Though only HMM and profile HMM are explained in this section, a lot of variants and extensions of HMMs have also been developed and applied to various problems in bioinformatics. For example, a special kind of HMMs have been applied to finding gene-coding regions in DNA sequences and stochastic context-free grammar (an extension of HMM) have been applied to prediction of RNA secondary structures [7].

5   String Kernel

Support vector machines (SVMs) have been widely applied to various problems in artificial intelligence, pattern recognition and bioinformatics since the SVM was proposed by Cortes and Vapnik in 1990's [5]. In this section, we overview methods for applying SVMs to classification of biological sequences. In particular, we overview *kernel functions* (to be explained below) for biological sequences.

5.1   Support Vector Machine and Kernel Function

SVMs are basically used for binary classification. Let POS and NEG be the sets of *positive examples* and *negative examples* in a training set, where each example is represented as a point in d-dimensional Euclidean space. Then, an SVM finds a hyperplane h such that the distance between h and the closest point is the maximum (i.e., the margin is maximized) under the condition that all points in POS lie above h, all points in NEG lie below h (see Fig. 6). Once this h is obtained, we can infer that a new test data z is positive (resp. negative) if z lies above h (resp. below h). If there does not exist h which completely separates POS from NEG, an SVM finds h which maximizes the *soft margin*, where we omit details of the soft margin (see [5,6]).

In order to apply an SVM effectively, it is important to design a *kernel function* which is suited to an application problem. Consider the case of classification of biological sequences. Since a sequence is not a point in Euclidean space, we can not directly apply SVMs to sequences. We should find a mapping from the space of sequences to the d-dimensional Euclidean space. Such a mapping is an example of a kernel function. Kernel functions can also be used in principal component analysis (PCA) and canonical correlation analysis (CCA) [6,40].

We consider a space $\mathcal{X}$ of objects. For example, $\mathcal{X}$ can be a set of DNA/protein sequences (Fig. 7). We also consider a *feature map* Φ from $\mathcal{X}$ to $\mathcal{R}^d$, where $d \in \{1, 2, 3, \ldots\}$ (we can even consider infinite dimensional space (Hilbert space) instead of $\mathcal{R}^d$). Then, we define a kernel K from $\mathcal{X} \times \mathcal{X}$ to $\mathcal{R}$ by

$$K(x, x') = \Phi(x) \cdot \Phi(x'),$$

where $a \cdot b$ is the inner product between vectors a and b. $K(x, x')$ is regarded as a measure of similarity between x and x'. It is known that if a function K from $\mathcal{X} \times \mathcal{X}$ to $\mathcal{R}$ is symmetric (i.e., $K(x, x') = K(x', x)$) and positive semi-definite (i.e., $\sum_{i=1}^{n} \sum_{j=1}^{n} a_i a_j K(x_i, x_j) \geq 0$ holds for any $n > 0$, for any $(a_1, \ldots, a_n) \in \mathcal{R}$ and any $(x_1, \ldots, x_n) \in \mathcal{R}^n$), K is a valid kernel (i.e., there exists some $\Phi(x)$ such that $K(x, x') = \Phi(x) \cdot \Phi(x')$).

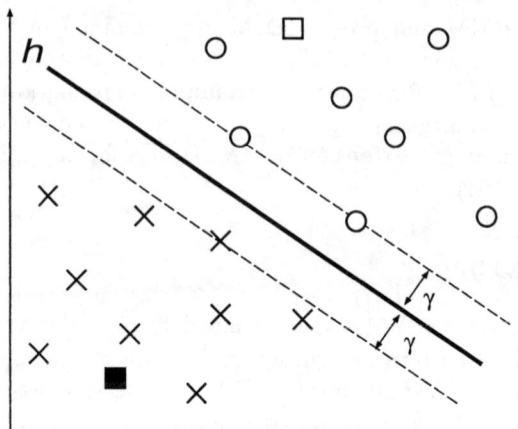

Fig. 6. SVM finds hyperplane h with the maximum margin γ such that positive examples (denoted by circles) are separated from negative examples (denoted by crosses). In this case, a new example denoted by white square (resp. black square) is inferred as positive (resp. negative)

5.2   Spectrum Kernel and Its Variants

One of the simplest kernel functions for sequences is the *spectrum kernel* [20]. Let k be a positive integer. Then, we define a feature map $\Phi_k(s)$ from a set of sequences over $\mathcal{A}$ to $\mathcal{R}^{\mathcal{A}^k}$ by

$$\Phi_k(s) = (occ(t,s))_{t \in \mathcal{A}^k},$$

where $occ(t,s)$ denotes the number of occurrences of substring t in string s. Then, the *k-spectrum kernel* is defined as $K(s,s') = \Phi_k(s) \cdot \Phi_k(s')$. Though the number of dimensions of $\mathcal{R}^{\mathcal{A}^k}$ is large, we can compute $K(s,s')$ efficiently (in $O(kn)$ time) using data structure named *suffix trees* without computing $\Phi_k(s)$ [20]. Here, we consider the case of $k = 2$ and $\mathcal{A} = \{A, C\}$. Then, we have $\Phi_2(s) = (occ(AA, s), occ(AC, s), occ(CA, s), occ(CC, s))$. Thus, for example, we have $K(ACCAC, CCAAAC) = 4$ since $\Phi_2(ACCAC) = (0,2,1,1)$ and $\Phi_2(CCAAAC) = (2,1,1,1)$.

The spectrum kernel was extended to allow small mismatches (the *mismatch kernel*) [21]. For k-mer $t = t[1]\ldots t[k]$, let $N_{(k,m)}(t)$ be the set of k-length sequences each of which differs from t at most m-positions. For example, $N_{(3,1)}(ACG) = \{ACG, CCG, GCG, TCG, AAG, AGG, ATG, ACA, ACC, ACT\}$ for $\mathcal{A} = \{A, C, G, T\}$. We define $\phi_{(k.m)}(t)$ for $t \in \mathcal{A}^k$ by

$$\phi_{(k,m)}(t) = (\phi_u(t))_{u \in \mathcal{A}^k},$$

where $\phi_u(t) = 1$ if $t \in N_{(k,m)}(u)$, otherwise $\phi_u(t) = 0$. Then, we define the feature map $\Phi_{(k,m)}(s)$ of the mismatch kernel by

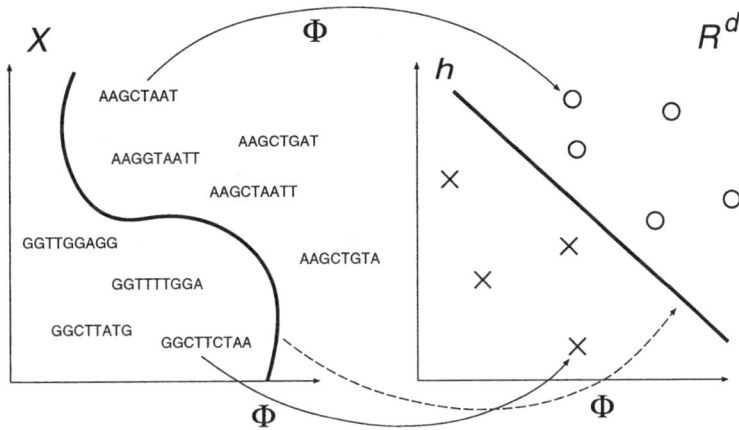

Fig. 7. Feature map Φ from sequence space $\mathcal{X}$ to d-dimensional Euclidean space $\mathcal{R}^d$. Φ maps each sequence in $\mathcal{X}$ to a point in $\mathcal{R}^d$

$$\Phi_{(k,m)}(s) = \sum_{i=1}^{|s|-k+1} \phi_{(k,m)}(s[i \ldots i+k-1]).$$

It should be noted that $\Phi_{(k,0)}$ coincides with the feature map of the spectrum kernel.

There is another way to extend the spectrum kernel. The *motif kernel* was proposed using a set of motifs in place of a set of short substrings [2]. Let $\mathcal{M}$ be a set of motifs and $occ_M(m,s)$ denote the number of occurrences of motif $m \in \mathcal{M}$ in sequence s. Then, we define the feature map $\Phi_M(s)$ by

$$\Phi_M(s) = (occ_M(m,s))_{m \in \mathcal{M}}.$$

Since the number of motifs may be very large, an efficient method is employed for searching motifs [2].

5.3 SVM-Pairwise

As mentioned in Section 2, the score obtained by the Smith-Waterman algorithm (SW-score) is widely used as a standard measure of similarity between two protein sequences. Therefore, it is reasonable to develop kernels based on the SW-score (i.e., $\max_{i,j} F[i][j]$). Liao and Noble proposed a simple method to derive a feature vector using the SW-score [23]. For two sequences s and s', let $sw(s,s')$ denote the SW-score between s and s'. Let $S = \{s_1, \ldots, s_n\}$ be a set of sequences used as training data, where some sequences are used as positive examples and the others as negative examples. For each sequence s (s may not be in S), we define a feature vector $\Phi_{SW}(s)$ by

$$\Phi_{SW}(s) = (sw(s,s_i))_{s_i \in S}.$$

Then, the kernel is simply defined as $\Phi_{SW}(s) \cdot \Phi_{SW}(s')$. In order to apply this kernel to analysis of real sequence data, some normalization procedures are required. Details of normalization procedures are given in [23].

5.4   SVM-Fisher Kernel

It is reasonable to try to combine HMM and SVM. The *SVM-Fisher kernel* is one of such kernels. To use the SVM-Fisher kernel, we first train a profile HMM with each positive training data set using the Baum-Welch algorithm. Let m be the number of match states in the profile HMM. Given sequence s, $E_i(a)$ denotes the expected number of times that $a \in \mathcal{A}$ is observed in the i-th match state for s, $e_i(a)$ denotes the emission probability for $a \in \mathcal{A}$, and θ_{al} is the coordinate corresponding to a of the l-th ($l \in \{1, \ldots, 9\}$) Dirichlet distribution (see [13] and [7] for the details about the Dirichlet distribution in HMMs). It is known that $E_i(a)$ can be computed using the Forward and Backward algorithms [7, 13]. Then, the feature vector $\Phi_F(s)$ is defined by

$$\Phi_F(s) = \left(\sum_{a \in \mathcal{A}} E_i(a) \left[\frac{\theta_{al}}{e_i(a)} - 1 \right] \right)_{(l,q_i) \in \{1, \ldots, 9\} \times Q_{MATCH}}.$$

Using the *Gaussian RBF kernel* [6], the SVM-Fisher kernel is defined as

$$K(s, s') = \exp\left(-\frac{|\Phi_F(s) - \Phi_F(s')|^2}{2\sigma^2} \right),$$

where the width σ is the median Euclidean distance in the feature space from any positive example to the nearest negative example.

5.5   Marginalized Kernel

Tsuda *et al.* proposed the *marginalized kernel*, based on the expectation with respect to hidden variables [35]. The marginalized kernel is defined in a very general way so that various types of kernels can be derived depending on application areas.

Let x be a visible variable (or a tuple of visible variables) in some finite set $\mathcal{X}$. Let h be a hidden variable (or a tuple of hidden variable) in some finite set $\mathcal{H}$. Suppose we have a kernel function $K_Z(z, z')$ between two combined variables $z = (x, h)$ and $z' = (x', h')$. Then, the marginalized kernel is defined by

$$K(x, x') = \sum_{h \in \mathcal{H}} \sum_{h' \in \mathcal{H}} P(h|x)P(h'|x')K_Z(z, z').$$

Since $P(h|x)$ is a posterior distribution and thus is unknown in general, it should be estimated from the data. It is not difficult to see that $K(x, x')$ is a valid kernel (i.e., positive semi-definite) if $K_Z(z, z')$ is a valid kernel.

Now, we define the marginalized count kernel using HMM. Let $s = s[1] \ldots s[k]$ be a sequence over $\mathcal{A}$. Suppose that $s[i]$ is emitted at state $q_{\pi[i]}$ of a fixed HMM

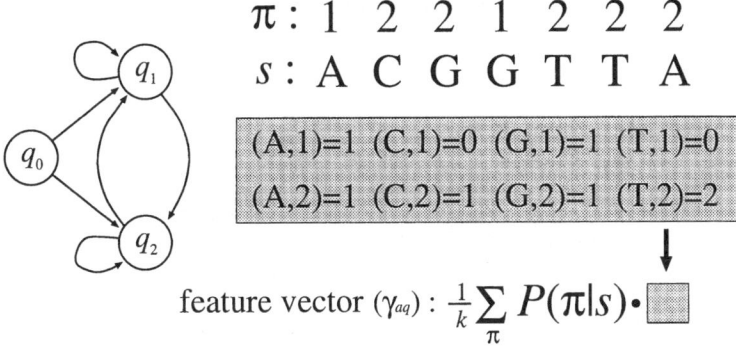

Fig. 8. Illustration of the marginalized count kernel. Each element of a feature vector corresponds to the number of occurrences of a combination of symbol and state. The value of each element is obtained by taking weighted sum of the numbers over all paths π

and thus we have a sequence of states $\pi = \pi[1] \dots \pi[k]$. Then, we define z by a pair of s and π (i.e., $z = (s, \pi)$). We define the *count kernel* $K_Z(z, z')$ for z and z' as

$$K_Z(z, z') = \sum_{a \in \mathcal{A}} \sum_{q \in Q} c_{aq}(z) c_{aq}(z'),$$

where $c_{aq}(z)$ denotes the frequency of occurrences of a pair (a, q) in z. A vector of $c_{aq}(z)$ (i.e., $(c_{aq}(z))_{(a,q) \in \mathcal{A} \times Q}$) is considered as a feature vector $\Phi(z)$. This $c_{aq}(z)$ can be rewritten as

$$c_{aq}(z) = \frac{1}{k} \sum_{i=1}^{k} \delta(s[i], a) \delta(q_{\pi[i]}, q),$$

where $\delta(x, x') = 1$ if $x = x'$, otherwise $\delta(x, x') = 0$.

Assuming that we know the posterior probability $P(\pi|s)$, we define the *marginalized count kernel* as

$$K(s, s') = \sum_{\pi} \sum_{\pi'} P(\pi|s) P(\pi'|s') K_Z(z, z'),$$

where the summation is taken over all possible state sequences and $k = |s|$ can be different from $k' = |s'|$. This kernel is rewritten as

$$K(s, s') = \sum_{a \in \mathcal{A}} \sum_{q \in Q} \gamma_{aq}(s) \gamma_{aq}(s'),$$

where $\gamma_{aq}(s)$ denotes the marginalized count (see Fig. 8) defined by

$$\gamma_{aq}(s) = \frac{1}{k} \sum_{\pi} P(\pi|s) \sum_{i=1}^{k} \delta(s[i], a) \delta(q_{\pi[i]}, q)$$

$$= \frac{1}{k} \sum_{i=1}^{k} P(q_{\pi[i]} = q|s) \delta(s[i], a).$$

It should be noted that linearity of expectations is used to derive the last equality. As described in Section 4, $P(q_{\pi[i]} = q|s)$ can be computed using the Forward and Backward algorithms.

5.6   Local Alignment Kernel

Since a kernel function is considered to be a measure of similarity, it is reasonable to try to use the SW-score as a kernel function. However, it is known that the SW-score is not a valid kernel [32]. On the other hand, it is known that the score obtained using *a pair HMM* is a valid kernel under some condition [9, 38], where a pair HMM is a variant of HMMs which outputs a pairwise alignment in place of a sequence for a usual HMM [7]. Based on this fact, the *local alignment kernel* (LA-kernel, in short) is proposed [32].

Recall that the score of a pairwise (local) alignment (s', t') is given by

$$score(s', t') = \sum_{i=1}^{l} f(s'[i], t'[i]).$$

Let $\Pi(s, t)$ be the set of all possible local alignments between sequences s and t. We define the local alignment kernel $K_{LA}^{(\beta)}(s, t)$ by

$$K_{LA}^{(\beta)}(s, t) = \sum_{(s', t') \in \Pi(s, t)} \exp(\beta \cdot score(s', t')),$$

where $\beta \geq 0$ is a constant to be adjusted depending on applications and training data sets. It is proved that $K_{LA}^{(\beta)}(s, t)$ is a valid kernel under reasonable conditions [32]. $K_{LA}^{(\beta)}(s, t)$ can also be considered as the score obtained by applying the Forward algorithm to a pair HMM and two sequences s, t. Furthermore, $K_{LA}^{(\beta)}(s, t)$ can be computed efficiently using the dynamic programming technique as in the Forward algorithm [32].

Here, we note that the SW-score can be written as

$$sw(s, t) = \max_{(s', t') \in \Pi(s, t)} score(s', t') = \frac{1}{\beta} \log \left(\max_{(s', t') \in \Pi(s, t)} \exp(\beta \cdot score(s', t')) \right).$$

From this and the definition of the LA-kernel, it follows that

$$\lim_{\beta \to +\infty} \frac{1}{\beta} \ln K_{LA}^{(\beta)}(s, t) = sw(s, t).$$

This equation clarifies the relationship between the LA-kernel and the SW-score [32]. It is also interesting to note that the LA-kernel is defined without introducing a feature map. The feature space will be infinite because the number of possible alignments is infinite if we consider all sequence pairs.

5.7   Comparison of String Kernels

We saw several kernels for measuring similarities between sequences. These kernels are classified into four classes (see also Fig. 9).

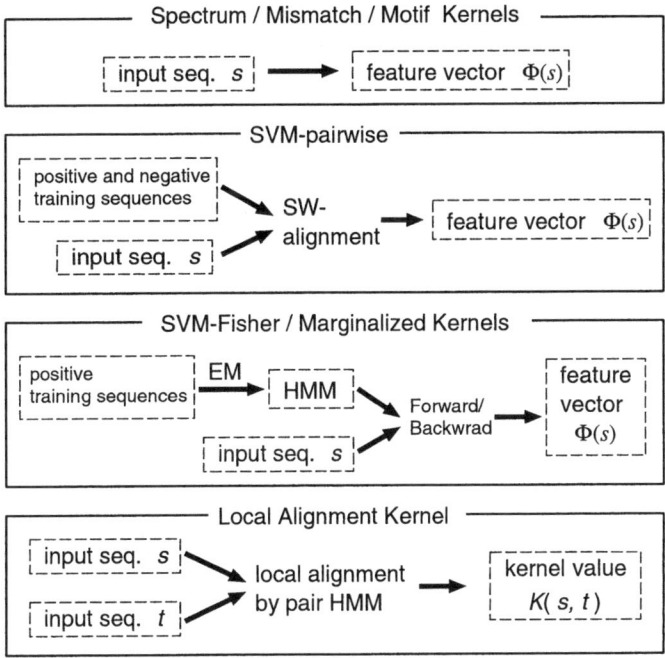

Fig. 9. Comparison of string kernels

(i) spectrum kernel, mismatch kernel, motif kernel
A feature vector is directly computed from an input sequence (though efficient algorithms are employed to compute kernel functions without computing feature vectors).
(ii) SVM-pairwise
A feature vector is computed from an input sequence and sequences in the training data set.
(iii) SVM-Fisher, marginalized count kernel
An HMM is trained using positive training data set. Then, a feature vector is extracted from the HMM with an input sequence.
(iv) local alignment kernel
The value of the kernel function is directly computed from two input sequences without computing feature vectors.

Kernels in class (i) (especially, spectrum kernel) have a merit that kernel values can be computed very efficiently. Kernels in classes (ii) and (iv) require longer time (especially in training phase) because dynamic programing algorithms take quadratic time. In order to compute kernel values in class (iii), it is required to train HMMs, where the Baum-Welch algorithm is usually employed to train these HMMs. Therefore, the performance may depend on how HMMs are trained.

These kernels except the marginalized count kernel were experimented with the benchmark data set for detecting remote homology at the SCOP superfamily level [2, 13, 21, 23, 32]. In order to apply kernel methods to remote homology detection, we develop some methods for combining the results from multiple SVMs since an SVM can classify only two classes (i.e., positive and negative). For that purpose, there are two approaches: (a) simply selecting the class for which the corresponding SVM outputs the highest score, (b) using majority votes from multiple SVMs. In the case of remote homology detection, the former approach (a) is usually used [2, 13, 21, 23, 32]. In this approach, we first construct an SVM for each class, where sequences in the class are used as positive examples and sequences not in the class are used as negative examples. Then, we apply a test sequence to each SVM and the SVM with the highest score is selected.

The results of experiments with the benchmark data set suggest that kernel based methods are in general better than a simple HMM search or a simple homology search using the SW-score. The results also suggest the following relation:

$$\text{motif kernel} \succ \text{LA-kernel} \succ \text{SVM-pairwise} \succ \text{mismatch kernel}$$
$$\succ \text{spectrum kernel} \succ \text{SVM-Fisher kernel,}$$

where $x \succ y$ means that the performance of x is better than that of y. However, some of these experiments are performed separately and the performance is significantly affected by tuning of parameters. Therefore, it is not so clear which kernel is the best. It seems that the performances also depend on applications and data sets.

Though the performance of kernel methods are better than SW-search for the benchmark data set, kernel methods require a substantive number of sufficiently different sequences as training data. However, only a few tens of superfamilies have enough number of sequences. Therefore, homology search using the SW-algorithm or its variants is still very useful in practice.

6   Graph Kernel

Inference of properties of *chemical compounds* is becoming important in bioinformatics as well as in other fields because it has potential applications to *drug design*. In order to process chemical compounds in computers, chemical compounds are usually represented as labeled graphs. Therefore, it is reasonable to develop kernels to measure similarities between labeled graphs. However, to my knowledge, only a few kernels have been developed. In this section, we review the marginalized graph kernel [8, 16], which is a marginalized kernel for graphs. It should be noted that other types of graph kernels [8, 17] and some extensions of the marginalized graph kernel [24] were proposed.

A *labeled graph* $G = (V, E)$ is defined by a set of vertices V, a set of undirected edges $E \subseteq V \times V$, and a labeling function l from V to $\mathcal{A}$, where $\mathcal{A}$ is the set of atom types (i.e., $\mathcal{A} = \{$H,O,C,N,P,S,Cl,$\ldots\}$). Though we only consider labels of vertices for simplicity in this paper, the methods can be extended for cases where labels of edges are taken into account. For graph G, V^k denotes the set of

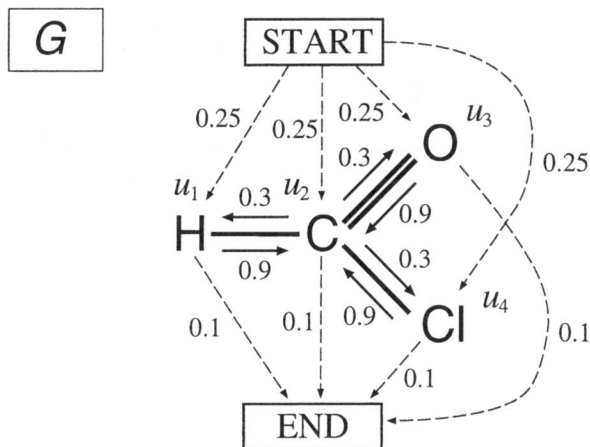

Fig. 10. Example probability distribution on a graph, where $(1 - P_q(v))P_a(u|v)$ is shown for each solid arrow. For $\pi = u_1 u_2 u_3$, $l(\pi) = $ (H,C,O) and $P(\pi) = 0.25 \cdot 0.9 \cdot 0.3 \cdot 0.1$. For $\pi' = u_2 u_4 u_2 u_3$, $l(\pi') = $ (C,Cl,O,C) and $P(\pi') = 0.25 \cdot 0.3 \cdot 0.9 \cdot 0.3 \cdot 0.1$

sequences of k vertices, and V^* denotes the set of all finite sequences of vertices (i.e., $V^* = \bigcup_{k=1}^{\infty} V^k$). The labeling function l can be extended for sequences of vertices by letting $l(\pi) = (l(\pi[1]), l(\pi[2]), \ldots, l(\pi[k]))$ for each element $\pi = \pi[1]\pi[2]\ldots\pi[k] \in V^k$. If $\pi \in V^k$ satisfies the property that $(\pi[i], \pi[i+1]) \in E$ for all $i = 1, \ldots, k-1$, π is called a *path*.

Here we consider probability distributions on paths (see Fig. 10). For each $\pi \in V^*$, we define $P(\pi)$ by

$$P(\pi) = P_0(\pi[1]) \cdot \left(\prod_{i=2}^{k} P_a(\pi[i]|\pi[i-1]) \right) \cdot P_q(\pi[k])$$

where $P_0(v)$, $P_a(u|v)$ and $P_q(v)$ denote an initial probability distribution on V ($\sum_{v \in V} P_s(v) = 1$), a transition probability distribution on $V \times V$ ($\sum_{u \in V} P_a(u|v) = 1$ for each $v \in V$) and a stopping probability distribution on V, respectively. For $(v, u) \notin E$, $P_a(u|v) = 0$ must hold. Letting $P_s(v) = P_0(v)P_q(v)$ and $P_t(u|v) = (1 - P_q(v))P_a(u|v)P_q(u)/P_q(v)$, we can rewrite $P(\pi)$ as

$$P(\pi) = P_s(\pi[1]) \prod_{i=2}^{k} P_t(\pi[i]|\pi[i-1]).$$

It should be noted that $P(\pi) = 0$ if π is not a path.

We assume that there exists a kernel function (i.e., a positive semi-definite function) $K_Z : A^* \times A^* \to \mathcal{R}$. In the simplest case, we can use the Dirac kernel [16] (see Fig. 11) defined by

$$K_Z(l, l') = \begin{cases} 1 \text{ if } l = l', \\ 0 \text{ otherwise,} \end{cases}$$

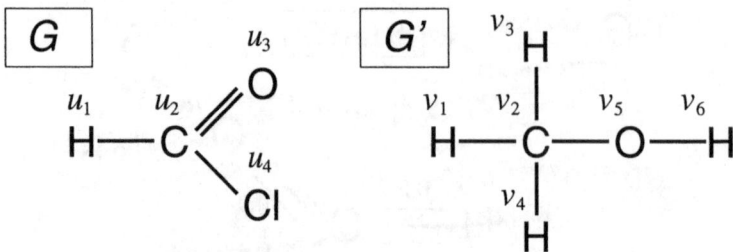

Fig. 11. Example of a pair of graphs. For paths $\pi = u_1 u_2 u_3$ of G and $\pi' = v_1 v_2 v_5$ of G', $l(\pi) = l(\pi') = $ (H,C,O) holds, from which $K_Z(l(\pi), l(\pi')) = 1$ follows. For paths $\pi'' = u_1 u_2 u_3 u_2 u_4$ of G and $\pi''' = v_1 v_2 v_5 v_2 v_1$ of G', $l(\pi'') = $ (H,C,O,C,Cl) and $l(\pi''') = $ (H,C,O,C,H) hold, from which $K_Z(l(\pi''), l(\pi''')) = 0$ follows

where it might be possible to develop kernel functions including chemical properties.

Now, we define the marginalized graph kernel [16]. Let $G = (V, E)$ and $G' = (V', E')$ be labeled graphs. Let P and P' be probability distributions on V^* and $(V')^*$, respectively. Then, the marginalized graph kernel is defined as:

$$K(G, G') = \sum_{(\pi, \pi') \in V^* \times (V')^*} P(\pi) P'(\pi') K_Z(l(\pi), l(\pi')),$$

where G and G' correspond to x and x' respectively and are omitted in the right hand side of this formula.

The above definition involves a summation over an infinite number of paths. However, it can be computed efficiently using matrix inversions if K_Z satisfies some property [8]. Here, we assume that K_Z is the Dirac kernel. Let $\pi = u_1 u_2 \ldots u_k$ and $\pi' = v_1 v_2 \ldots v_k$ be paths of G and G' such that $K_Z(l(\pi), l(\pi')) = 1$. Let Π be the set of such pairs of paths. We define $\gamma(\pi, \pi')$ by

$$\gamma(\pi, \pi') = P(\pi) \cdot P'(\pi').$$

Then, we have

$$K(G, G') = \sum_{(\pi, \pi') \in \Pi} \gamma(\pi, \pi').$$

Here, we define $\gamma_s(v, v')$ and $\gamma_t((u, u')|(v, v'))$ by

$$\gamma_s(v, v') = P_s(v) \cdot P'_s(v'),$$
$$\gamma_t((u, u')|(v, v')) = P_t(u|v) \cdot P_t(u'|v').$$

If we define the $|V| \cdot |V'|$ dimensional vector $\gamma_s = (\gamma_s(v, v'))_{(v,v') \in V \times V'}$ and the $(|V| \cdot |V'|) \times (|V| \cdot |V'|)$ transition matrix $\Gamma_t = (\gamma_t((u, u')|(v, v')))_{(u,u',v,v') \in V \times V' \times V \times V'}$, we have:

$$\sum_{(\pi, \pi') \in \Pi, |\pi| = |\pi'| = k} \gamma(\pi, \pi') = \gamma_s^t (\Gamma_t)^{k-1} \mathbf{1},$$

where γ_s^t is the transposed matrix of γ_s and $\mathbf{1}$ is the $|V| \cdot |V'|$ dimensional vector with all elements equal to 1. As in proving $1 - x = 1 + x + x^2 + x^3 + \ldots$ for $0 < x < 1$, we can prove the following:

$$
\begin{aligned}
K(G, G') &= \sum_{k=1}^{\infty} \left(\sum_{(\pi, \pi') \in \Pi, |\pi| = |\pi'| = k} \gamma(\pi, \pi') \right) \\
&= \sum_{k=1}^{\infty} \gamma_s^t \, (\Gamma_t)^{k-1} \, \mathbf{1} \\
&= \gamma_s^t \, (I - \Gamma_t)^{-1} \, \mathbf{1},
\end{aligned}
$$

where I denotes the identity matrix and $(I - \Gamma_t)^{-1}$ denotes the inverse matrix of $(I - \Gamma_t)$.

7 Conclusion

We overviewed fundamental computational and statistical methods in bioinformatics and recent advances in kernel methods for bioinformatics. Kernel methods have been a very active and exciting field in the last few years. As seen in this paper, a variety of kernel functions were developed for analyzing sequence data in a few years, where fundamental techniques in bioinformatics were efficiently combined with support vectors machines.

Though we focused on string kernels and graph kernels, kernel methods have been applied to other problems in bioinformatics, which include analysis of gene expression data [19, 27], analysis of phylogenetic profiles [39], analysis of metabolic pathways [40], prediction of protein subcellular locations [30], prediction of protein secondary structures [37], classification of G-protein coupled receptors [15], and inference of protein-protein interactions [3, 10]. Though we focused on SVMs, kernel functions can also be used with other methods, which include principal component analysis (PCA) and canonical correlation analysis (CCA) [6, 40]. More details and other application of kernel methods in bioinformatics can also be found in [33].

Huge amount of various types of biological data are being produced everyday. Therefore, it is needed to develop more efficient and flexible methods for extracting important information behind those data. Kernel methods will be one of key technologies for that purpose. More and more studied should be done for development of other kernel functions as well as improvement of support vector machines and other kernel based methods.

Acknowledgements

This work was partially supported by a Japanese-French SAKURA grant named "Statistical and Combinatorial Analysis of Biological Networks". The author would like to thank Jean-Philippe Vert and other members of that project, through which he learned much about kernel methods.

References

1. Bailey, T. L. and Elkan, C., Fitting a mixture model by expectation maximization to discover motifs in biopolymers, *Proc. Second International Conf. on Intelligent Systems for Molecular Biology*, 28-36, 1994.
2. Ben-Hur, A. and Brutlag, D., Remote homology detection: a motif based approach, *Bioinformatics*, 19:i26-i33, 2003.
3. Bock, J. R. and Gough, D. A., Predicting protein-protein interactions from primary structure, *Bioinformatics*, 17:455-460, 2001.
4. Brazma, A., Jonassen, I., Eidhammer, I. and Gilbert, D., Approaches to the automatic discovery of patterns in biosequences, *Journal of Computational Biology*, 5:279-305, 1998.
5. Cortes, C. and Vapnik, V., Support vector networks, *Machine Learning*, 20:273-297, 1995.
6. Cristianini, N. and Shawe-Taylor, J., *An Introduction to Support Vector Machines and Other Kernel-Based Learning Methods*, Cambridge Univ. Press, 2000.
7. Durbin, R., Eddy, S., Krogh, A. and Mitchison, G., *Biological Sequence Analysis. Probabilistic Models of Proteins and Nucleic Acids*, Cambridge University Press, 1998.
8. Gärtner, T., Flach, P. and Wrobel, S., On graph kernels: Hardness results and efficient alternatives, *Proc. 16th Annual Conf. Computational Learning Theory* (LNAI 2777, Springer), 129-143, 2003.
9. Haussler, D., Convolution kernels on discrete structures, Technical Report, UC Santa Cruz, 1999.
10. Hayashida, M., Ueda, N. and Akutsu, T., Inferring strengths of protein-protein interactions from experimental data using linear programming, *Bioinformatics*, 19:ii58-ii65. 2003.
11. Henikoff, A. and Henikoff, J. G., Amino acid substitution matrices from protein blocks, *Proc. Natl. Acad. Sci. USA*, 89:10915-10919, 1992.
12. Hourai, Y., Akutsu, T. and Akiyama, Y., Optimizing substitution matrices by separating score distributions, *Bioinformatics*, 20:863-873, 2004.
13. Jaakola, T., Diekhans, M. and Haussler, D., A discriminative framework for detecting remote protein homologies, *Journal of Computational Biology*, 7:95-114, 2000.
14. Kann, M., Qian, B. and Goldstein, R. A., Optimization of a new score function for the detection of remote homologs, *Proteins: Structure, Function, and Genetics*, 41:498-503, 2000.
15. Karchin, R., Karplus, K. and Haussler, D., Classifying G-protein coupled receptors with support vector machines, *Bioinformatics*, 18:147-159, 2002.
16. Kashima, J., Tsuda, K. and Inokuchi, A., Marginalized kernels between labeled graphs, *Proc. 20th Int. Conf. Machine Learning*, 321-328, AAAI Press, 2003.
17. Kondor, R. I. and Lafferty. J. D., Diffusion kernels on graphs and other discrete input spaces, *Proc. 19th Int. Conf. Machine Learning*, 315-322, AAAI Press, 2002.
18. Lawrence, C. E., Altschul, S. F., Boguski, M. S., Liu, J. S., Neuwald, A. F. and Wootton, J. C., Detecting subtle sequence signals: a Gibbs sampling strategy for multiple alignment, *Science*, 262:208-214, 1993.
19. Lee, Y. and Lee, C-K., Classification of multiple cancer types by multicategory support vector machines using gene expression data, *Bioinformatics*, 19:1132-1139, 2003.
20. Leslie, C., Eskin, E. and Noble, W. E., The spectrum kernel: a string kernel for svm protein classification, *Proc. Pacific Symp. Biocomputing 2002*, 564-575, 2002.

21. Leslie, C., Eskin, E., Cohen, A., Weston, J. and Noble, W. E., Mismatch string kernels for discriminative protein classification, *Bioinformatics*, 20:467-476, 2004.
22. Levitt, M., Gernstein, M., Huang, E., Subbiah, S. and Tsai, J., Protein folding: The endgame, *Annual Review of Biochemistry*, 66:549-579, 1997.
23. Liao, L. and Noble, W. S., Combining pairwise sequence similarity and support vector machines for detecting remote protein evolutionary and structural relationships, *Journal of Computational Biology*, 10:857-868, 2003.
24. Mahé, P., Ueda, N., Akutsu, T., Perret, J-L. and Vert, J-P., Extensions of marginalized graph kernels, *Proc. 21st Int. Conf. Machine Learning*, 552-559, AAAI Press, 2004.
25. Moult, J., Fidelis, K., Zemla, A. and Hubbard, T., Critical assessment of methods for protein structure prediction (CASP)-round V, *Proteins: Structure, Function, and Genetics*, 53, 334-339, 2003.
26. Mount, D. W., *Bioinformatics: Sequence and Genome Analysis*, Cold Spring Harbor Laboratory Press, 2001.
27. Mukherjee, S. *et al.*, Estimating dataset size requirements for classifying DNA microarray data, *Journal of Computational Biology*, 10:119-142, 2003.
28. Murzin, A. G. *et al.*, SCOP: A structural classification of proteins database for the investigation of sequences and structures, *Journal of Molecular Biology*, 247:536-540, 1995.
29. Notredame, C., Recent progresses in multiple sequence alignment: A survey, *Pharmacogenomics*, 3:131-144, 2002.
30. Park, K-J. and Kanehisa, M., Prediction of protein subcellular locations by support vector machines using compositions of amino acids and amino acid pairs, *Bioinformatics*, 19:1656-1663, 2003.
31. Pevzner, P. A. *Computational Molecular Biology. An Algorithmic Approach*, The MIT Press, 2000.
32. Saigo, H., Vert, J-P., Ueda, N. and Akutsu, T., Protein homology detection using string alignment kernels, *Bioinformatics*, 20:1682-1689, 2004.
33. Schölkopf, B, Tsuda, K. and Vert, J-P., *Kernel Methods in Computational Biology*, MIT Press, 2004.
34. Thompson, J., Higgins, D. and Gibson, T., CLUSTAL W: Improving the sensitivity of progressive multiple sequence alignment through sequence weighting position-specific gap penalties and weight matrix choice, *Nucleic Acids Research*, 22:4673-4390, 1994.
35. Tsuda, K., Kin, T. and Asai, K., Marginalized kernels for biological sequences, *Bioinformatics*, 18:S268-S275, 2002.
36. Wang, L. and Jiang, T., On the complexity of multiple sequence alignment, *Journal of Computational Biology*, 1:337–348, 1994.
37. Ward, J. J., McGuffin, L. J., Buxton, B. F. and Jones, D. T., Secondary structure prediction with support vector machines, *Bioinformatics*, 19:1650-1655, 2003.
38. Watkins, C., Dynamic alignment kernels, *Advances in Large Margin Classifiers*, 39-50, MA, MIT Press, 2000.
39. Vert, J-P., A tree kernel to analyse phylogenetic profiles, *Bioinformatics*, 18:S276-S284, 2002.
40. Yamanishi, Y., Vert, J-P., Nakaya, A. and Kanehisa, M., Extraction of correlated gene clusters from multiple genomic data by generalized kernel canonical correlation analysis, *Bioinformatics*, 19:i323-i330, 2003.

Indexing and Mining Audiovisual Data

Pierre Morizet-Mahoudeaux[1] and Bruno Bachimont[1,2]

[1] Department of Computer Science and Engineering,
UMR-CNRS 6599 - Heudiasyc,
University of Technology of Compiègne, France
[2] Research and Experiment Department,
Institut National de l'Audiovisuel, France
pmorizet@hds.utc.fr

Abstract. In this paper we present a review of recent research and development works, which have been developed in the domain of indexing
and mining audio-visual document. We first present the characteristics
of the audio-visual documents and the outcomes of digitising this kind
of documents. It raises several important issues concerning the new definition of what is a document, what is indexing and what are the numeric principles and technologies available for performing indexing and
mining tasks. The analysis of these issue let us introduce the notion
of temporal and multimedia objects, and the presentation of the three
steps for indexing multimedia documents. It includes the clear distinction between descriptors and indexing. Finally we introduce the MPEG-7
paradigm, which sets the technical environment for developing indexing
applications; Then we shortly review current developments, based on
the text mining, the XML-Schema, and the event description interface
approaches.

1 Introduction

1.1 Motivation

Indexing document has been an important task from the time, when we began
to collect document in libraries, and other administration offices. It has become
a technological challenge with the increase of document production, which has
followed the computer development. It is now of strategic importance for companies, administrations, education and research centres to be able to handle and
manage the morass of documents being produced each day, worldwide. Document structuring languages such as XML, search engines, and other automatic
indexing engines has been the subject of numerous research and development
in the last years. We will not go further in the discussion of the needs for general document indexing work. We will focus on the more specialised domain of
audio-visual documents.

Audio visual documents call for several specific action: archiving, legal deposit, restoring, and easy access allowing [5, 6, 7].

S. Tsumoto et al. (Eds.): AM 2003, LNAI 3430, pp. 34–58, 2005.

Table 1. Radio and TV Broadcasting Archives since 1995(*source INA, 2003*)

Radio programs	TV programs
575 000 (hours)	535 000 hours

Table 2. Legal deposit (professional archives are partially included in legal deposit) (source INA 2003)

Hours of TV	Hours of Radio
430 000 hours	500 000 hours

For the task of archiving, almost each country has an institute, an administration or a company, which is in charge of recording, registering and storing the flow of radio and TV programs, which are broadcast each day. The table 1 gives the figures of the Professional Archives of the Audio-visual National Institute (INA, France). They correspond to a total of 1.1 million hours of radio and TV broadcasting, or approximately 70 000 hours a year of audio and audio-visual programs (for the French broadcasting systems) since 1995.

The legal deposit task corresponds to information concerning their broadcasting content given by the radio and TV broadcasting companies. This information is used, for example, to pay the corresponding right to the concerned professionals (authors, actors, composers, etc.). The figures of the legal deposit at INA is given in table 2.

It corresponds to a total of 930 000 hours of broadcasting, registered on 2,5 millions documents covering 113-km of shelf space (8-km / year). It would take 133 years for watching or listening all archives.

Audio-visual document have been stored on some physical support, which may degrade or be destroyed over time. So it is necessary to develop technologies and numerous effort to maintain and even restore, what belongs to our cultural patrimony.

Storing is of no use if we cannot access what has been stored. There is a need for accessing audio-visual documents just to re-view old document, or to build a new production form previous ones, or to develop specific studies. Accessing the right audio-visual document has become a real challenge in the morass of already stored documents. This is the most demanding effort in developing new and efficient technologies in audio-visual indexing and mining.

1.2   Outcomes of Digitised Audio-Visual Documents Production

The consequence of digitising audio-visual document can be sum up by three outcomes : the dematerialisation (annihilation) of content, the integration of several media on the same medium, and the digitisation of temporal objects [4].

The classical notion of document has been built in the context, where the recording media was the same as the retrieval media (restitution media) : the paper that I read is the same as the paper that I store. In the numerical context of annihilation of content, the storing media (hard disk) is not the same as the retrieval media (the screen, or the printed paper). A device has interfered in between to rebuild the reading document from the stored document. The core of the problems linked to the publication of contents lays at the foundation of the numerical document. For this reason, the outcome of the evolution from the paper-based document to the digitised document corresponds to the evolution of the classical indexing for information retrieval to indexing for electronic publication.

Before the era of digitised document each medium was limited to a dedicated support, without interaction with other media. The audio-visual information, recorded on a magnetic tape or a silver film, was not linked to any other information (texts, graphs, ...). Conversely, it was difficult to mix text and good quality pictures (separate pages in a book) and even more text with audio-visual. When they are transformed into digitised data, media can more easily be mixed. Besides technical problems, this new state raises new fundamental difficulties concerning writing and reading multimedia: how to integrate different medium in a writing process although it is dedicated for a reading usage? In this context, indexing becomes a reading instrumentation. Rather than information retrieval it is aimed at organising information of its reading.

Audio and audio-visual objects impose their rhythmic and reading sequence, they are temporal objects. They are built in a duration dimension instead of a spatial dimension as a text would be. They call for revisiting what is indexing. In the analogue context, audio-visual indexing corresponds to the identification of a document (cataloguing) and a global description of its content (what it is about), without a smaller level of description. This level is not need, merely because there is no means to read a portion of the analogue record, without reading all the record. The digitised record allows a random access to the content, which calls for revisiting the indexing issues.

So we come up to three major issues:

- What is a document? We will define the different types of documents, and we will introduce the notion of meta-data.
- What is indexing? We will define three types of indexing: conceptual indexing, document indexing, and content-based indexing.
- What are the numeric multimedia possibilities? What are the difficulties raised by temporal object, image, or audio-visual flow indexing? What are the different levels of indexing, according to its nature and the index (can we index a sound by a word, for example).

2   Document

2.1   What Is a Document ?

Definition: a document is a *content* instituted by a *publication act*, written down a medium, which possesses a *spatial* and *temporal delimitation*.

The words used in this definition call for some more precise explanation about their meaning in the scope of this paper.

- Content: a content is a pattern written down a medium, which can be meaningfully interpreted by a person or a community.
  Sometimes the word content is not used to express the interpretable pattern, but its meaning, which is the result of interpretation. The notion of "containing" is all that permits to put the content on some handling format, and the tools, which allow to handle this format. For example, the content could be a written text, including the letters shape, the page layout etc. The containing would be the paper, he ink, and tools for printing, hard-copying etc.
- Publication act: a meaningful material pattern is a document whenever it becomes available to some public. This availability gives to the material pattern the state of an *interpretable* pattern.
- Spatial delimitation: to become a document, it is necessary to know where the content begins and where it ends, what belongs to it and what does not.
- Temporal delimitation: the meaningful material pattern of a document must remain the same, whatever the time of its consultation or reading. The modification of its content gives rise to a new publication.
  A content becomes a document only when it is fixed by a given intention and it becomes available to some reader. Modifying the content is not re-publishing it. An already published book cannot be modified. It must be re-edited.

Finally a document is written down a medium. The document medium articulation varies along the technology used to elaborate the support and the writing process used. This articulation determines the type of document and its properties. It can be described according to six characteristics

- The recording medium: a document is the material writing of a content. Consequently, the recording medium is the writing medium. This medium is in charge of keeping up, and saving the written content. For example, the recording medium of a book is the paper, it is a magnetic tape, or a silver film for an audio-visual document or a movie, its is the randomly accessible memory for a digitised information.
- The recording pattern: it is the pattern, which is used to write down the content on the material medium. For example, it is a typography of an alphabet for a book, a magnetic signal for a video, a binary code for numerical documents.
- The appropriation medium: the ultimate aim of a document is to be accessed by some reader. Thus, a document can be red, referred to, viewed on the appropriate medium. It is on this medium that the reader can appropriate the content. An appropriation medium can be the screen of a monitor, the paper of a book, the loud-speaker, etc.
- The appropriation physical set: The physical medium lays out the content. To be red by the user, the content must be presented in a physical pattern, which is compatible with the physical medium. For example from the magnetic signal (recording pattern) of a video tape (recording medium), the TV set (appropriation medium) rebuilds a visual signal (the colour pixels on the

screen), which can be viewed by the viewer. It can be sum up by the following scheme :

magnetic signal (recording pattern) → video-tape (recording medium) → TV set (appropriation medium) → visual signal (colour pixels on the screen).

- The semiotic appropriation form: the presentation displayed on the appropriation medium follows a structure or a scheme, such that it can be directly understandable by the user. Consequently, this form is the appropriation form, which allows the user to appropriate the content. The appropriation form corresponds to a form, which can be interpreted by the user to the extent where it belongs to an already known semiotic register. If a document calls for several semiotic appropriation forms, we will say that the document is a multimedia document. Audio-visual is multimedia since it calls up images, music, noise and speech. Images can also be multimedia if it contains texts and iconic structures.

- The appropriation modality: the appropriation semiotic form concerns one or several perceptive modalities. If there are several perceptive modalities, the document is multi-modal. Audio-visual documents are multi-modal, since they call for the eyesight and the hearing.

Traditionally we are used to textual paper-based documents. However this kind of document is a special case since :

1. the recording medium and the appropriation medium are the same: the medium used for reading is the same as the medium used for storing,
2. the recording form and the appropriation form are the same: what we read is what has been put on the medium.

The paper-based document became a special case when we had to consider another kind of document, the temporal documents. In this case we must distinguish the different semiotic appropriation forms:

- Static and spatial appropriation forms: all the interpretable structures are presented to the reader at the same time. The way (the order) of reading are not imposed to the user. Even if the structure of the document suggests a canonical way of reading, it is not a necessary condition of reading.
- Temporal and dynamic appropriation forms: the interpretable structures are presented successively to the user, according to an rhythm imposed by the document. The order and the rhythm of the document constitute the meaning of the document.

This second case corresponds to audio and audio-visual documents. They record a temporal flow to preserve and to re-build its meaning. However, this kind of document raise the following problems:

1. the recording form must be hardware, thus it must be spatial. This is the only way to preserve the temporal information, since it cannot be stored in the content.

2. the semiotic form is temporal, which means that the temporality is intrinsic to the understandability of the document. The document must carry the temporality by itself.

From this, we can deduce that the recording medium does not equal the appropriation medium, and that the recording form does not equal the appropriation form.

Consequently, it is mandatory to have a process to rebuild the temporal form of a temporal document from its record. This process must be a mechanical one, that is to say, a process to re-build a temporal flow from a static and hardware components ordering. For example, the magnetic signal of a video tape, which is static, lets drive the video tape-recorder or the TV set to rebuild a physical appropriation form. The semiotic appropriation form can then merge with the physical appropriation form.

Thus we must distinguish the recording form from the content, because it is not self-readable. It is not aimed at to be red, but to be played by some mechanical means, which will rebuild the temporal form of the document. The recorded form can be accessed only by the means of a reading device, a *player*, which can decode this form to rebuild the document.

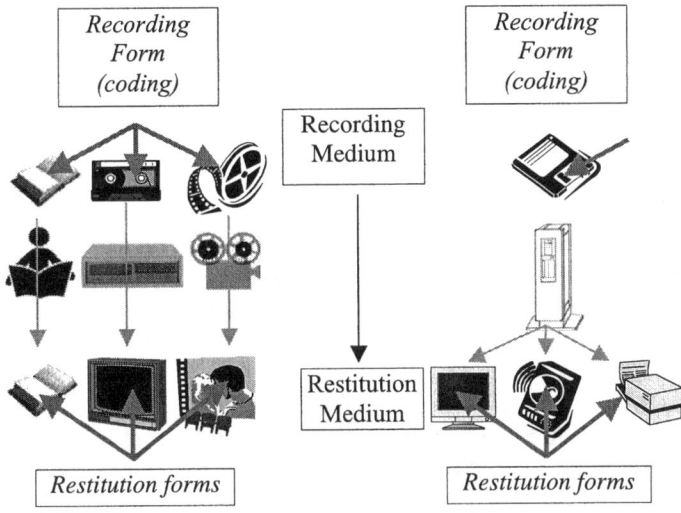

Fig. 1. The documentary dimensions

Once we have introduced this notion of a mechanical means, to play the document from its record, digitizing is just a change in the coding and the technology. So, it seems as if the digitizing does not change what we new about temporal documents. However, we will see in the next section, that this change of representation will bring much more modification.

To conclude this section, we can ask where lies the true nature of a document ? It seems that the appropriation forms are the real deposit of the document. The dimensions linked to the record characterize rather the resources to rebuild the document than the document itself. So we come to the conclusion that temporal document exists only during its temporal progress, and that the recording medium is not a document: it is a resource. A movie is movie only at the time when it is viewed in the cinema or broadcasted on the TV channel. It is not a paradox, but just the conclusion of the temporal nature of the document. The movie, recorded on a silver film, or the audio-visual document registered on the video tape are not documents. They are tools and resources, that we can use to access the document.

The viewed document is always the result of a (computed) transformation. What we consult is not what is recorded, but the output of its transformation by a computation. Thus a document is linked to the computing process, which rebuilds it and the information, which parameters and drive the rebuilding. This information describe what is necessary for matching the rebuilding with the viewed objective. It is thus meta data, information about the document, which makes it useful for a given rebuilding. Meta data makes it possible to use and exploit information. They are a generalisation of index and information retrieval concepts.

Finally, meta data must be created simultaneously with the document, and not afterwards like index in general. They are integrated to the content, such that we can say that meta data are data.

3   Indexing

3.1   What Is Indexing in General ?

According to the AFNOR standard indexing is:

Definition: Describing and characterising a document by the representation of the concepts contained in the document, and recording the concepts in some organised file, which can be easily accessed. Files are organised as paper or digitised sheets, indices, tables, catalogues, etc., queries are handled by these files.

This definition concerns textual documents, it must be generalised. For this generalisation, we will introduce later the notion of descriptors. First let's try to define indexing in its general accceptation, without the context of any computer based process. The main objective of indexing is to make information accessible, by the means of an index. Indexing is the process by which the content of a document is analysed, in order to be expressed in a form, which allows content accessing and handling. The word indexing means altogether the process and its result. Thus indexing is the description of a document for the purpose of a given use.

Indexing can be typically divided in two steps:

- A conceptual analyse step: the document is analysed for concept extraction.
- A documentary expressing step: concepts are translated into a documentary language with tools such as thesaurus, classification, etc.

This last step is important. The type of index is determined by the type of document handling, which is pursued. Typically the main considered handling is information retrieval: to find where is the searched information and to extract the corresponding documents from the documents collection. Indexing has two purposes: on the one hand, it must be exploitable to determine where is the searched information, and on the other hand it must permit to fetch this information. In the library, for example, each book is referred to by a category determining its content, and a quotation determining its place on a given shelf. Besides, index cards contain all books descriptions. When a user looks for books dealing with a given query, the librarian refers to the cards to find out, which books correspond to the query, and where they are. Indexing was used to find out the relevant information (the books), and its localisation (the shelf). Index cards have been built for an easy handling by the librarian.

So, to build an efficient indexing, we must first define the level of accuracy, which is needed for the application. Accuracy is determined by two characteristics : firstly it corresponds to the richness of the concepts and descriptors used for indexing, secondly it corresponds to the precision of information localisation in the described documents. The first one is called *acuteness* of the description and the second one is called *granularity* of the description.

Acuteness depends on the wanted faithfulness of the research results. It is defined by:

- The concepts repository
- The structure used to articulate indices in the indexing. Usually, the structure is Boolean.

Granularity depends on the wanted handling facility of information contained in the document. For a given set of contents; we call the *manipulation unit*, the smallest directly accessible and manageable entity. For example the manipulation unit for a text is the alphabetic character, and it is the pixel for an image. However it is not useful to localise information more precisely than the manipulation unit, which contains it. It is not necessary to know where, in a given unit, lies the searched information, since it will not be accessible by the content accessing system. For example, the manipulation unit is the *book* or the *video-tape* for the librarian or archivist. It is the *page* or the *scene* for the reader. However, the documentary system of the reader is the book, it is not the library.

3.2   Outcomes of Digitising: Granularity and Digitising

The massive digitising of content has had many consequences on indexing. Digitising may have a more or less impact on indexing, depending on the way it is managed. We can distinguish two approaches : digitising the *physical support* of appropriation, and digitising the *semiotic support* of appropriation.

Digitising the physical support means that the content format has been digitised. The digital unit is arbitrary, and there is no direct link left between the digital unit and the document manipulation unit. On the one hand, the document interpretation cannot induce the nature and value of the digital unit. On the other hand the modification of one unit may not modify the interpretation of the document. For example, a given pixel is a digital unit, which has an arbitrary link with the image to which it belongs. Moreover, the modification of a pixel will not significantly affect the image. Five wrong pixels will not modify the meaning of an image output on a screen.

Digitising the semiotic support means that a link between each unity and the content interpretation has been defined. The link may be arbitrary, in the sense that its linguistic meaning is arbitrary, but it is systematic. The modification of one unit will modify the meaning. For example the alphabet characters are discrete units of the written form. Although they have an arbitrary link with the meaning, the modification of one alphabetic character, may modify the meaning of a document. What would be the value of a screen, which would modify five alphabetic characters on each page?

We will discuss later on the multimedia aspects of digitising, however, we can consider now the example of the compression and digitising MPEG standard for audiovisual documents. MPEG-1 and MPEG-2 specify compression and digitising standard based on the pixel unit, and exploiting the redundancy of information linked to each pixel. This information concerns luminance and chrominance, and it has no link with the interpretation of the documents. On the contrary, the MPEG-4 standard analyses the audiovisual flow as a set of objects linked by spatio-temporal relations. For example, the television screen background is a distinct object of the broadcasted flow. From a certain point of view, this object is a significant sign, and can be used accordingly.

Whatever the aspect of digitising is concerned, be it physical or semiotic, we can define all arbitrary needed levels of granularity for digitised manipulation unit. This possibility tremendously increases the complexity of indexing: the manipulation unit was implicit in the traditional case (the book or the document). Digitising imposes to explicitly define the part of document, which corresponds to the searched information.

Indices are not only structured according to the logical and conceptual relations, which exist between the descriptors that they use. They are also linked by the relations, which link the described parts of a content. Indices can be based on markup languages for digitised documents.

3.3   Content-Based Indexing

As we have seen above, digitising has open new possibilities for defining manipulation unit, and has open the way to articulate content-based indexing with the document structure. Digitising has also open new possibilities, which have widen the field to works on indexing. Effectively, traditionally, the document content is indexed by linguistic concepts expressed with a controlled vocabulary. However, the digital media can handle any binary representation. Consequently it is not more necessary to limit indices to linguistic ones. For example, for several years, studies have concerned non-linguistic indices for images or sounds. The question is then whether we can index a document content by images or sounds, following the natural intuition of indexing images by images and sounds by sounds.

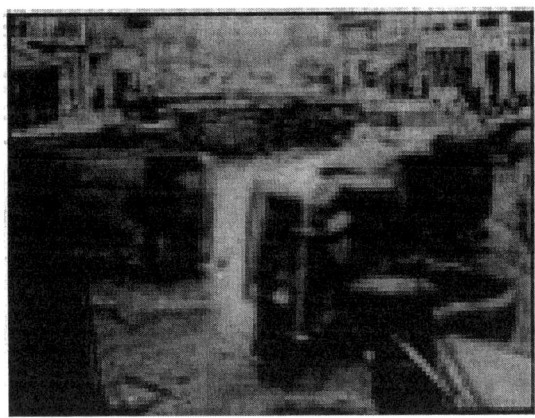

Fig. 2. What does show this image: a storm, a criminal attempt, a riot ?

This intuition is based upon an analogy with textual information retrieval. A text is roughly composed of strings separated by the space character. Each string is more or less a word. This property is very important, since words have a meaning, even out of the context prescribed by the functional linguistic system (the meaning of a word can be defined independently of its use in a sentence). Consequently, if we build a request with words, out of context, to find out the textual segments, which contains them, we obtain parts of documents which have a potential link with the query. For textual documents:

- Queries are built with words (strings built with alphabetic characters).
- The system performs a comparison with patterns (strings, words, . . .) in the text, separated by spaces or punctuation characters.

Of course, this process may be improved to lower the noise (documents, which do not have a relationship with the query, mainly because the context has changed or reduced the meanings of words of the query), and to improve the silence (by expanding the query with words of the same meaning as those in the query, in the concerned context).

This approach can be extended by analogy to audio-visual documents. Thus, for audiovisual documents content indexing we must make the following assumptions :

- Queries built with sounds or images make it possible to find similar documents based on a distance measurements between images or sounds. The information retrieval is based on a similarity process.
- We can index a document content with image-indices or sound-indices.

The first assumption is reasonably possible to implement, but not necessary useful. The second assumption does not hold. In fact, the first assumption does not refer to the exact notion of index, but rather to that of descriptors.

3.3.1   Descriptors *Versus* Indices

Images interpretation is not realised in the same way as linguistic interpretation. Images are analogue representation of a real world. They are signs (or signals). However they send back to what it means through an equivalent perceptive form. They are a "sign that shows". Concepts, expressed by words, are arbitrary representation of the real world: the link between a word and its meaning is arbitrary and conventional. In this sense, a concept is a "sign that says".

The main problem with images, and with "signs that show" is that they show without specifying what they show. They do not prescribe a signification. This is not the case with concepts. They are expressed by words, extracted from a language, from which they inherit the systematic properties. The concept prescribes a meaning, because it belongs to a system of opposition and differences, which gives a content to it out of any context. There is no such system for images or sounds. So we have to precisely make the distinction between the notion of *descriptors* for an image or a sound, and the indices, which will permit its qualification. We can introduce now the two following definitions:

- A descriptor is a piece of information extracted from a document by automatic means. It is close to the physical content of the document.
- An index is a position or a value given in the scope of an interpretative system, and associated to the management of a set of documents, i.e. a document collection.

A descriptor is not an index, to the extent that two descriptors containing different values of the same kind of information can refer to the same interpretation of documents. For example, two different colour histograms do not mean that the images from which they have been extracted are significantly different. Descriptors are extracted information, they do not correspond to any category. Conversely, two different indices or concepts refer to two different interpretations of the contents.

The available audio-visual descriptors are :

- Iconic descriptors.
- Key-frames.
- Descriptors of the digital signal (texture, histograms, ...)
- Descriptors computed from descriptors of the digital signal.

These fact are confirmed by the documentary practice. In the audio-visual industry, contents are accompanied along their live cycle by textual documents, which prescribe their meaning. Since they have no meaning by themselves, audio-visual documents are put into a textual universe, which builds the meaning they will carry out with their audio-visual manifestation. They are letters of intention, project description, scripts, conductors, mounting notes, etc. The archives comment the contents to give them a meaning, which will be used for retrieval.

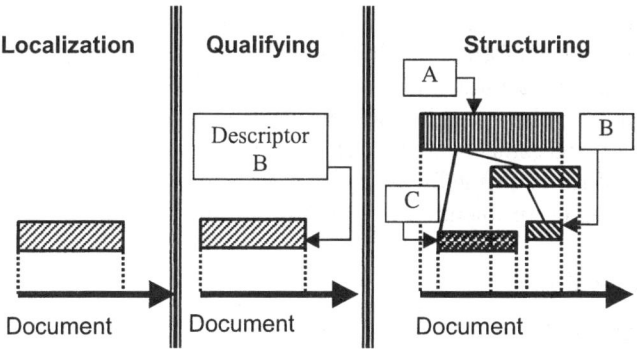

Fig. 3. The three steps of indexing

3.4   Three Types of Indexing

Now we can sum up what we have seen about indexing. From its first beginning, to its recent mutation following the computer introduction, we can distinguish three types of indexing :

- Conceptual indexing : the content is qualified by a concept, which describes what the document is about. Concepts can belong to more or less complex and organised structures. They can be simple lists of terms, thesaurus, or even ontology. The organisation is linguistic or logic. Recent research in this domain concern how to use artificial intelligence, and knowledge representation for developing indexing tools.
- Structural indexing : these indices describe how two indexed segments of the document are linked. It concerns the layout of the document and its structure. It focuses mainly on the way to articulate qualification and localisation.
- Content-based indexing : rather than indexing it is content-based description. It concerns the extraction of characteristics. It makes it possible to link a document content, according to some distance measurement.

Finally, indexing can be decomposed into three steps, which represent the functions that can be assigned to indexing :

- Localisation: where the descriptors are, It permits to know where is information according to manipulation units.
- Qualifying: what do they concern, It builds the links between what we are searching and the interpretation of what has been localised.
- Structuring; how they are linked one another. This articulation permits to intersect qualification and localisation in the scope of an index structure.

4   Multimedia Indexing

We have introduced above the notion of a multimedia document as a document calling for several semiotic appropriation forms. Audio-visual is multimedia since it calls up images, music, noise and speech. Such a document mobilizes several semiotic appropriation forms. In addition, if it contains several perceptive modalities, the document is multi-modal. Audio-visual documents are multi-modal, since they call for the eyesight and the hearing. We have seen also that one consequence of digitizing is that it allows to consider as much semiotic units as necessary. With multimedia we must take into account new objects, which modify the indexing problem: the temporal objects.

4.1   Temporal Objects

Temporal objects are contents, the semiotic restitution form of which is dynamic or temporal. Consequently they enforce the order and the rhythm of reading. They have a duration, which prevent to consider then in one glance. We need time to consult their content. They are not randomly meaningfully readable. However, in the digital context, some of these problems can be resolved.

In an analog context, reading tools are physical devices, which restitute their temporal form from a spatial and coded record. These tools are dedicated and specialised, and prevent random access to any part of a temporal object. In a numerical context, digitising provides tools for signal processing (compression, scripting, watermarking). In addition, digitised temporal contents can be integrated into a computer information system for exchange and management [9, 10, 11, 12, 13].

4.2   Computer Information Systems

Digitising is a process, which results in content transformation, by applying techniques issued from signal processing, pattern recognition, and more generally applied mathematics. Computerisation concerns exchanging and handling contents, by applying techniques issued from document engineering, software engineering, and more generally symbolic computing. In the case of digitising, the content is a physical object (the light encoded in the pixels, a sound wave), which is processed by the numerical application of mathematic laws. In the case of computerisation, the content is an information, a computing object, which is handled by symbol processing. This is essentially the computerisation, which modifies the indexing approach for audio-visual objects. They mainly concern :

- The integration of the documentation and the documents line : the production of a temporal object is complex, and thus is realised in distinct steps, each of which containing its own documentation : production (scripts, story-board, . . .), broadcasting (TV magazines, TV conductors, . . .), archiving (notes, annexes, dots). The computerisation allows the integration of all documents on the same support. It allows also to exchange the corresponding information, along the audio-visual object life cycle. The content is built up, broadcasted, and archived carrying along its documentation, which is enriched and adapted along its life cycle.
- Document and documentation link : segments of the document and its documentation can be linked, thanks to the digital support.

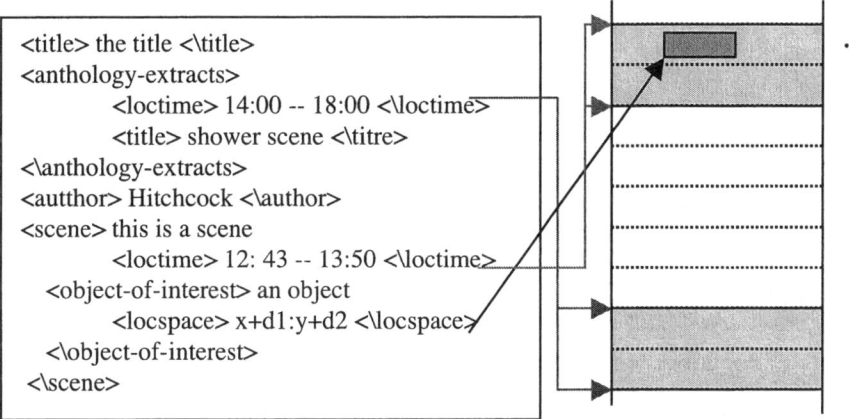

```
<title> the title <\title>
<anthology-extracts>
        <loctime> 14:00 -- 18:00 <\loctime>
        <title> shower scene <\titre>
<\anthology-extracts>
<autthor> Hitchcock <\author>
<scene> this is a scene
        <loctime> 12: 43 -- 13:50 <\loctime>
    <object-of-interest> an object
        <locspace> x+d1:y+d2 <\locspace>
    <\object-of-interest>
<\scene>
```

Fig. 4. The document information is not in the document, and its organisation is not that of the described document

- Integration of the document and the documentation : the document and the documentation are on the same support and the documentation is mandatory for exploiting the document.

To conclude, the main drawback of computerisation is simple, but fundamental : the coexistence on the same support of the content and documentary information. However, coexistence does not mean inclusion. Meta data are integrated in and linked with the content, but not included in it. Markup are not in the document by itself, but in a separated document (notes, review). The indexed document and its indices are linked, however the description order may be different from the order of the segments in the document. We give an example to illustrate this aspect in figure 4.

5 MPEG-7: Multimedia Content Description Interface

The *Motion Picture Expert Group* (MPEG) is a committee of experts in charge of proposing technological standards for the audio-visual and hypermedia. Its work has mainly concerned audio and video objects compression. The standards MPEG-1, MPEG-2, and MPEG-4 allow the broadcasting on the network of audio-visual contents, which could not be transmitted otherwise. MPEG-7 does not concern data compression but content description. The addressed problem is not signal digitising but content exchanging by communicating document descriptions, which allow their identification and exploitation.

5.1 General Description of MPEG-7

MPEG-7 stands for Multimedia Content Description Interface. It is a new standard for the description of multimedia content, designed to assist content-based access to multimedia data. The standard defines three kinds of information that comprise the description :

- Creation and usage information. It regards mostly textual information, commonly known as metadata or metainfo.
- Structural information expresses low-level and machine-oriented description. It describes content in the form of signal segments and their properties.
- Semantic information concerns the conceptual aspects to express high-level and human oriented information. They deal with semantic entities, such as objects, events and concepts.

5.2   Structural Information of MPEG-7

MPEG-7 specifies a standard set of *Descriptors* that can be used to describe various types of multimedia information. I specifies also a riche set of pre-defined structures of Descriptors and their relationships, as well as ways to define one's own structures. These structures are called *Description Schemes*. Defining Description Schemes is done by using a special language, the *Description Definition Language* (DLL), which is also part of the standard. The information structures available are :

- Features: they concern all what we need to express for describing the document (authors, scenes, segments, ...)
- Descriptors: they are the formal representation of a feature,
- Schemata description: they correspond to structures linking two different descriptors or other schemata descriptors. To a certain extent, they are an adaptation to MPEG-7 of the notion of DTD of XML, or of Schema of XML-Schema
- The *Description Definition Language* (DLL), to create descriptors and description schemata. It is an extension of XML-Schema

Figure 5 explains a hypothetical MPEG-7 chain in practice. The circular boxes depict tools that are doing things, such as encoding or decoding, whereas the square boxes represent static elements, such as a description. The dotted boxes in the figure encompass the normative elements of the MPEG-7 standard. There can be other streams from content to user; these are not depicted here. Furthermore, it is understood that there might be cases where a binary efficient representation of the description is not needed, and a textual representation would suffice. Thus, the use for the encoder and decoder is optional.

5.3   MPEG-7 Basic Descriptors and Schemata

MPEG-7 proposes standards for the sound schemata, the video schemata, and the multimedia schemata.

5.3.1   Sound Schemata

Audio schemata are designed to allow the expression of information about the sound signal, which can be extracted with tools available today. They concern :

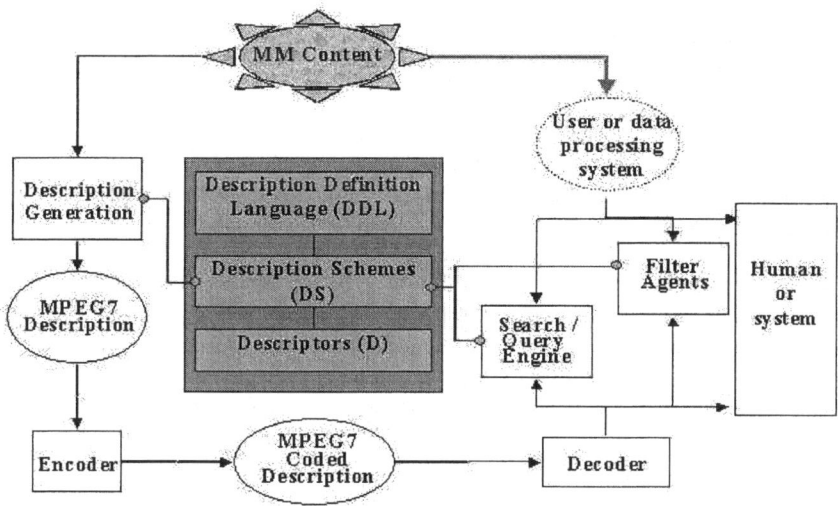

Fig. 5. An abstract representation of possible applications using MPEG-7

- sounds effects.
- the quality in tone of music instruments. The scheme describes the perceptive properties with a reduced number of descriptors, such as "richness", "attack", ...
- the speech : it is described by a combination of sounds and words, which allows to find unknown words of a given vocabulary with the associated sounds.
- the melodies : the scheme is designed to allow query by analogy, specially with an aria whistled or hummed by the user.
- low-level descriptions (temporal envelope, spectral representation, harmonics, ...).

A "silence" descriptor permits to describe a silent content.

5.3.2   Video Schemata

Video and visual schemata are more elaborated and complex. The mainly concern the following aspects :

- Basic descriptors to localise, with a variable accuracy, a part of a visual or video content. For example, they can return a 2D coordinate system, which can be typical of a given or several frames. In the last case it allows the comparison of positions between different frames.
- Colour descriptors: quantisation, colour space, prevailing colour, ...
- Texture: partition of homogeneous texture area, histograms, ...,
- Patterns: area analysis, edges representation, three dimensions patterns,
- Movements: camera movement, trajectory, movement analysis, ...

- Localisation: spatio-temporal localisation of a video sequence as a "pipe" or spatio-temporal region,
- Face recognition.

5.3.3   Multimedia Schemata

This last set is the richest and the most complex. In addition, it takes explicitly into account documentary, editorial, and conceptual information, which are necessary for the hypermedia description. The main proposed structures are :

- Content management: MPEG-7 elements describe the content creation, its production, its encoding, the coding and files formats,
- Content description: it concerns the structural and semantical aspects. The description of the semantical content uses conceptual description, based on the "real world", which is close to human understanding of multimedia information.
- Browsing and content accessing: summary structures, as well as partitions or decompositions are available. "Variations" are the description of different resources, which represent variants of the same content depending of the context. For example, the linguistic variants of the same audio-visual program.
- Content organisation: for the description of the organisation of collections of objects, events or content segments.
- User interaction: it concerns user preferences or profile for content reading. They can be used with the "variation" schemata to propose user-adapted content (the user language for example).

5.4   Example: Description Scheme of the Video Mounting Transitions

To conclude this section, we give an example of the specification of a description scheme concerning the transitions between mounted video segments [8]. First, we must define the syntax. It is written thanks to the DDL, based on the XML Schema as follows :

```
<!-- ############################################-->
<!-- Definition of Transition DS -->
<!-- ############################################-->
<complexType name="TransitionType">
  <complexType>
    <extension base="mpeg7:VideoSegmentType">
      <sequence>
        <element type="GradualEvolution"
                 type="mpeg7:GradualEvolutionType"
                 minOccurs="0"/>
        <element name="SpatioTemporalLocator"
                 type="mpeg7:SpatioTemporalLocatorType"
                 minOccurs="0"/>
```

```
</sequence>
<attribute name="editingLevel" use="optional">
  <simpleType base="string">
    <enumeration value="global"/> <!--Or InterShot-->
    <enumeration value="composition"/>
```

Secondly, the semantic concepts are defined as in table 3.

Table 3. Definition of the semantic concepts of a video mounting transition

TransitionType	Describes a transition realised between two edited video segments during an editing process. Three different types of transitions are distinguished based on the value of the attribute editingLevel: global transitions, composition transitions, and internal transitions. Three different types of transitions are also distinguished based on the value of the attribute evolution: cuts, analog cuts, and gradual transitions.
GradualEvolution	Describes the transition when it is a gradual (optional). It does not apply to transitions that are cuts and analog residual cuts.

6   Current Approaches

We will present three current approaches to audio-visual document indexing. The first refers to the classical text mining approach. Although it does not bring new concepts in indexing, it remains the most developed approach for the present time. It is mainly due to its efficiency, and its facility of use. We will shortly present some recent approaches, and will not go further in detailed description. Other approaches use spatio-temporal description and object oriented models of multimedia data bases. We invite the reader to use the bibliographical references given at the end of the paper [16, 17, 18, 19, 27, 28, 29, 30, 31, 32]. The second approach is mainly based on the XML Schema tools, which is a very promising approach. The last one, is based on an prototype, which has been developed at INA.

6.1   Text Mining

6.1.1   Statistical Analysis Approaches

Indexing is based on the computation of the number of occurrences of words (strings) in the document. It makes the assumption that the document can be represented by the strings, which have the highest number of occurrences. The number of occurrences is standardised by the total number of words in the collection of documents.

Let N be the total number of documents and idf_i the number of documents where the string i appears.

$$tr_i = \log \frac{N - idf_i}{idf_i}$$

denotes the level of discrimination of the documents by this string.

It is preferable to take into account the distribution of words in one document as well as the distribution of words in the collection of documents. Let N be the total number of documents, $tf_{i,j}$, the number of occurrences of the word w_i in the document D_j, and n_j the total number of different words in D_j. We compute two parameters :

$$P_{1_{i,j}} = (1 + \log tf_{i,j}) \frac{1}{\sqrt{(1 + \log tf_{1,j})^2 \ldots (1 + \log tf_{n_j,j})^2}}$$

$$P_{2_{i,j}} = (1 + \log tf_{i,j}) \log \frac{N}{df_i}$$

where, df_i is the number of documents, where the word w_i appears. P_1 represents the relevance of representing one document D_j by the word w_i, and P_2 represents the selectivity of the word w_i in the collection of documents. We usually compute a combination of P_1, and P_2 to take advantage of both characteristics .

This basic notion is completed by the statistical distribution of strings in the documents or linguistic approaches to compute the weight of strings.

$$index_i : d_k(weight_{i_k}) : d_l(weight_{i_l}) : d_m weight_{i_m})$$

To reduce the number of indices, and to widen their scope of representation, words are reduced to their roots by stemming algorithms.

6.1.2   Text Mining with Meta-knowledge

In this approach, the statistical computation of words weight is linked with knowledge about the semantic relationships, with exist in the vocabulary. They can be, for example, the words, which surround a given word, the situation of the word in the document, or in some part of the document (the paragraph, for example), or an ontology of the concepts supported by the words [3]. In this last case the ontology is also used for organising the domain is themes and indexing is linked with the themes. organisation.

6.1.3   Text Mining with SOM

These approaches are based on the works developed by Kohonen, known as the *Self Organisation Maps*. Instead of computing statistical distribution of words, its is possible to use their distribution on a neural network map. In this approach the position of words (respectively documents) on a map is computed depending on their respective contribution to the neurones, which recognise documents (respectively word). Figure 7 presents some known results, which have been presented in the litterature [14, 15, 20, 21, 22, 23].

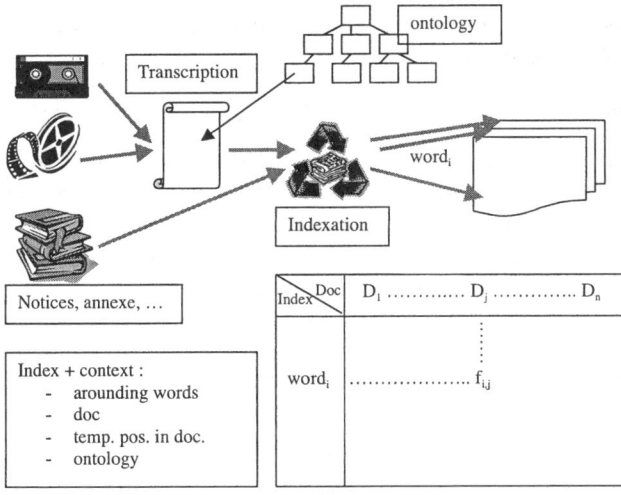

Fig. 6. Indexing is driven by knowledge about the words taxonomy

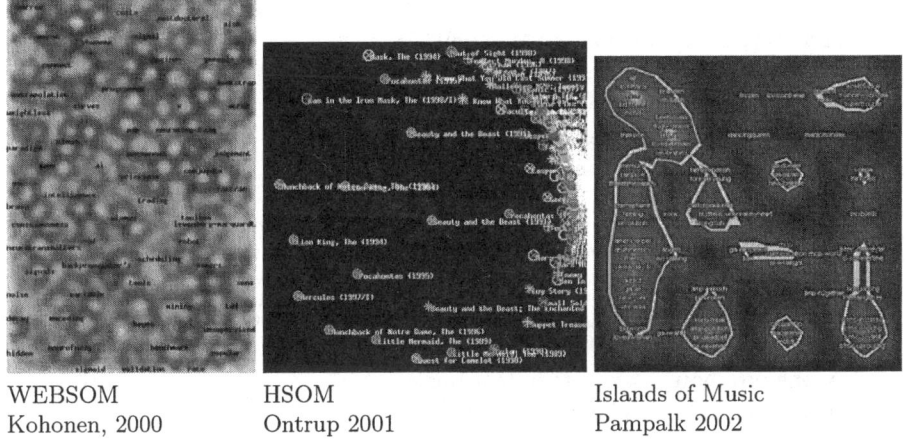

WEBSOM	HSOM	Islands of Music
Kohonen, 2000	Ontrup 2001	Pampalk 2002

Fig. 7. Words and documents are organised on the maps according to their respective distance

6.2 XML-Schema and Databases

Numerous approaches for digitization, storage and retrieval of audiovisual information and its associated data are based on XML schema and the MPEG-7 standard [2]. In their approach of bridging XML-Schema and relational database, I. Varlamis and M. Vazirgiannis define a XML-Schema for describing documents, objects and relations [24, 25]. The XML-Schema file contains five different types of subelements.

- xsd:element: They define the name and type of each XML element. For example the statement

```
<xsd:element name = "AudioVisual" type = " AudioVisualDS " />
```

defines that XML files may contain an element named *AudioVisual* with complex content and as described elsewhere in the XML-Schema.
- xsd:attribute: They describe the name and type of attributes of an XML element. They may contain an attribute **use** with the value **required**, which states that these attributes are mandatory for this XML element. They can be of simple (integer, float, string, etc.) or complex type (i.e. enumerations, numerical range etc.). For example, in the following statements, the first xsd:attribute definition states that the *Trackleft* attribute may take an integer value, whereas the second xsd:attribute, noted *AVType* may take a value the format of which is described elsewhere in the XML-Schema.

```
<xsd:attribute name = "TrackLeft" type =" xsd:integer" use="required"/>
<xsd:attribute name = "AVType" type = "AVTypeD" use="required"/>
```

- xsd:simpleType: They define new datatypes that can be used for XML attributes. For example :

```
<xsd:simpleType name = "AVTypeD" >
    <xsd:restriction base = "string">
        <xsd:enumeration value = "Movie" />
        <xsd:enumeration value = "Picture" />
    </xsd:restriction>
</xsd:simpleType>
```

- xsd:attributeGroup: They group xsd:attribute definitions that are used by many XML elements.
- xsd:complexType: They represent the various entities of the metadata model. They contain:
  - one ore more <xsd:attribute> tags
  - one ore more<xsd:element> tags

Here follows the complete definition of the internal structure of the Audiovisual XML element :

```
<xsd:element name="AudioVisual type=" AudioVisualDS " />
<xsd:complexType name="AudioVisualDS">
    <xsd:attribute name="id" type=" ID use="required />
    <xsd:attribute name="AVType" type="AVTypeD" use="required"/>
    <xsd:sequence>
<xsd:element maxOccurs="1" minOccurs="0"name="Syntactic" type="SyntacticDS" />
<xsd:element maxOccurs="1" minOccurs="0"name="Semantic" type="SemanticDS" />
<xsd:element maxOccurs="1" minOccurs="0" ref="MetaInfoDS" />
    </xsd:sequence> </xsd:complexType>
<xsd:simpleType name="AVTypeD">
    <xsd:restriction base="string">
```

```
    <xsd:enumeration value="Movie" />
    <xsd:enumeration value="Picture" />
    <xsd:enumeration value="Document" />
</xsd:restriction> </xsd:simpleType>
```

The AudioVisual element :

- has two attributes ("id", which is a number and "AVType", which can take one of the values Movie, Picture, or Document)
- may contain two sub-elements namely Syntactic and Semantic (with their sub-elements)
- may contain e reference to a MetaInfoDS element

The structure of the XML Schema file contains the definition of the various entities and some supportive structure, and the description of the structure of the database commands.

The extension elements are:

- DBCommand
- DBInsert, DBUpdate
- DBDelete
- DBReply
- DBSelect

Finally, for mapping XML-SCHEMA into a Relational schema, the XML-Schema file that contains information about structure of the exchanged XML documents is used to generate the relational database structures. Then, XML documents are parsed to contruct the appropriate SQL commands.

6.3   Audio-Visual Event Description Interface (INA)

The AEDI can be seen as an XML language adapted to XML constraints. It permits to express description schemata, which define the n dimensional structure of a given type of an audio-visual document [1, 9, 10, 11]. It is a representation model which include meta-data linked to the production of an audio-visual document. It permits the expression of description schemata, which defines the n dimensional structure of an audio-visual document. The meta-data, which are produced by the AEDI model are linked to the content of the audio-visual documents.

The AEDI model has been implemented in the MIPE environment (*Multimedia Indexing Publishing Environment*), which is an editor/composer/publisher environment [1]. MIPE permits browsing document such as summary, index, textual transcriptions, including typical images of an video sequence. These navigation tools allow the direct access to the original documents by following the links available. It is also possible to access only a part of a document.

The MIPE prototype is composed of several main modules.

- The *ontology* defines the semantics of concepts used for describing the audio-visual contents. It is mainly used as a browsing document.
- The *description scheme* defines the classes of objects available for the description of documents, and the structural relations between classes. It allows to build reasoning on description.
- The *AEDI description* defines the documents segments, which have been indexed and builds the descriptors instances corresponding to the classes defined in the description scheme.
- The *covering texts* (notices, transcriptions, scripts, copyrights, ...), are XML encoded and linked to some AEDI description by Hypertext links. For example the text/sound can be aligned according to a transcription.
- The *audio-visual document* is a specific temporal selection in one or several video or audio files.

7   Conclusion

We have seen that the main outcome of audio-visual document digitizing is the integration of all documents linked to a video production line on the same support.

The main consequence is a revisiting of the definition of indexing, which generalizes the text indexing definition. By breaking the document integrity and putting all documents on the same support it becomes possible to define indices linked to the semantical objects, which compose an audio-visual document. The most important property of these objects is that they can be temporal objects.

The development of marked-up languages has open the possibility of developing indexing based on a semantical document description. It also made it possible to propose effective computer-based systems, which can implement actual application.

References

[1] Gwendal Auffret, Jean Carrive, Olivier Chevet, Thomas Dechilly, Remi Ronfard, and Bruno Bachimont, Audiovisual-based Hypermedia Authoring - using structured representations for efficient access to AV documents, in ACM Hypertext, 1999

[2] G. Akrivas, S. Ioannou, E. Karakoulakis, K. Karpouzis,Y. Avrithis, A.Delopoulos, S. Kollias, M. Vazirgiannis, I.Varlamis. An Intelligent System for Retrieval and Mining of Audiovisual Material Based on the MPEG-7 Description Schemes. European Symposium on Intelligent Technologies, Hybrid Systems and their implementation on Smart Adaptive Systems (EUNITE), Spain, 2001.

[3] Bachimont B. et Dechilly T., Ontologies pour l'indexation conceptuelle et structurelle de l'audiovisuel, Eyrolles, dans Ingénierie des connaissances 1999-2001.

[4] Bachimont B., Isaac A., Troncy R., Semantic Commitment for Designing Ontologies : a Proposal. 13th International Conference EKAW'02, 1-4 octobre 2002, Siguenza, Espagne

[5] Bachimont B. Indexation multimédia, in Assistance intelligente à la recherche d'information, édité par Eric Gaussier et Marie-Hélène Stefanini,, Hermès, 2002

[6] Bachimont B. "audiovisual indexing and automatic analysis: problems and perspectives from an archiving point of view" Imagina 2002, Monaco, 12 february 2002

[7] Bruno Bachimont. Le document audiovisuel, le numérique, ses usages et son archivage. Le document multimédia en sciences du traitement de l'information. Ecole thématique du CNRSGDR I3, Documents et évolution. Cépaduès-Editions, tome 1, p. 111-128,2000.

[8] Bachimont B., (1998), MPEG-7 and Ontologies: an editorial perspective, Virtual Systems and Multimedia 98, Gifu, Japan, Oct. 1998.

[9] Carrive, J., Pachet, F., Ronfard, R. (1998). Using Description Logics for Indexing Audiovisual Documents. International Workshop on Description Logics (DL'98), Trento, Italy, ITC-Irst pp.116-120, 1998.

[10] Carrive J., Pachet F., Ronfard R. (2000b), Logiques de descriptions pour l'analyse structurelle de film, in Ingéniérie des Connaissances, évolutions récentes et nouveaux défis, Charlet J., Zacklad M., Kassel G., Bourigault D. (ed.), Eyrolles, pp. 423-438.

[11] Carrive J., Pachet F., Ronfard R. (2000a), Clavis: a temporal reasoning system for classification of audiovisual sequences, in proceedings of the Content-Based Multimedia Access (RIAO'2000), Paris, France, April 12-14, pp. 1400-1415.

[12] Gwenaël Durand, P. Faudemay, Cross-indexing and access to mixed-media contents, Proc. CBMI01 International Workshop on Content-Based Multimedia Indexing, Brescia, Italy, September 2001.

[13] M. Erwig, R. H. Gueting, M. Schneider, M. Vazirgiannis. Spatio-Temporal Data Types: An Approach to Modeling and Querying Moving Objects in Databases, GeoInformatica Journal 3(3), Kluwer Publishers, 1999.

[14] T. Kohonen, S. Kaski, K. Lagus, J. Salojärvi, J. Honkela, V. Paatero, and A. Saarela. (2000) Self Organization of a Massive Document Collection. IEEE Transactions on Neural Networks, Special Issue on Neural Networks for Data Mining and Knowledge Discovery, volume 11, number 3, pages 574-585. May 2000.

[15] Lagus, K. (2000) Text Mining with the WEBSOM. Acta Polytechnica Scandinavica, Mathematics and Computing Series no. 110, Espoo 2000, 54 pp. D.Sc.(Tech) Thesis, Helsinki University of Technology, Finland. URL http://www.cis.hut.fi/krista/thesis/

[16] Lespinasse K. and Bachimont B. (2001). Is Peritext a Key for Audiovisual Documents ? The Use of Texts Describing Television Programs to Assist indexing. CICLing2001, Mexico, Springer-Verlag. conference: CICLing2001.

[17] T. Markousis, D. Tsirikos, M. Vazirgiannis, G. Stavrakas. A Client-Server Design for Interactive Multimedia Documents based on Java, in Elsevier - Computer Communications Journal, 2000.

[18] I. Mirbel B. Pernici T. Sellis S. Tserkezoglou, M. Vazirgiannis. Checking Temporal Integrity of Interactive Multimedia Documents, in Very Large Data Bases journal,9(2): 111-130, 2000.

[19] I. Mirbel, B. Pernici, M. Vazirgiannis. Temporal Integrity Constraints in Interactive Multimedia Documents, in the proceedings of IEEE-International Conference on Multimedia Computing and Systems (ICMCS '99), Florence, Italy, June 1999.

[20] J. Ontrup and H. Ritter, Text Categorization and Semantic Browsing with Self-Organizing Maps on non-euclidean Spaces, Proceedings of PKDD-01 5th European Conference on Principles and Practice of Knowledge Discovery in Databases, pp. 338-349, ed. L. De Raedt and A. Siebes, publ. Springer LNAI 2168, 2001

[21] J. Ontrup and H. Ritter, Hyperbolic Self-Organizing Maps for Semantic Navigation, Advances in Neural Information Processing Systems 14, 2001

[22] E. Pampalk, A. Rauber, and D. Merkl, Content-based Organization and Visualization of Music Archives, Proceedings of the ACM Multimedia 2002, pp 570-579, Juan les Pins, France, December 1-6, 2002.

[23] E. Pampalk, A. Rauber, D. Merkl, Using Smoothed Data Histograms for Cluster Visualization in Self-Organizing Maps, Proceedings of the Intl Conf on Artificial Neural Networks (ICANN 2002), pp. 871-876, August 27.-30. 2002, Madrid, Spain

[24] I. Varlamis, M. Vazirgiannis, P. Poulos. Using XML as a medium for describing, modifying and querying audiovisual content stored in relational database systems, International Workshop on Very Low Bitrate Video Coding (VLBV). Athens 2001.

[25] I. Varlamis, M. Vazirgiannis. Bridging XML-Schema and relational databases. A system for generating and manipulating relational databases using valid XML documents, in the proceedings of ACM Symposium on Document Engineering, Nov. 2001, Atlanta, USA

[26] I. Varlamis, M. Vazirgiannis. Web document searching using enhanced hyperlink semantics based on XML, proceedings of IDEAS '01, Grenoble, France.

[27] M. Vazirgiannis D. Tsirikos, Th.Markousis, M. Trafalis, Y. Stamati, M. Hatzopoulos, T. Sellis. Interactive Multimedia Documents: a Modeling, Authoring and Rendering approach, in Multimedia Tools and Applications Journal (Kluwer Academic Publishers), 2000.

[28] M. Vazirgiannis, Y. Theodoridis, T. Sellis. Spatio-Temporal Composition and Indexing for Large Multimedia Applications, in ACM/Springer-Verlag Multimedia Systems Journal, vol. 6(4), 1998.

[29] M. Vazirgiannis, C. Mourlas. An object Oriented Model for Interactive Multimedia Applications, The Computer Journal, British Computer Society, vol. 36(1), 1/1993.

[30] M. Vazirgiannis. Multimedia Data Base Object and Application Modeling Issues and an Object Oriented Model, in Multimedia Database Systems: Design and Implementation Strategies, Kluwer Academic Publishers, 1996, Pages: 208-250.

[31] E.Veneau, R.Ronfard, P.Bouthemy, From Video Shot Clustering to Sequence Segmentation, Fifteenth International Conference on Pattern Recognition (ICPR'2000), Barcelona, september 2000.

[32] D. Vodislav, M. Vazirgiannis. Structured Interactive Animation for Multimedia Documents, Proceedings of IEEE Visual Languages Symposium, Seattle, USA, September 2000.

Relevance Feedback Document Retrieval Using Support Vector Machines

Takashi Onoda[1], Hiroshi Murata[1], and Seiji Yamada[2]

[1] Central Research Institute of Electric Power Industry,
Communication & Information Laboratory, 2-11-1 Iwado Kita,
Komae-shi, Tokyo 201-8511, Japan
{onoda, murata}@criepi.denken.or.jp
[2] National Institute of Informatics, 2-1-2 Hitotsubashi,
Chiyoda-ku, Tokyo 101-8430, Japan
seiji@nii.ac.jp
http://research.nii.ac.jp/~seiji/index-e.html

Abstract. We investigate the following data mining problems from the document retrieval: From a large data set of documents, we need to find documents that relate to human interest as few iterations of human testing or checking as possible. In each iteration a comparatively small batch of documents is evaluated for relating to the human interest. We apply active learning techniques based on Support Vector Machine for evaluating successive batches, which is called *relevance feedback*. Our proposed approach has been very useful for document retrieval with relevance feedback experimentally. In this paper, we adopt several representations of the Vector Space Model and several selecting rules of displayed documents at each iteration, and then show the comparison results of the effectiveness for the document retrieval in these several situations.

1   Introduction

As the Internet technology progresses, accessible information by end users is explosively increasing. In this situation, we can now easily access a huge document database through the WWW. However it is hard for a user to retrieve relevant documents from which he/she can obtain useful information, and a lot of studies have been done in information retrieval, especially document retrieval[1]. Active works for such document retrieval have been reported in TREC(Text Retrieval Conference)[2] for English documents, IREX(Information Retrieval and Extraction Exercise)[3] and NTCIR(NII-NACSIS Test Collection for Information Retrieval System)[4] for Japanese documents.

In most frameworks for information retrieval, a Vector Space Model (which is called VSM) in which a document is described with a high-dimensional vector is used[5]. An information retrieval system using a vector space model computes the similarity between a query vector and document vectors by cosine of the two vectors and indicates a user a list of retrieved documents.

S. Tsumoto et al. (Eds.): AM 2003, LNAI 3430, pp. 59–73, 2005.

In general, since a user hardly describes a precise query in the first trial, interactive approach to modify the query vector by evaluation of the user on documents in a list of retrieved documents. This method is called *relevance feedback*[6] and used widely in information retrieval systems. In this method, a user directly evaluates whether a document is relevant or irrelevant in a list of retrieved documents, and a system modifies the query vector using the user evaluation. A traditional way to modify a query vector is a simple learning rule to reduce the difference between the query vector and documents evaluated as relevant by a user.

In another approach, relevant and irrelevant document vectors are considered as positive and negative examples, and relevance feedback is transposed to a binary classification problem[7]. Okabe and Yamada[7] proposed a frame work in which relational learning to classification rules was applied to interactive document retrieval. Since the learned classification rules is described with symbolic representation, they are readable to our human and we can easily modify the rules directly using a sort of editor. For the binary classification problem, Support Vector Machines(which are called SVMs) have shown the excellent ability. And some studies applied SVM to the text classification problems[8] and the information retrieval problems[9].

Recently, we have proposed a relevance feedback framework with SVM as active learning and shown the usefulness of our proposed method experimentally[10]. Now, we are interested in which is the most efficient representation for the document retrieval performance and the learning performance, boolean representation, TF representation or TFIDF representation, and what is the most useful selecting rule for displayed documents at each iteration. In this paper, we adopt several representations of the Vector Space Model(which is called VSM) and several selecting rules of displayed documents at each iteration, and then show the comparison results of the effectiveness for the document retrieval in these several situations.

In the remaining parts of this paper, we explain a SVM algorithm in the second section briefly. An active learning with SVM for the relevance feedback, and our adopted VSM representations and selecting displayed documents rules are described in the third section. In the fourth section, in order to compare the effectiveness of our adopted representations and selecting rules, we show our experiments using a TREC data set of Los Angeles Times and discuss the experimental results. Eventually we conclude our work in the fifth section.

2   Support Vector Machines

Formally, the Support Vector Machine (SVM) [11] like any other classification method aims to estimate a classification function $f : \mathcal{X} \rightarrow \{\pm 1\}$ using labeled training data from $\mathcal{X} \times \{+1\}$. Moreover this function f should even classify unseen examples correctly.

In order to construct good classifiers by learning, two conditions have to be respected. First, the training data must be an unbiased sample from the same source(pdf) as the unseen test data. This concerns the experimental setup. Second, the size of the class of functions from which we choose our estimate f, the so-called capacity of the learning machine, has to be properly restricted according to statistical learning theory[11]. If the capacity is too small, complex discriminant functions cannot be approximated sufficiently well by any selectable function f in the chosen class of functions the learning machine is too simple to learn well. On the other hand, if the capacity is too large, the learning machine bears the risk of overfitting. In neural network training, overfitting is avoided by early stopping, regularization or asymptotic model selection[12, 13, 14, 15].

For SV learning machines that implement linear discriminant functions in feature spaces, the capacity limitation corresponds to finding a large margin separation between the two classes. The margin ϱ is the minimal distance of training points $(\mathbf{x}_1, y_1), \ldots, (\mathbf{x}_i, y_i), \mathbf{x}_i \in \mathbf{R}, y_i \in \{\pm 1\}$ to the separation surface, i.e. $\varrho = \min_{i=1,\ldots,\ell} \rho(\mathbf{z}_i, f)$, where $\mathbf{z}_i = (\mathbf{x}_i, y_i)$ and $\rho(\mathbf{z}_i, f) = y_i f(\mathbf{x}_i)$, and f is the linear discriminant function in some feature space

$$f(\mathbf{x}) = (\mathbf{w} \cdot \Phi(\mathbf{x})) + b = \sum_{i=1}^{\ell} \alpha_i y_i (\Phi(\mathbf{x}_i) \cdot \Phi(\mathbf{x})) + b, \qquad (1)$$

with $\mathbf{w}$ expressed as $\mathbf{w} = \sum_{i=1}^{\ell} \alpha_i y_i \Phi(\mathbf{x}_i)$. The quantity Φ denotes the mapping from input space $\mathcal{X}$ by explicitly. transforming the data into a feature space $\mathcal{F}$ using $\Phi : \mathcal{X} \to \mathcal{F}$. (see Figure 1). SVM can do so implicitly. In order to train and classify, all that SVMs use are dot products of pairs of data points $\Phi(\mathbf{x}), \Phi(\mathbf{x}_i) \in \mathcal{F}$ in feature space (cf. Eq. (1)). Thus, we need only to supply a so-called kernel function that can compute these dot products. A kernel function k allows to implicitly define the feature space (Mercer's Theorem, e.g. [16]) via

$$k(\mathbf{x}, \mathbf{x}_i) = (\Phi(\mathbf{x}) \cdot \Phi(\mathbf{x}_i)). \qquad (2)$$

By using different kernel functions, the SVM algorithm can construct a variety of learning machines, some of which coincide with classical architectures:

Polynomial classifiers of degree d:

$$k(\mathbf{x}, \mathbf{x}_i) = (\kappa \cdot (\mathbf{x} \cdot \mathbf{x}_i) + \Theta)^d,$$

where κ, Θ, and d are appropriate constants.
Neural networks(sigmoidal):

$$k(\mathbf{x}, \mathbf{x}_i) = \tanh(\kappa \cdot (\mathbf{x} \cdot \mathbf{x}_i) + \Theta),$$

where κ and Θ are appropriate constants.
Radial basis function classifiers:

$$k(\mathbf{x}, \mathbf{x}_i) = \exp\left(-\frac{\|\mathbf{x} - \mathbf{x}_i\|^2}{\sigma}\right),$$

where σ is an appropriate constant.

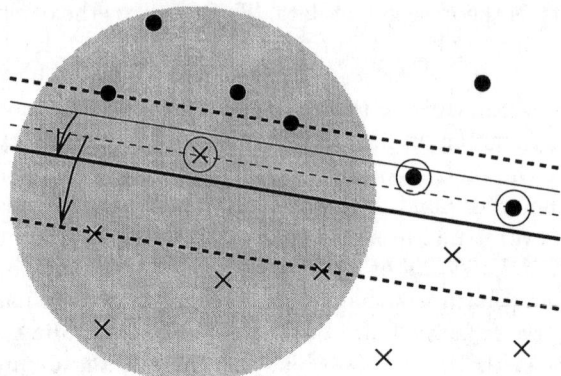

Fig. 1. A binary classification toy problem: This problem is to separate black circles from crosses. The shaded region consists of training examples, the other regions of test data. The training data can be separated with a margin indicated by the slim dashed line and the upper fat dashed line, implicating the slim solid line as discriminate function. Misclassifying one training example(a circled white circle) leads to a considerable extension(arrows) of the margin(fat dashed and solid lines) and this fat solid line can classify two test examples(circled black circles) correctly

Note that there is no need to use or know the form of Φ, because the mapping is never performed explicitly The introduction of Φ in the explanation above was for purely didactical and not algorithmical purposes. Therefore, we can computationally afford to work in implicitly very large (e.g. 10^{10}- dimensional) feature spaces. SVM can avoid overfitting by controlling the capacity and maximizing the margin. Simultaneously, SVMs learn which of the features implied by the kernel k are distinctive for the two classes, i.e. instead of finding well-suited features by ourselves (which can often be difficult), we can use the SVM to select them from an extremely rich feature space.

With respect to good generalization, it is often profitable to misclassify some outlying training data points in order to achieve a larger margin between the other training points (see Figure 1 for an example). This soft-margin strategy can also learn non-separable data. The trade-off between margin size and number of misclassified training points is then controlled by the regularization parameter C (softness of the margin). The following quadratic program (QP) (see e.g. [11, 17]):

$$\min \|\mathbf{w}\|^2 + C \sum_{i=1}^{\ell} \xi_i$$

$$\text{s.t.} \quad \rho(\mathbf{z}_i, f) \geq 1 - \xi_i \text{ for all } 1 \leq i \leq \ell \tag{3}$$

$$\xi_i \geq 0 \qquad \text{for all } 1 \leq i \leq \ell$$

leads to the SV soft-margin solution allowing for some errors.

In this paper, we use VSMs, which are high dimensional models, for the document retrieval. In this high dimension, it is easy to classify between relevant

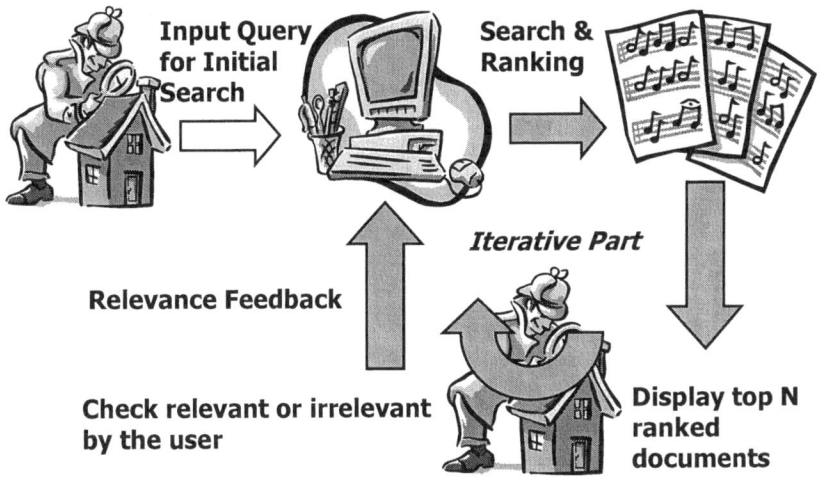

Fig. 2. Image of the relevance feedback documents retrieval: The gray arrow parts are made iteratively to retrieve useful documents for the user. This iteration is called feedback iteration in the information retrieval research area

and irrelevant documents. Therefore, we generate the SV hard-margin solution by the following quadratic program.

$$\min \quad \|\mathbf{w}\|^2$$
$$\text{s.t.} \quad \rho(\mathbf{z}_i, f) \geq 1 \text{ for all } 1 \leq i \leq \ell \tag{4}$$

3 Active Learning with SVM in Document Retrieval

In this section, we describe the information retrieval system using relevance feedback with SVM from an active learning point of view, and several VSM representation of documents and several selecting rules, which determine displayed documents to a user for the relevance feedback.

3.1 Relevance Feedback Based on SVM

Fig. 2 shows the concept of the relevance feedback document retrieval. In Fig. 2, the iterative procedure is the gray arrows parts. The SVMs have a great ability to discriminate even if the training data is small. Consequently, we have proposed to apply SVMs as the classifier in the relevance feedback method. The retrieval steps of proposed method perform as follows:

Step 1: **Preparation of documents for the first feedback:**
The conventional information retrieval system based on vector space model displays the top N ranked documents along with a request query to the user. In our method, the top N ranked documents are selected by

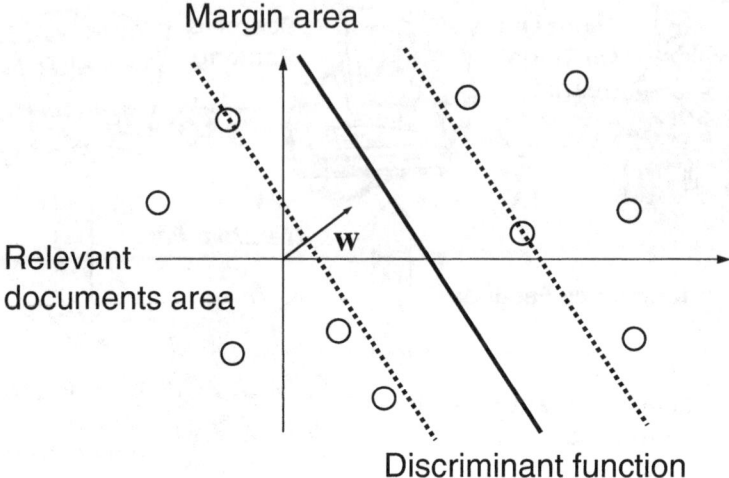

Fig. 3. The figure shows a discriminant function for classifying relevant or irrelevant documents: Circles denote documents which are checked relevant or irrelevant by a user. The solid line denotes a discriminant function. The margin area is between dotted lines

using cosine distance between the request query vector and each document vector for the first feedback iteration.

Step 2: **Judgment of documents:**
The user then classifiers these N documents into relevant or irrelevant. The relevant documents and the irrelevant documents are labeled. For instance, the relevant documents have "+1" label and the irrelevant documents have "-1" label after the user's judgment.

Step 3: **Determination of the optimal hyperplane:**
The optimal hyperplane for classifying relevant and irrelevant documents is determined by using a SVM which is learned by labeled documents(see Figure 3).

Step 4: **Discrimination documents and information retrieval:**
The documents, which are retrieved in the Step 1, are mapped into the feature space. The SVM learned by the previous step classifies the documents as relevant or irrelevant. Then the system selects the documents based on the distance from the optimal hyper plane and the feature of the margin area. The detail of the selection rules are described in the next section. From the selected documents, the top N ranked documents, which are ranked using the distance from the optimal hyperplane, are shown to user as the information retrieval results of the system. If the number of feedback iterations is more than m, then go to next step. Otherwise, return to Step 2. The m is a maximal number of feedback iterations and is given by the user or the system.

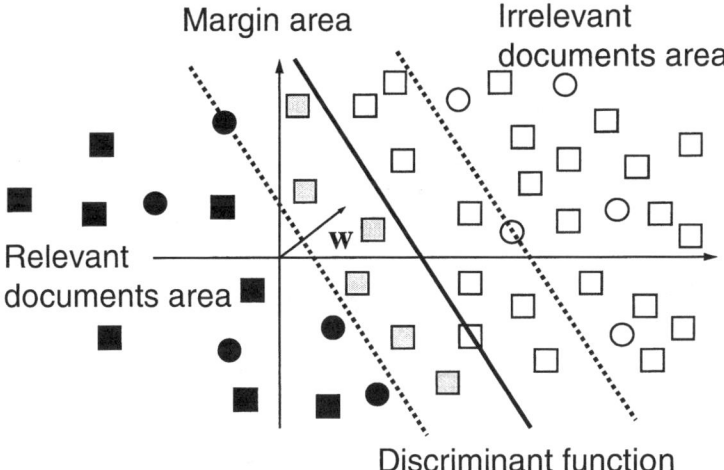

Fig. 4. The figure shows displayed documents as the result of document retrieval: Boxes denote non-checked documents which are mapped into the feature space. Circles denotes checked documents which are mapped into the feature space. The system displays the documents which are represented by black circles and boxes as the result of document retrieval to a user

Step 5: **Display of the final retrieved documents:**
    The retrieved documents are ranked by the distance between the documents and the hyper-plane which is the discriminant function determined by SVM. The retrieved documents are displayed based on this ranking(see Figure 4).

3.2   VSM Representations and Selection Rules of Displayed Documents

We discuss the issue of the term t_i in the document vector d_j. In the Information Retrieval research field, this term is called the term weighting, while in the machine learning research filed, this term is called the feature. t_i states something about word i in the document d_j. If this word is absent in the document d_j, t_i is zero. If the word is present in the document d_j, then there are several options. The first option is that this term just indicates whether this word i is present or not. This presentation is called boolean term weighting. The next option is that the term weight is a count of the number of times this word i occurs in this document d_j. This presentation is called the term frequency(TF). In the original Rocchio algorithm[6], each term TF is multiplied by a term $\log\left(\frac{N}{n_i}\right)$ where N is the total number of documents in the collection and n_i is the number of documents in which this word i occurs. This last term is called the inverse document frequency(IDF). This representation is called the term frequency-the inverse document frequency(TFIDF)[1]. The Rocchio algorithm is the original

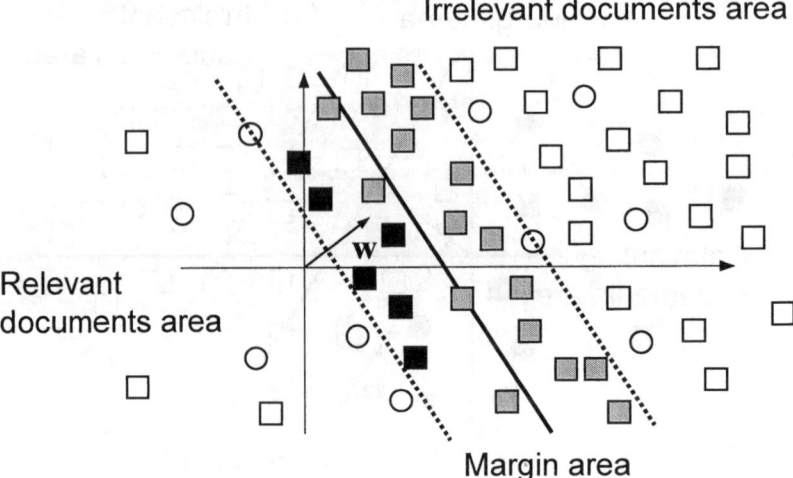

Fig. 5. Mapped non-checked documents into the feature space: Boxes denote non-checked documents which are mapped into the feature space. Circles denotes checked documents which are mapped into the feature space. Black and gray boxes are documents in the margin area. We show the documents which are represented by black boxes to a user for next iteration. These documents are in the margin area and near the relevant documents area

relevance feedback method. In this paper, we compare the effectiveness of the document retrieval and the learning performance among boolean term weighting, term frequency(TF) and term frequency inverse document frequency(TFIDF) representations for our relevance feedback based on SVM.

Next, we discuss two selection rules for displayed documents, which are used for the judgment by the user. In this paper, we compare the effectiveness of the document retrieval and the learning performance among the following three selection rules for displayed documents.

Selection Rule 1:
    The retrieved documents are mapped into the feature space. The learned SVM classifies the documents as relevant or irrelevant. The documents, which are discriminated relevant and in the margin area of SVM are selected. From the selected documents, the top N ranked documents, which are ranked using the distance from the optimal hyperplane, are displayed to the user as the information retrieval results of the system(see Figure 5). This rule is expected to achieve the most effective retrieval and keep the learning performance. This rule is our proposed one for the relevance feedback document retrieval.

Selection Rule 2:
    The retrieved documents are mapped into the feature space. The learned SVM classifies the documents as relevant or irrelevant. The documents,

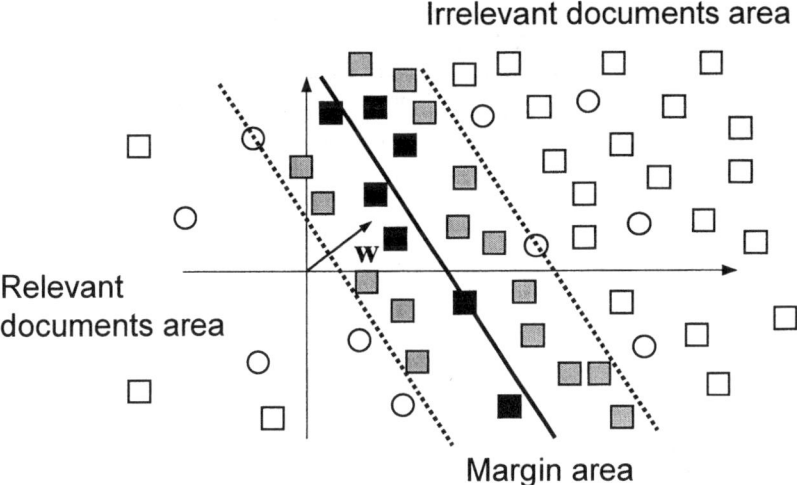

Fig. 6. Mapped non-checked documents into the feature space: Boxes denote non-checked documents which are mapped into the feature space. Circles denotes checked documents which are mapped into the feature space. Black and gray boxes are documents in the margin area. We show the documents which are represented by black boxes to a user for next iteration. These documents are near the optimal hyperplane

which are on the optimal hyperplane or near the optimal hyperplane of SVM, are selected. The system chooses the N documents in these selected documents and displays to the user as the information retrieval results of the system(see Figure 6). This rule should make the best learning performance from an active learning point of view.

4   Experiments

4.1   Experimental Setting

In the reference [10], we already have shown that the utility of our interactive document retrieval with active learning of SVM is better than the Rocchio-based interactive document retrieval[6], which is conventional one. This paper presents the experiments for comparing the utility for the document retrieval among several VSM representations, and the effectiveness for the learning performance among the several selection rules, which choose the displayed documents to judge whether a document is relevant or irrelevant by the user. The document data set we used is a set of articles in the Los Angeles Times which is widely used in the document retrieval conference TREC [2]. The data set has about 130 thousands articles. The average number of words in an article is 526. This data set includes not only queries but also the relevant documents to each query. Thus we used the queries for experiments.

We adopted the boolean weighting, TF, and TFIDF as VSM representations. The detail of the boolean and TF weighting can be seen in the section 3. We used TFIDF[1], which is one of the most popular methods in information retrieval to generate document feature vectors, and the concrete equation[18] of a weight w_t^d of a term t in a document d is in the following.

$$w_t^d = L \times t \times u \qquad\qquad (5)$$

$$L = \frac{1 + \log(tf(t,d))}{1 + \log(\text{average of } tf(t,d))} \qquad (tf)$$

$$t = \log\left(\frac{n+1}{df(t)}\right) \qquad (idf)$$

$$u = \frac{1}{0.8 + 0.2\frac{uniq(d)}{\text{average of } uniq(d)}} \qquad (\text{normalization})$$

The notations in these equation denote as follows:

- w^{d_t} is a weight of a term t in a document d,
- $tf(t,d)$ is a frequency of a term t in a document d,
- n is the total number of documents in a data set,
- $df(t)$ is the number of documents including a term t,
- $uniq(d)$ is the number of different terms in a document d.

In our experiments, we used two selection rules to estimate the effectiveness for the learning performance. The detail of these selection rules can be seen in the section 3.

The size N of retrieved and displayed documents at each iteration in the section 3 was set as twenty. The feedback iterations m were 1, 2, and 3. In order to investigate the influence of feedback iterations on accuracy of retrieval, we used plural feedback iterations.

In our experiments, we used the linear kernel for SVM learning, and found a discriminant function for the SVM classifier in this feature space. The VSM of documents is high dimensional space. Therefore, in order to classify the labeled documents into relevant or irrelevant, we do not need to use the kernel trick and the regularization parameter C(see section 2). We used LibSVM [19] as SVM software in our experiment.

In general, retrieval accuracy significantly depends on the number of the feedback iterations. Thus we changed feedback iterations for 1,2,3 and investigated the accuracy for each iteration. We utilized precision and recall for evaluating the retrieval performance of three document representations and two selection rules to display documents. The following equations are used to compute precision and recall. Since a recall-precision curve is investigated to each query, we used the average recall-precision curve over all the queries as evaluation.

$$precision = \frac{\text{The No. of retrieved relevant doc.}}{\text{The No. of retrieved doc.}},$$

$$recall = \frac{\text{The No. of retrieved relevant doc.}}{\text{The total No. of relevant doc.}}.$$

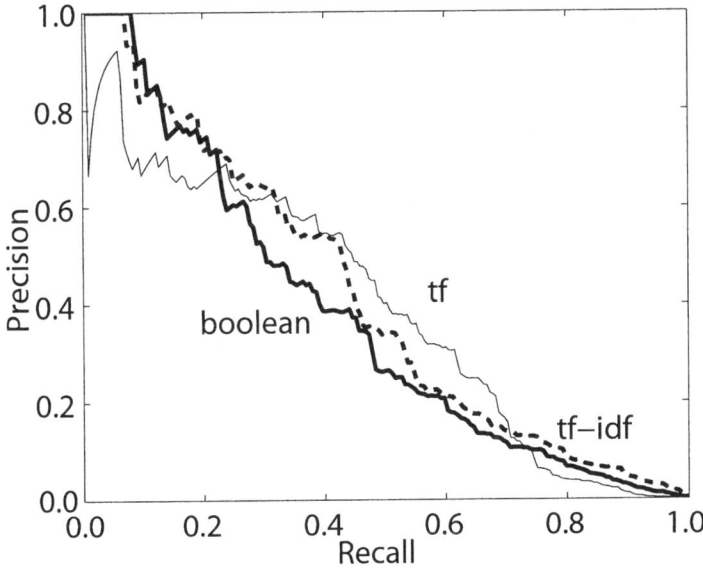

Fig. 7. The figure shows the retrieval effectiveness of SVM based feedback(using the selection rule 1) for the boolean, TF, and TFIDF representations: The lines show recall-precision performance curve by using twenty feedback documents on the set of articles in the Los Angeles Times after 3 feedback iterations. The wide solid line is the boolean representation, the broken line is TFIDF representation, and the solid line is TF representation

4.2 Comparison of Recall-Precision Performance Curves Among the Boolean, TF and TFIDF Weightings

In this section, we investigate the effectiveness for the document retrieval among the boolean, TF and TFIDF weightings, when the user judges the twenty higher ranked documents at each feedback iteration. In the first iteration, twenty higher ranked documents are retrieved using cosine distance between document vectors and a query vector in VSMs, which are represented by the boolean, TF and TFIDF weightings. The query vector is generated by a user's input of keywords. In the other iterations, the user does not need to input keywords for the information retrieval, and the user labels "+1" and "-1" as relevant and irrelevant documents respectively.

Figure 7 left side shows a recall-precision performance curve of our SVM based method for the boolean, TF and TFIDF weightings, after four feedback iterations. Our SVM based method adopts the selection rule 2. The thick solid line is the boolean weighting, the broken line is the TFIDF weighting, and the thin solid line is the TF weighting.

This figure shows that the retrieval performance of the boolean, TF, and TFIDF representations are almost same roughly. However, when we see this figure closely, the TFIDF representation is higher than that of the other two

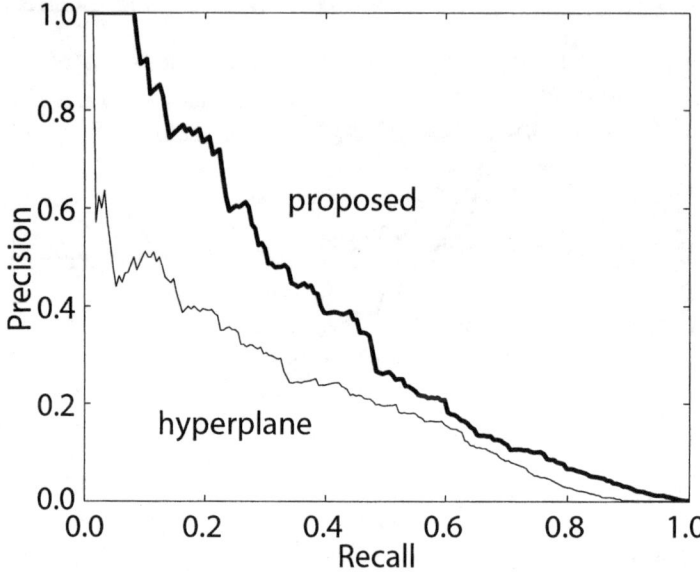

Fig. 8. The figure shows the retrieval effectiveness of SVM based feedback for the selection rule 1 and 2: The lines show recall-precision performance curves by using twenty feedback documents on the set of articles in the Los Angeles Times after 3 feedback iterations. The thin solid line is the selection rule 1, and the thick solid line is the selection rule 2

representations, i.e., the boolean and the TF representations. Consequently, in this experiment, we conclude that the TFIDF representation is a useful VSM representation for our proposed relevant feedback technique to improve the performance of the document retrieval.

4.3   Comparison of Recall-Precision Performance Curves Between the Selection Rule 1 and 2

Here, we investigate the effectiveness for the document retrieval between the selection rule 1 and 2, which are described in the section 3.

Figure 8 shows a recall-precision performance curves of the selection rule 1 and 2 for the boolean weightings, after four feedback iterations. The thin solid line is the selection rule 1, and the thick solid line is the selection rule 2. This figure shows that the precision-recall curve of the selection rule 1 is better than that of the selection rule 2. The selection rule 1 is our proposed method and the selection rule 2 denotes the selection of documents,which are on or near the hyperplane.In this experiment,we conclude that the our proposed selection rule is a useful selection for our proposed relevant feedback technique to improve the performance of the document retrieval.

Table 1 gives the average number of relevant documents in the twenty displayed documents for the selection rule 1 and 2 as a function of the number of

Table 1. Average number of relevant documents in the twenty displayed documents for the selection rule 1 and 2 using the boolean representation

No. of feedback iterations	Ave. No. of relevant documents	
	selection rule 1	selection rule 2
0	6.444	6.444
1	10.333	4.444
2	10.444	8.333
3	7.778	6.444

Table 2. Average total number of relevant documents for the selection rule 1 and 2 using the boolean representation

No. of feedback iterations	Ave. No. of relevant documents	
	selection rule 1	selection rule 2
0	6.444	6.444
1	16.778	10.889
2	27.222	19.222
3	35.000	25.667

iterations. In this table, iteration number 0 denotes the retrieval result based on cosine distance between the query vector and document vectors, which are represent by the TFIDF. We can see from the table 1 that the average number of relevant documents in the twenty displayed documents for the selection rule 1 is higher than that of the selection rule 2 at each iteration. After all, when the selection rule 2 is adopted, the user have to see a lot of irrelevant documents at each iteration. The selection rule 1 is effective to immediately put on the upper rank the special documents,which relate to the user's interesting. When the selection rule 1 is adopted, the user do not need to see a lot of irrelevant documents at each iteration. However, it is hard for the rule 1 to immediately put on the upper rank all documents, which relate to the user's interesting. In the document retrieval, a user do not want to get all documents, which relate to the user's interest. The user wants to get some documents, which relate to the user's interest as soon as possible. Therefore, we conclude that the feature of the selection rule 1 is better than that of the selection rule 2 for the relevance feedback document retrieval.

Table 2 gives the average total number of relevant documents for the selection rule 1 and 2 at each iteration. In this table, iteration number 0 denotes the retrieval result based on cosine distance between the query vector and document vectors, which are represent by the TFIDF. In table 2, the average number of relevant documents in the twenty displayed documents decreases at iteration number 3. We can see from table 2 that almost relevant documents can be found at the iteration number 3. This situation means that there are few relevant documents in the rest documents and it is difficult to find new relevant documents in the rest documents. Therefore, the average number of relevant documents in the twenty displayed documents decreases with the increase of the number of iterations.

5   Conclusion

In this paper, we adopt several representations of the Vector Space Model and several selecting rules of displayed documents at each iteration, and then show the comparison results of the effectiveness for the document retrieval in these several situations.

In our experiments, when we adopt our proposed SVM based relevance feedback document retrieval, the binary representation and the selection rule 1, where the documents that are discriminated relevant and in the margin area of SVM, are displayed to a user, show better performance of document retrieval. In future work, we will plan to analyze our experimental results theoretically.

References

1. Yates, R.B., Neto, B.R.: Modern Information Retrieval. Addison Wesley (1999)
2. TREC: (http://trec.nist.gov/)
3. IREX: (http://cs.nyu.edu/cs/projects/proteus/irex/)
4. NTCIR: (http://www.rd.nacsis.ac.jp/ntcadm/)
5. Salton, G., McGill, J.: Introduction to modern information retrieval. McGraw-Hill (1983)
6. Salton, G., ed. In: Relevance feedback in information retrieval. Englewood Cliffs, N.J.: Prentice Hall (1971) 313–323
7. Okabe, M., Yamada, S.: Interactive document retrieval with relational learning. In: Proceedings of the 16th ACM Symposium on Applied Computing. (2001) 27–31
8. Tong, S., Koller, D.: Support vector machine active learning with applications to text classification. In: Journal of Machine Learning Research. Volume 2. (2001) 45–66
9. Drucker, H., Shahrary, B., Gibbon, D.C.: Relevance feedback using support vector machines. In: Proceedings of the Eighteenth International Conference on Machine Learning. (2001) 122–129
10. Onoda, T., Murata, H., Yamada, S.: Interactive document retrieval with active learning. In: International Workshop on Active Mining (AM-2002), Maebashi, Japan (2002) 126–131
11. Vapnik, V.: The Nature of Statistical Learning Theory. Springer (1995)
12. Bishop, C.: Neural Networks for Pattern Recognition. Clarendon Press, Oxford (1995)
13. Murata, N., Yoshizawa, S., Amari, S.: Network information criterion - determining the number of hidden units for an artificial neural network model. IEEE Transactions on Neural Networks 5 (1994) 865–872
14. Onoda, T.: Neural network information criterion for the optimal number of hidden units. In: Proc. ICNN'95. (1995) 275–280
15. Orr, J., Müller, K.R., eds.: Neural Networks: Tricks of the Trade. LNCS 1524, Springer Verlag (1998)

16. Boser, B., Guyon, I., Vapnik, V.: A training algorithm for optimal margin classifiers. In Haussler, D., ed.: 5th Annual ACM Workshop on COLT, Pittsburgh, PA, ACM Press (1992) 144–152
17. Schölkopf, B., Smola, A., Williamson, R., Bartlett, P.: New support vector algorithms. Neural Computaion **12** (2000) 1083 – 1121
18. Schapire, R., Singer, Y., Singhal, A.: Boosting and rocchio applied to text filtering. In: Proceedings of the Twenty-First Annual International ACM SIGIR. (1998) 215–223
19. Kernel-Machines: (http://www.kernel-machines.org/)

Micro View and Macro View Approaches
to Discovered Rule Filtering

Yasuhiko Kitamura[1], Akira Iida[2], and Keunsik Park[3]

[1] School of Science and Technology, Kwansei Gakuin University,
2-1 Gakuen, Sanda, Hyogo 669-1337, Japan
ykitamura@ksc.kwansei.ac.jp
http://ist.ksc.kwansei.ac.jp/~kitamura/index.htm
[2] Graduate School of Engineering, Osaka City University,
3-3-138, Sugimoto, Sumiyoshi-ku, Osaka, 558-8585
iida@kdel.info.eng.osaka-cu.ac.jp
[3] Graduate School of Medicine, Osaka City University,
1-4-3, Asahi-Machi, Abeno-ku, Osaka, 545-8585
kspark@msic.med.osaka-cu.ac.jp

Abstract. A data mining system tries to semi-automatically discover knowledge by mining a large volume of raw data, but the discovered knowledge is not always novel and may contain unreasonable facts. We try to develop a discovered rule filtering method to filter rules discovered by a data mining system to be novel and reasonable ones by using information retrieval technique. In this method, we rank discovered rules according to the results of information retrieval from an information source on the Internet. In this paper, we show two approaches toward discovered rule filtering; the micro view approach and the macro view approach. The micro view approach tries to retrieve and show documents directly related to discovered rules. On the other hand, the macro view approach tries to show the trend of research activities related to discovered rules by using the results of information retrieval. We discuss advantages and disadvantages of the micro view approach and feasibility of the macro view approach by using an example of clinical data mining and MEDLINE document retrieval.

1 Introduction

The active mining [1] is a new approach to data mining, which tries to discover "high quality" knowledge that meets users' demand in an efficient manner by integrating information gathering, data mining, and user reaction technologies. This paper argues the discovered rule filtering method [3,4] that filters rules obtained by a data mining system based on documents retrieved from an information source on the Internet.

Data mining is an automated method to discover useful knowledge for users by analyzing a large volume of data mechanically. Generally speaking, conventional methods try to discover significant relations among attributes in the statistic sense from a large number of attributes contained in a given database, but if we pay

S. Tsumoto et al. (Eds.): AM 2003, LNAI 3430, pp. 74–91, 2005.
© Springer-Verlag Berlin Heidelberg 2005

attention to only statistically significant features, we often discover rules that have been known by the user. To cope with this problem, we are developing a discovered rule filtering method that filters a large number of rules discovered by a data mining system to be novel ones to the user. To judge whether a rule is novel or not, we utilize information sources on the Internet and try to judge the novelty of rule according to the search result of document retrieval that relates to the discovered rule.

In this paper, we first discuss the principle of integrating data mining and information in Section 2, and we show the concept and the process of discovered rule filtering using an example of clinical data mining in Section 3. We then show two approaches toward discovered rule filtering; the micro view approach and the macro view approaches in Section 4. In Section 5, we show an evaluation of the macro view approach. Finally we conclude this paper with our future work in Section 6.

2 Integration of Data Mining and Information Retrieval

Data mining process can be defined to discover significant relations among attributes from a large volume of data set $D(\subseteq A_1 \times A_2 \times \ldots \times A_n)$ where A_i $(1 \leq i \leq n)$ is an attribute of data. For simplicity of discussion, we assume each attribute value is 0 or 1. Hence, data mining process can be viewed as a function $dm(D) \subseteq R = \{<A_{c1}, A_{c2}, \ldots, A_{cp} \rightarrow A_d>\}$ which takes a data set D as an input and produces a set of rules representing relations among attributes. As methods to produce such a set of rules, we normally use statistical methods that consider precision and/or recall measure. When we try to discover novel rules, we often sacrifice the recall measure.

On the other hand, information retrieval process can defined to count the co-occurrences of the specified keywords from a large volume of document set $D' \subseteq B_1 \times B_2 \times \ldots \times B_m$ where B_j $(1 \leq j \leq m)$ is a keyword. Hence, information retrieval process can be viewed as a function $ir(D', \{B_{k1}, B_{k2}, \ldots, B_{kq}\}) \in$ **Int** which takes a set of keywords as an input and produces the number of co-occurrences of the keywords, where **Int** is a set of integer. Practically, the function produces a list of documents which contain the keywords rather than just the number of co-occurrences.

Now what can we get by integrating data mining and information retrieval. If we have a proper function $c(A_i) = B_j$ that associate an attribute A_i in data mining process with a keyword B_j in information retrieval process, we can associate the result of data mining with that of information retrieval. For example, let us assume that we have a rule $<A_{c1}, A_{c2}, \ldots, A_{cp} \rightarrow A_d>$ as a result of data mining. We can get the number k that is the number of co-occurrences when the keywords in the discovered rule are used for information retrieval. Formally it is given as $ir(D', \{c(A_{c1}), c(A_{c2}), \ldots, c(A_{cp})\}) = k$. Then, we can rank discovered rules according to k. If k is large, it is probable that the discovered rule has been known. On the other hand, if k is small, it is probable that the discovered rule is novel.

Some information retrieval systems accept additional keywords and parameters. For example, a document retrieval system accepts a parameter that specifies range of publication as its input. By utilizing this function, we can recognize whether discovered rules deal with a latest research topic or not.

3 Discovered Rule Filtering

As a target of data mining, we use a clinical examination database of hepatitis patients, which is offered by the Medical School of Chiba University, as a common database on which 10 research groups cooperatively work in our active mining project [5]. Some groups have already discovered some sets of rules. For example, a group in Shizuoka University analyzed sequential trends of the relation between a set of blood test data (GPT), which represents a progress of hepatitis, and other test data and has already discovered a number of rules, as one of them is shown in Fig. 1.

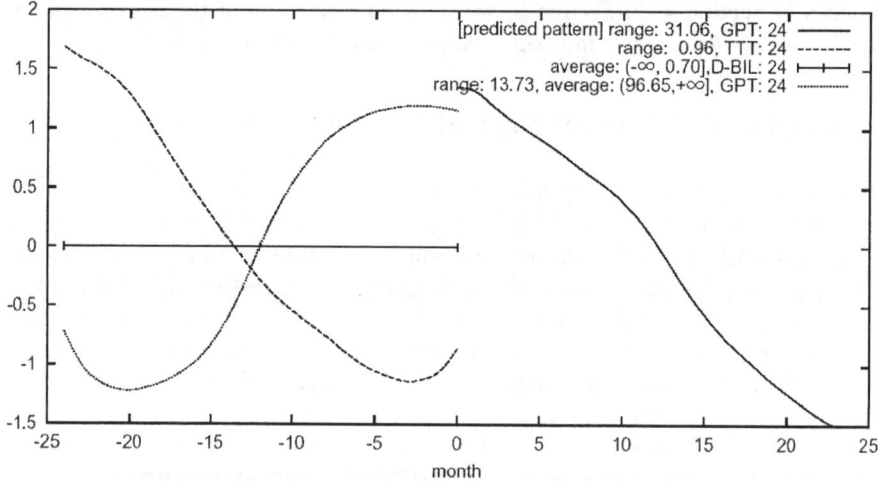

Fig. 1. An example of discovered rule

This rule shows a relation among GPT (Glutamat-Pyruvat-Transaminase), TTT (Thymol Turbidity Test), and D-BIL (Direct Bilirubin) and means "If, for the past 24 months, D-BIL stays unchanged, TTT decreases, and GPT increases, then GPT will decrease for the following 24 months." A data mining system can semi-automatically discover a large number of rules by analyzing a set of given data. On the other hand, discovered rules may include ones that are known and/or uninteresting to the user. Just showing all of the discovered rules to the user may result in putting a burden on her. We need to develop a method to filter the discovered rules into a small set of unknown and interesting rules to her. To this end, in this paper, we try to utilize information retrieval technique from the Internet.

When a set of discovered rules are given from a data mining system, a discovered rule filtering system first retrieves information related to the rules from the Internet and then filter the rules based on the result of information retrieval. In our project, we aim at discovering rules from a hepatitis database, but it is not easy to gather information related to hepatitis from the Internet by using naïve search engines because the Web information sources generally contain a huge amount of various and noisy information. We instead use the MEDLINE (MEDlars on LINE) database as the target of retrieving information, which is a bibliographical database (including abstracts) that covers more than 4000 medical and biological journals that have been published in about 70 countries. It has already stored more than 11 million documents since 1966. PubMed (http://www.ncbi.nlm.nih.gov/entrez/query.fcgi) is a free MEDLINE search service on the Internet run by NCBI (National Center for Biotechnology Information). By using the Pubmed, we can retrieve MEDLINE documents by submitting a set of keywords just like an ordinary search engine.

A discovered rule filtering process takes the following steps.

Step 1: Extracting keywords from a discovered rule

At first, we need to find a set of proper keywords to retrieve MEDLINE documents that relate to a discovered rule. Such keywords can be acquired from a discovered rule, the domain of data mining, and the interest of the user. These are summarized as follows.

● **Keywords related to attributes of a discovered rule.** These keywords represent attributes of a discovered rule. For example, keywords that can be acquired from a discovered rule shown in Fig. 1 are GPT, TTT, and D-BIL because they are explicitly shown in the rule. When abbreviations are not acceptable for the Pubmed, they need to be converted into normal names. For example, TTT and GPT should be converted into "thymol turbidity test" and "glutamic pyruvic transaminase" respectively.

● **Keywords related to a relation among attributes.** These keywords represent relations among attributes that constitute a discovered rule. It is difficult to acquire such keywords directly from the rule because, in many cases, they are not explicitly represented in the rule. They need to be included manually in advance. For example, in the hepatitis data mining, "periodicity" should be included when the periodicity of attribute value change is important.

● **Keywords related to the domain.** These keywords represent the purpose or the background of the data mining task. They should be included in advance as the common keywords. For hepatitis data mining, "hepatitis" is the keyword.

● **Keywords related to the user's interest.** These keywords represent the user's interest in the data mining task. They can be acquired directly by requesting the user to input the keywords.

Step 2: Gathering MEDLINE documents efficiently

We then perform a sequence of MEDLINE document retrievals. For each of discovered rules, we submit the keywords obtained in Step 1 to the Pubmed system [2]. However, redundant queries may be submitted when many of discovered rules are similar, in other words common attributes constitute many rules. The Pubmed is a popular system that is publicly available to a large number of researchers over the world, so it is required to reduce the load to the system. Actually, too many requests from a user lead to a temporal rejection of service to her. To reduce the number of submissions, we try to use a method that employs a graph representation, as shown in Fig. 2, to store the history of document retrievals. By referring to the graph, we can gather documents in an efficient way by reducing the number of meaningless or

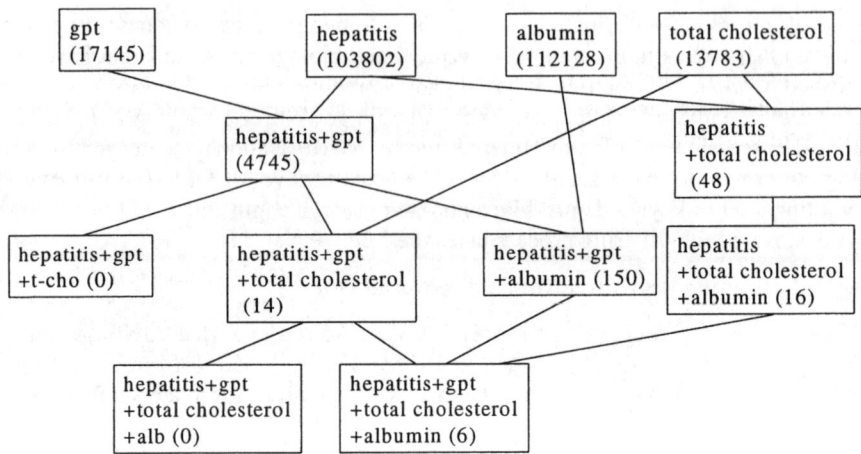

Fig. 2. A graph that represents document retrieval history

redundant keyword submissions. The graph in Fig. 2 shows pairs of submitted key-words and the number of hits. For example, this graph shows that a submission includ-ing keywords "hepatitis," "gpt," and "t-cho" returns nothing. It also shows that the combination of "hepatitis" and "gpt" is better than the combination of "hepatitis" and "total cholesterol" because the former is expected to have more returns than the latter.

Step 3: Filtering Discovered Rules

We filter discovered rules by using the result of MEDLINE document retrieval. More precisely, based on a result of document retrieval, we rank discovered rules. How to rank discovered rules by using the result of document retrievals is a core method of discovered rule filtering.

Basically the number of documents hit by a set of keywords shows the correlation of the keywords in the MEDLINE database, so we can assume that the more the num-ber of hits is, the more the combination of attributes represented by the keywords is commonly known in the research field. We therefore use a heuristic such that "If the number of hits is small, the rule is novel." We discuss the detail in the next section.

The published month or year of document can be another hint to rank rules. If many documents related to a rule are published recently, the rule may contain a hot topic in the field.

Step 4: Estimating User's Preference

Retrieving documents by simply submitting keywords obtained in Step 1 may pro-duce a wide variety of documents. They may relate to a discovered rule, but may not to the user's interest. To deal with this problem, we may request the user to input additional keywords that represent her interest, but this may put a burden to her. Relevance feedback is a technique that indirectly acquires the preference of the user. In this technique, the user just feedbacks "Yes" or "No" to the system depending on whether she has interest in a document or not. The system uses the feedbacks as a clue to analyze the abstract of the document and to automatically find keywords that show the user's interest, and uses them for further document retrievals.

4 Two Approaches to Discovered Rule Filtering

How to filter discovered rules according to the search result of MEDLINE document retrieval is a most important issue of this work. We have two approaches; the micro view approach and the macro view approach, to realize discovered rule filtering.

4.1 Micro View Approach

In the micro view approach, we retrieve and show documents related to a discovered rule directly to the user.

By using the micro view approach, the user can obtain not only novel rules discovered by a data mining system, but also documents related to the rules. By showing a rule and documents related to the rule at once, the user can get more insights on the rule and may have a chance to start a new data mining task. In our preliminary experiment, at first we showed a discovered rule alone, shown in Figure 1, to a medical doctor and received the following comment (Comment 1). The doctor seems to take the discovered rule as a commonly known fact.

> **Comment 1:** "TTT shows an indicator of the activity of antic body. The more active the antic bodies are, the less active the hepatitis is and therefore the amount of GPT decreases. This rule can be interpreted by using well known facts."

We then retrieved related documents by using the rule filtering technique. The search result with keywords "hepatitis" and "TTT" was 11 documents. Among them, there was a document, shown in Fig. 3, in which the doctor shows his interest as mentioned in a comment (Comment 2).

> **Comment 2:** "This document discusses that we can compare type B virus with type C virus by measuring the TTT value of hepatitis virus carriers (who have not contracted hepatitis). It is a new paper published in 2001 that discusses a relation between TTT and hepatitis, but it reports only a small number of cases. The discovered rule suggests the same symptom appears not only in carriers but also in patients. This rule is important to support this paper from a standpoint of clinical data."

The effect shown in this preliminary examination is that the system can retrieve not only a new document related to a discovered rule but also a new viewpoint to the rule, and gives a chance to invoke a new mining process. In other words, if the rule alone is shown to the user, it is recognized just as a common fact, but if it is shown with a related document, it can motivate the user to analyze the amount of TTT depending on the type of hepatitis by using a large volume of hepatitis data. We hope this kind of effect can be found in many other cases.

However, it is actually difficult to retrieve appropriate documents rightly related a rule because of the low performance of information technique. Especially, when a rule is simple as it is composed of a small number of attributes, the IR system returns a noisy output, documents including a large number of unrelated ones. When a rule is complicated as it is composed of a large number of attributes, it returns few documents.

1: Hepatol Res 2001 Sep;21(1):67–75

Comparison of clinical laboratory liver tests between asymptomatic HBV and HCV carriers with persistently normal aminotransferase serum levels.

Murawaki Y, Ikuta Y, Koda M, Kawasaki H.

Second Department of Internal Medicine, Tottori University School of Medicine, 683–8504, Yonago, Japan

We examined the clinicopathological state in asymptomatic hepatitis C virus (HCV) carriers with persistently normal aminotransferase serum levels in comparison with asymptomatic hepatitis B virus (HBV) carriers. The findings showed that the thymol turbidity test (TTT) values and zinc sulfate turbidity test (ZTT) values were significantly higher in asymptomatic HCV carriers than in asymptomatic HBV carriers, whose values were within the normal limits. Multivariate analysis showed that the independent predictor of serum TTT and ZTT levels was the HCV infection. In clinical state, simple and cheap tests such as TTT and ZTT are useful for mass screening to detect HCV carriers in medical check–ups of healthy workers.

PMID: 11470629 [PubMed – as supplied by publisher]

Fig. 3. A document retrieved

To see how the micro view approach works, we performed a preliminary experiment of discovered rule filtering. We used 20 rules obtained from the team in Shizuoka University and gathered documents related to the rules from the MEDLINE database. The result is shown in Table 1.

In this table, "ID" is the ID number of rule and "Keywords" are extracted from the rule and are submitted to the Pubmed. "No" shows the number of submitted keywords. "Hits" is the number of documents returned. "Ev" is the evaluation of rule by a medical doctor. He evaluated each rule, which was given in a form depicted in Fig. 1, and categorized into 2 classes; R (reasonable rules) and U (unreasonable rules).

This result tells us that it is not easy to distinguish reasonable or known rules from unreasonable or garbage ones by using only the number of hits. It shows a limitation of micro view approach.

To cope with the problem, we need to improve the performance of micro view approach as follows.

As we can see, except Rule 13, rules with hits more than 0 are categorized in reasonable rules, but a number of reasonable rules hit no document. It seems that the number of submitted keywords affects the number of hits. In other words, if a rule is complex with many keywords, the number of hits tends to be few.

Table 1. The preliminary experiment of discovered rule filtering

ID	Ev.	Hits	No.	Keywords
1	R	6	4	hepatitis, gpt, t–cho, albumin
2	U	0	4	hepatitis b, gpt, t–cho, chyle
3	U	0	4	hepatitis c, gpt, lap, hemolysis
4	R	0	5	hepatitis, gpt, got, na, lap
5	R	0	6	hepatitis, gpt, got, ttt, cl, (female)
6	U	0	5	hepatitis, gpt, ldh, hemolysis, blood group a
7	R	7	4	hepatitis, gpt, alb, jaundice
8	R	9	3	hepatitis b, gpt, creatinine
10	R	0	4	hepatitis, ttt, t–bil, gpt
11	U	0	4	hepatitis, gpt, alpha globulin, beta globulin
13	U	8	4	hepatitis, hemolysis, gpt, (female)
14	U	0	4	hepatitis, gpt, ttt, d–bil
15	U	0	3	hepatitis, gpt, chyle
17	R	0	5	hepatitis, gpt, ttt, blood group o, (female)
18	R	2	3	hepatitis c, gpt, t–cho
19	R	0	6	hepatitis, gpt, che, ttt, ztt, (male)
20	R	0	5	hepatitis, gpt, lap, alb, interferon
22	U	0	7	hepatitis, gpt, ggtp, hemolysis, blood group a, (female), (age 45–64)
23	U	0	4	hepatitis b, gpt, got, i–bil
27	U	0	4	hepatitis, gpt, hemolysis, i–bil

(1) Accurate Document Retrieval. In our current implementation, we use only keywords related to attributes contained in a rule and those related to the domain, and the document retrieval is not accurate enough and often contains documents unrelated to the rule. To improve the accuracy, we need to add adequate keywords related to relations among attributes. These keywords represent relations among attributes that constitute a discovered rule. It is difficult to acquire such keywords directly from the rule because, in many cases, they are not explicitly represented in the rule. They need to be included manually in advance. For example, in the hepatitis data mining, "periodicity" should be included when the periodicity of attribute value change is important.

(2) Document Analysis by Applying Natural Language Processing Methods. Another method is to refine the results by analyzing the documents using natural language processing technique. Generally speaking, information retrieval technique only retrieves documents that contain the given keyword(s) and does not care the context in which the keyword(s) appear. On the other hand, natural language processing technique can clarify the context and can refine the result obtained by information retrieval technique. For example, if a keyword is not found in the same sentence in which another keyword appears, we might conclude that the document does not argue a relation between the two keywords. We hence can improve the accuracy of discovered rule filtering by analyzing whether the given keywords are found in a same sentence. In addition, if we can analyze whether the sentence argues the conclusion of the document, we can further improve the accuracy of rule filtering.

4.2 Macro View Approach

In the macro view approach, we try to roughly observe the trend of relation among keywords. For example, the number of documents in which the keywords co-occur approximately shows the strength of relation among the keywords. We show two methods based on the macro view approach.

(1) Showing Research Activities Based Pair-Wise Keyword Co-occurrence Graph
Fig. 4, 5, and 6 show keyword co-occurrence graphs. In each graph, a node represents a keyword and the length of edge represents the inverse of the frequency of co-occurrences of keywords connected by the edge. The number attached to the edge represents the frequency of co-occurrence. Hence, the more documents related to a pair keywords are retrieved from the Pubmed, the closer the keywords are in the graph.

For example, Fig. 4 shows that the relation between any pair among ALB, GPT, and T-CHO is strong. Fig. 5 shows that the relation between T-CHO and GPT is strong, but that between chyle and either of T-CHO and GPT is rather weak. Fig. 6 shows that the relations among GPT, female, and G-GTP are strong, but the relation between hemolysis and G-GTP and those between "blood group a" and the other keywords are weak.

We then form clusters of keywords by using the Hierarchical Clustering Scheme [7]. As a strategy to form clusters, we adopt the complete linkage clustering method (CLINK). In the method, the distance between clusters A and B is defined as the longest among the distances of every pair of a keyword in cluster A and a keyword in cluster B. The method initially forms a cluster for each keyword. It then repeats to merge clusters within a threshold length into one or more clusters.

We can regard keywords in a cluster are strongly related and research activities concerning the keywords have been done much, so we have a hypothesis to filter rules in the macro view method as follows.

[Hypothesis] (Macro View Approach)

1. The number of clusters concerning a known rule is 1.
2. The number of clusters concerning an unknown rule is 2.
3. The number of clusters concerning a garbage rule is more than 3.

Rule with only one cluster are regarded as known rules because a large number of papers concerning every pair of keywords in the rule have been published. Rules with two clusters are regarded as unknown rules. This is because research activities concerning keywords in each cluster have been done much, but those crossing the clusters have not been done. Rule with more than two clusters are regarded as garbage rules. Such a rule is too complex to understand because keywords are partitioned into many clusters and the rule consists of many unknown factors.

For example, if we set the threshold of CLINK to be 1 (the frequency of co-occurrences is 1), the rule in Fig. 4 is regarded as a known rule because all the keywords are merged into a single cluster. Keywords in Fig. 5 are merged into two clusters; one cluster consists of GPT and T-CHO and another consists of chyle only. Hence, the rule is judged to be unknown. Keywords in Fig. 6 are merged into 3

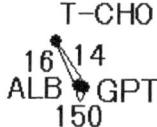

Fig. 4. The keyword co-occurrence graph of rule including GPT, ABL, and T-CHO

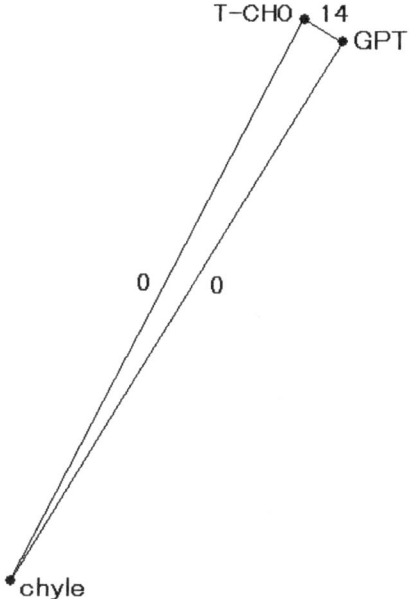

Fig. 5. The keyword co-occurrence graph of rule including GPT, T-CHO, and chyle

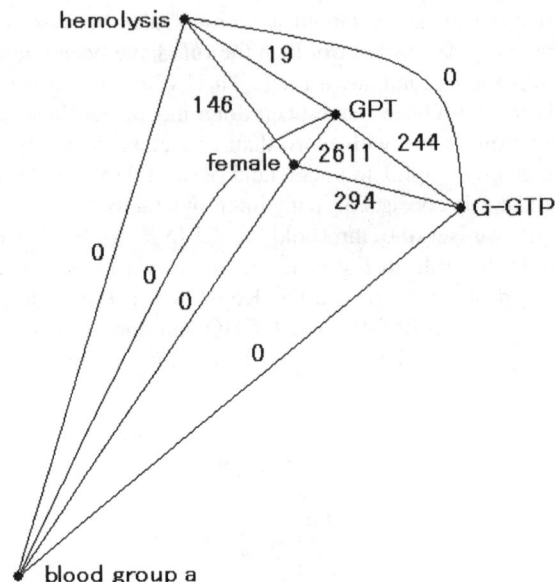

Fig. 6. The keyword co-occurrence graph of rule including GPT, G-GTP, hemolysis, female and "blood group a"

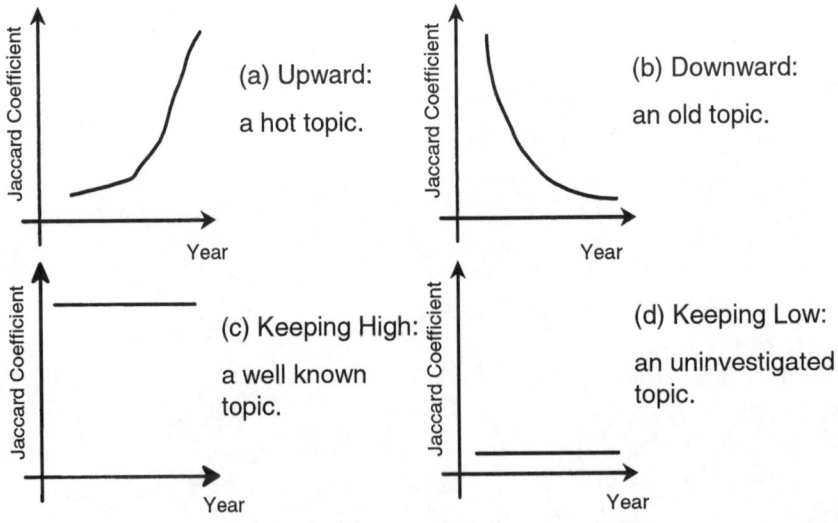

Fig. 7. Yearly trends of the Jaccard co-efficient

clusters as GPT, G-GTP, and female form a cluster and each of hemolysis and "blood group a" forms an individual cluster.

As a conclusion, the graph shape of reasonable rules looks different from that of unreasonable rules. But, when given a graph, how to judge whether the rule is reasonable or not is our future work.

(2) The yearly trend of research activities

The MEDLINE database contains bibliographical information of bioscience articles, which includes the year of publication, and the Pubmed can retrieve the information according to the year of publication. By observing the yearly trend of publication, we can see the change of research activity.

Generally speaking, the number of documents contained in the MEDLINE database increases rapidly year by year, so the number of documents hit by most sets of keywords increases. Hence, we use the Jaccard coefficient as an alternative to measure the yearly trend of publication. Given keywords K_1, K_2, ..., K_n, its Jaccard coefficient is defined as

$$\frac{h(K_1, K_2, \ldots, K_n)}{h(K_1) + h(K_2) + \cdots + h(K_n)}$$

where $h(L)$ is the number of documents hit by the set of keywords L. The Jaccard coefficient is a measure to show the strength of association among multiple keywords.

For example, we can have the following interpretations as shown in Fig. 7.

(a) If the Jaccard co-efficient moves upward, the research topic related to the keywords is hot.

(b) If the Jaccard co-efficient moves downward, the research topic related to the keywords is terminating.

(c) If the Jaccard co-efficient keeps high, the research topic related to the keyword is commonly known.

(d) If the Jaccard co-efficient keeps low, the research topic related to the keyword is not known. Few researchers show interest in the topic.

To evaluate a feasibility of this method, we submitted 4 queries to the MEDLINE database and show the results in Fig. 8 through Fig. 11.

(a) "hcv, hepatitis" (Fig.8)

The Jaccard co-efficient has been increasing since 1989. In 1989, we have an event of succeeding HCV cloning. HCV is a hot topic of hepatitis research.

(b) "smallpox, vaccine" (Fig.9)

The Jaccard co-efficient has been decreasing. In 1980, the World Health Assembly announced that smallpox had been eradicated. Recently, we see the number turns to be increasing because discussions about smallpox as a biochemical weapon arise.

(c) "gpt, got" (Fig.10)

The Jaccard co-efficient stays high. GPT and GOT are well known blood test measure and they are used to diagnose hepatitis. The relation between GPT and GOT is well known in the medical domain.

(d) "albumin, urea nitrogen" (Fig.11)

The Jaccard co-efficient stays low. The relation between albumin and urea nitrogen is seldom discussed.

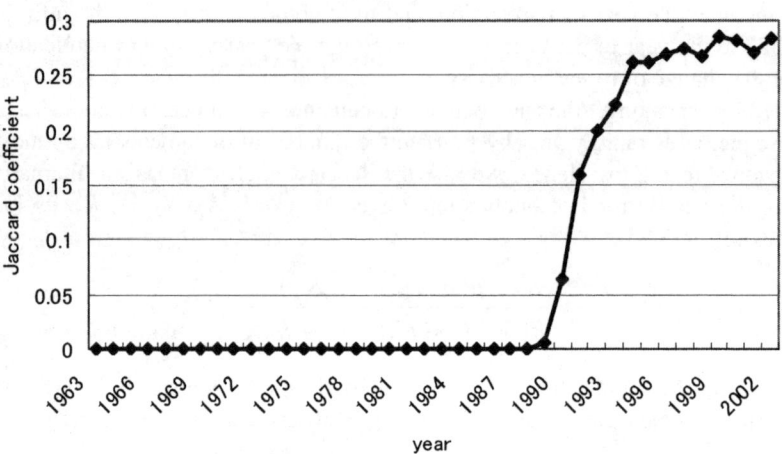

Fig. 8. The yearly trend of the Jaccard co-efficient concerning "hcv" and "hepatitis"

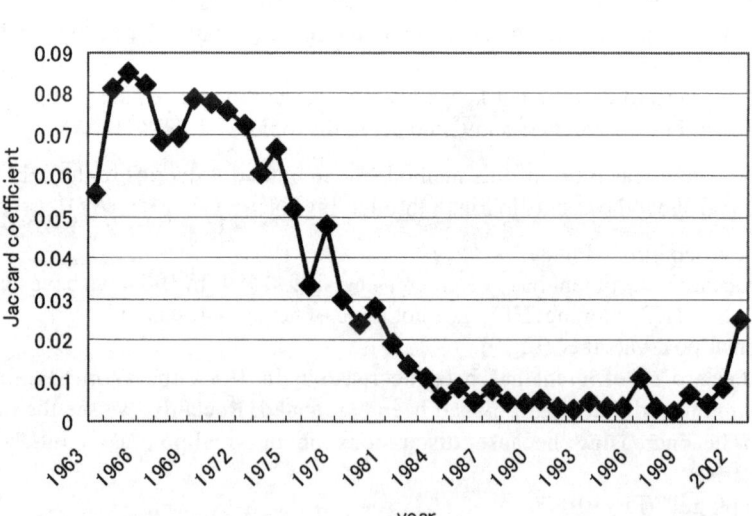

Fig. 9. The yearly trend of the Jaccard co-efficient concerning "snallpox" and "vaccine"

To show feasibility in the hepatitis data mining domain, we measured the yearly trend of Jaccard co-efficient of "hepatitis" and each of five representative hepatitis viruses (hav, hbv, hcv, hdv, and hev) and show the results in Fig. 12. We also show the history of hepatitis virus discovery in Table 2. There is apparently a co-relation between the Jaccard co-efficient and the discovery time of hepatitis viruses. In hepatitis research activities, works on hbv and hcv are major and especially those on hcv rapidly increase after its discovery.

gpt got

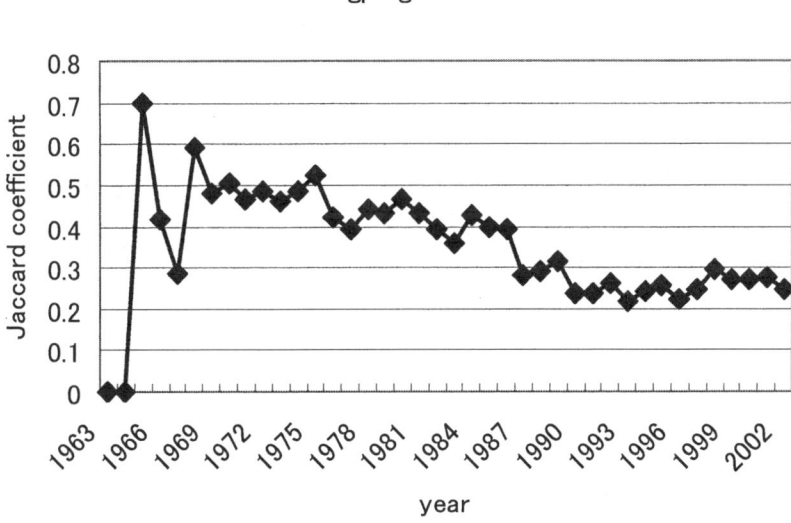

Fig. 10. The yearly trend of the Jaccard co-efficient concerning "gpt" and "got"

album in urea nitrogen

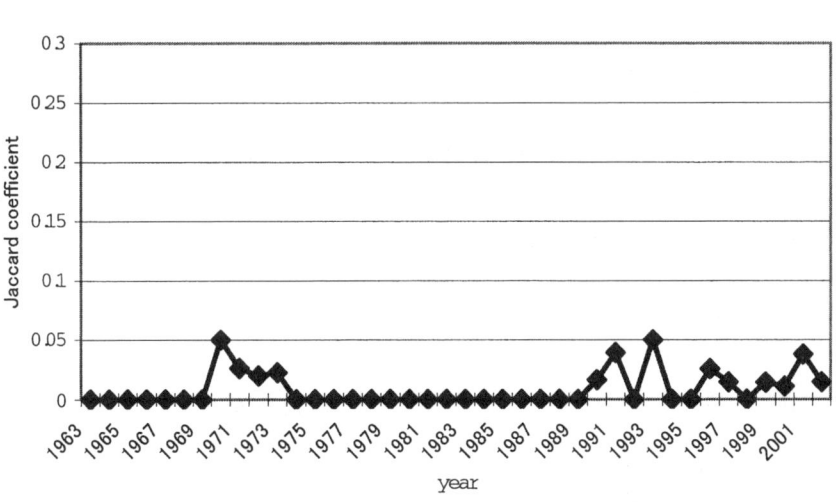

Fig. 11. The yearly trend of the Jaccard co-efficient concerning "albumin" and "urea nitrogen"

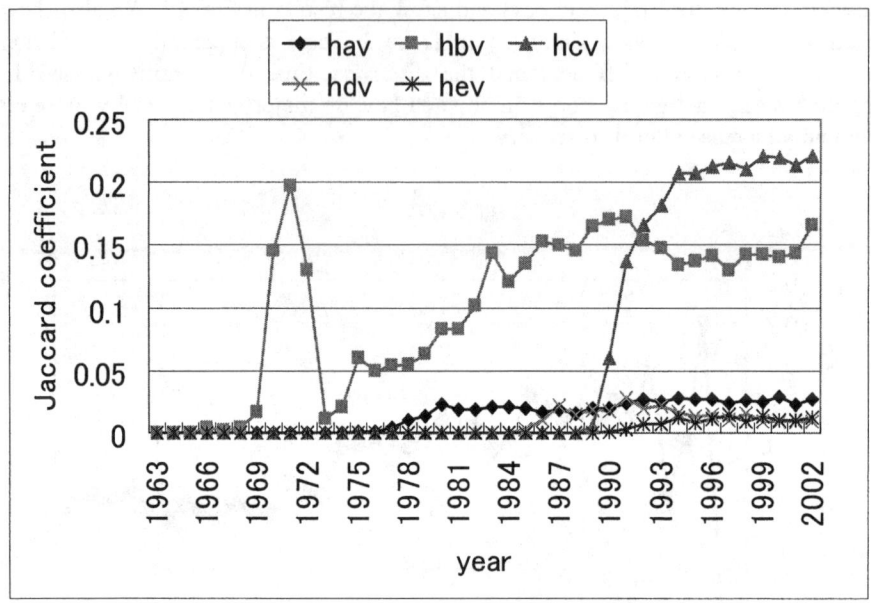

Fig. 12. The yearly trend of the Jaccard co-efficient concerning hepatitis viruses

Table 2. History of hepatitis viruses discovery

1965	Discovery of Australian antigen. This is the first step toward hbv discovery. (B.S. Blumberg)
1973	Discovery of hav. (S.M. Feinstone)
1977	Discovery of delta antigen. This is the first step toward hdv discovery. (M. Rizzetto)
1983	Detection of hev by reverse transcription-polymerase chain reaction. (M.S. Balayan)
1989	Success of cloning hcv. (Q.L. Choo)

From above results, the yearly trends well correspond with historical events in the medical domain, and can be a measure to know the research activities.

5 Evaluation of Macro View Approach

We performed an evaluation of the macro view approach by the questionnaire method. We first made a questionnaire shown in Fig. 13. 20 items are made from rules discovered by the data mining group in Shizuoka University [6] by extracting keywords from the rules. We sent out the questionnaire to 47 medical students in Osaka City University. The students were just before the state examination to be a medical doctor, so we suppose they are knowledgeable about the medical knowledge in text books.

Q: How do you guess the result when you submit the following keywords to the Pubmed system? Choose one among A, B, and C.

A (Known): Documents about a fact that I know are retrieved.
B (Unknown): Documents about a fact that I do not know are retrieved.
C (Garbage): No document is retrieved.

(1) [A B C] ALT and TTT
(2) [A B C] TTT, Direct-Bilirubin, and ALT
(3) [A B C] ALT, Total-Cholesterol, and Hepatitis C
(4) ....

Fig. 13. Questionnaire sent out to medical students

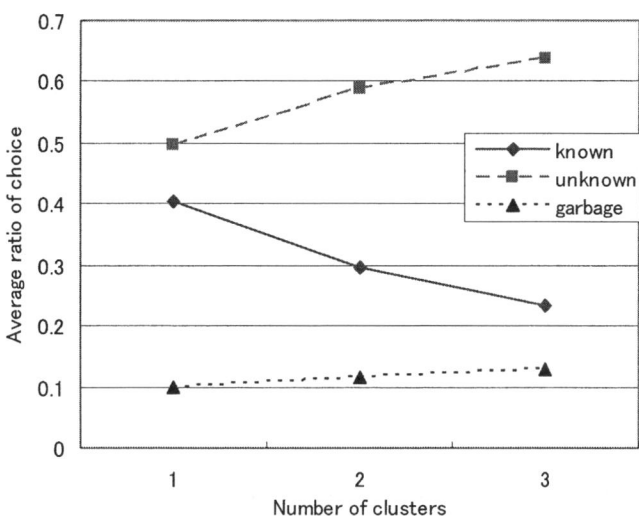

Fig. 14. The relation between the number of clusters and the evaluation of medical experts

We verify the hypothesis of the macro view method by using the result of the questionnaire. We show the relation between the number of clusters and the average ratio of choice in Fig. 14. The threshold of CLINK is 1. At the risk level of 5%, the graph shows two significant relations.

- As the number of clusters increases, the average ratio of "unknown" increases.
- As the number of clusters increases, the average ratio of "known" decreases.

The result does not show any significant relation about "garbage" choice because the number of students who chose "garbage" is relatively small to the other choices and does not depend on the number of clusters. We suppose the medical students hesitate to judge that a rule is just garbage.

The hypotheses of the macro view approach are partly supported by this evaluation. The maximum number of clusters in this examination is 3. We still need to examine how medical experts judge rules with more than 4 clusters.

6 Summary

We discussed a discovered rule filtering method which filters rules discovered by a data mining system into novel ones by using the IR technique. We proposed two approaches toward discovered rule filtering; the micro view approach and the macro view approach and showed merits and demerits of micro view approach and feasibility of macro view approach.

Our future work is summarized as follows.

- We need to find a clear measure to distinguish reasonable rules from unreasonable one, which can be used in the macro view method. We also need to find a measure to know the novelty of rule.
- We need to improve the performance of micro view approach by adding keywords that represent relations among attributes and by using natural language processing techniques. The improvement of micro view approach can contribute the improvement of macro view approach.
- We need to implement the macro view method in a discovered rule filtering system and apply it to an application of hepatitis data mining.

Acknowledgement

This work is supported by a grant-in-aid for scientific research on priority area by the Japanese Ministry of Education, Science, Culture, Sports and Technology.

References

1. H. Motoda (Ed.), Active Mining: New Directions of Data Mining, IOS Press, Amsterdam, 2002.
2. R. Baeza-Yates and B. Ribeiro-Neto, Modern Information Retrieval, Addison Wesley, 1999.
3. Y. Kitamura, K. Park, A. Iida, and S. Tatsumi. Discovered Rule Filtering Using Information Retrieval Technique. Proceedings of International Workshop on Active Mining, pp. 80-84, 2002.
4. Y. Kitamura, A. Iida, K. Park, and S. Tatsumi, Discovered Rule Filtering System Using MEDLINE Information Retrieval, JSAI Technical Report, SIG-A2-KBS60/FAI52-J11, 2003.

5. H. Yokoi, S. Hirano, K. Takabayashi, S. Tsumoto, Y. Satomura, Active Mining in Medicine: A Chronic Hepatitis Case – Towards Knowledge Discovery in Hospital Information Systems -, Journal of the Japanese Society for Artificial Intelligence, Vol.17, No.5, pp.622-628, 2002. (in Japanese)
6. M. Ohsaki, Y. Sato, H. Yokoi, and T. Yamaguchi, A Rule Discovery Support System for Sequential Medical Data – In the Case Study of a Chronic Hepatitis Dataset -, Proceedings of International Workshop on Active Mining, pp. 97-102, 2002.
7. S. C. Johnson, Hierarchical Clustering Schemes, Psychometrika, Vol.32, pp.241-254, 1967.

Mining Chemical Compound Structure Data Using Inductive Logic Programming

Cholwich Nattee[1], Sukree Sinthupinyo[1], Masayuki Numao[1],
and Takashi Okada[2]

[1] The Institute of Scientific and Industrial Research, Osaka University,
8-1 Mihogaoka, Ibaraki, Osaka, 567-0047, Japan
{cholwich, sukree, numao}@ai.sanken.osaka-u.ac.jp
[2] Department of Informatics, School of Science and Technology,
Kwansei Gakuin University, 2-1 Gakuen-cho,
Sanda, Hyogo, 669-1323, Japan
okada-office@kwansei.ac.jp

Abstract. Discovering knowledge from chemical compound structure data is a challenge task in KDD. It aims to generate hypotheses describing activities or characteristics of chemical compounds from their own structures. Since each compound composes of several parts with complicated relations among them, traditional mining algorithms cannot handle this kind of data efficiently. In this research, we apply Inductive Logic Programming (ILP) for classifying chemical compounds. ILP provides comprehensibility to learning results and capability to handle more complex data consisting of their relations. Nevertheless, the bottleneck for learning first-order theory is enormous hypothesis search space which causes inefficient performance by the existing learning approaches compared to the propositional approaches. We introduces an improved ILP approach capable of handling more efficiently a kind of data called multiple-part data, i.e., one instance of data consists of several parts as well as relations among parts. The approach tries to find hypothesis describing class of each training example by using both individual and relational characteristics of its part which is similar to finding common substructures among the complex relational instances. Chemical compound data is multiple-part data. Each compound is composed of atoms as parts, and various kinds of bond as relations among atoms. We then apply the proposed algorithm for chemical compound structure by conducting experiments on two real-world datasets: mutagenicity in nitroaromatic compounds and dopamine antagonist compounds. The experiment results were compared to the previous approaches in order to show the performance of proposed approach.

1 Introduction

Inductive learning of first-order theory from examples is interesting because first-order representation provides comprehensibility to the learning results and capability to handle more complex data consisting of relations. Yet, the bottleneck

S. Tsumoto et al. (Eds.): AM 2003, LNAI 3430, pp. 92–111, 2005.

for learning first-order theory is enormous hypothesis search space. Moreover, heuristic functions applied in the existing ILP approaches use only quantitative information to select an appropriate candidate, i.e., using only the number of training examples covered without considering the quality. This makes existing approaches sometimes perform worse than propositional approaches. Except from defining heuristic function, language bias is one of techniques used in order to reduce the search space. It is widely used in many ILP systems. However, this research focuses on proposing a heuristic function.

We introduce a novel learning approach focusing on a kind of data called *multiple-part data*, i.e., one instance of data consists of several parts as well as relations among parts. The objective of learning from multiple-part data is to find hypothesis for describing class of each example by using part characteristics individually and characteristics of relations among parts. This is similar to finding common substructures among instances in the same class.

Though the existing first-order theory learning approaches can handle this kind of data due to the power of first-order representation, there is a limitation in efficiency of results since numerous parts within one example make the search space become larger but contains similar hypothesis candidates. Thus, the search heuristics cannot lead to good hypotheses. In order to solve this problem, we propose an approach that weights each part according to its characteristics correlating to parts from other examples in the same class. This makes parts with common characteristics be given higher weights than the uncommon parts, and makes the search heuristics discriminate more efficiently. We adopt this weighting technique from the concept of multiple-instance learning which is an extended two-class propositional learning approach for data that are unable to be labeled individually, albeit several instances of data are gathered and labeled as a group. Each positive group may consist of both positive and negative instances. Nevertheless, the multiple-instance learning aims to learn to predict instances not groups, thereby rendering itself similar to supervised learning with noises in positive examples. Most learning algorithms for multiple-instance data solve this ambiguity by using similarity of data within the feature space to find the area where several instances from various positive groups are located together and negative group instances are far. This method is modified and used as the weighting technique to evaluate each part of the multiple-part data containing similarity among parts before incorporating the weights into search heuristics to find hypothesis that may consist of relations among parts.

To evaluate the proposed approach, we conducted an experiment on SAR studies for chemical compound structures. This is a promising process because the knowledge discovered will be useful for developing new drugs. These studies aim to predict the activity of compound from its structure. In recent years, the advance in High Throughput Screening (HTS) technology has produced vast amount of SAR data. Therefore, once the rules to predict activities of existing SAR data are found, it will significantly help screening process. SAR data represented by chemical compound structure can be categorized as multiple-part data. Because we aim to find substructures that predict activity of a compound, we apply the proposed system to learn hypotheses from this kind of data. We compare the learning results with the previous approaches in order to evaluate the performance.

This paper is mainly divided into two parts. We first introduce the multiple-part data, and describe the proposed approach. Then, we conduct the experiments for SAR studies on two chemical compound datasets. The experiment results are compared to the existing approaches to evaluate its performance. Finally, we conclude the paper and consider our future works.

2   Background

2.1   FOIL

FOIL [1] is a top-down ILP system which learns function-free Horn clause definitions of a target predicate using background predicates. Learning process in FOIL starts with training examples containing all positive and negative examples. The algorithm used in FOIL for constructing a function-free Horn clause consists of two main loops. In outer loop, a Horn clause partially covering the examples is constructed, and covered examples are removed from the training set. While in inner loop, partially developed clauses are iteratively refined by adding a literal one by one. Heuristic function is used to select the most appropriate clause. FOIL maintains covered examples in the form of *tuple* which is the substitutions (i.e., bindings of variables) of the clause under given example. Multiple tuples can be generated from one example.

FOIL uses a heuristic function based on the information theory for assessing usefulness of a literal. It provides effective guidance for clause construction. Purpose of this heuristic function is to characterize a subset of the positive examples. From the partial developing clause below

$$R(V_1, V_2, \ldots, V_k) \leftarrow L_1, L_2, \ldots, L_{m-1}$$

training tuples covered by this clause are denoted as T_i. The information required for T_i is calculated from T_i^+ and T_i^- which denote positive and negative tuples covered by the clause, respectively.

$$I(T_i) = -\log_2 \frac{|T_i^+|}{|T_i^+| + |T_i^-|} \tag{1}$$

If a literal L_m is selected and added, a new set of covered tuples T_{i+1} is created, then similar formula is given as

$$I(T_{i+1}) = -\log_2 \frac{|T_{i+1}^+|}{|T_{i+1}^+| + |T_{i+1}^-|} \tag{2}$$

From above, a heuristic used in FOIL is calculated as an amount of information gained when applying a new literal L_m;

$$Gain(L_i) = |T_i^{++}| \times (I(T_i) - I(T_{i+1})) \tag{3}$$

T_i^{++} is the positive tuples included in T_i and extended in T_{i+1}. This heuristic function is used over all candidate literals, and the literal with the largest value is selected and added to the partial developed clause in inner loop.

2.2   Multiple-Instance Learning

For the supervised learning problem, we try to design and create algorithms that are able to generate model from training examples to predict correct labels of unseen data, and each instance of training examples has to be labeled beforehand. However, this framework may not be suitable for some applications. Dietterich et al. then proposed the extended framework for supervised learning to handle more ambiguities called *Multiple-Instance Learning* [2]. The motivation behind this extended framework came from the drug activity prediction problem that aims to find the molecule that can bind well to the target protein. In the chemical process, chemists can conduct the experiment to check whether the given molecule binds well, nevertheless, one molecule may have several shapes or conformations. Therefore, we do not know which shape binds well, then, there is a proposition to use machine learning techniques to find the appropriate conformation for the target protein. This problem is different from the supervised learning that in the training examples, we know only which molecule binds well but we want to find which conformation of molecule binds well. In the new framework, unlabeled instances are grouped into a bag labeled as positive or negative. A positive bag contains at least one positive instance, otherwise labeled as negative. This framework is shown in Fig. 2 which can be compared to the supervised learning framework in Fig. 1. From this set-up, the target concept can be found from the area in the feature space that instances from various positive bags locating together, and that area is far from the instance from negative bags as shown in Fig. 3. Dietterich et al. proposed an algorithm that tries to find target concept by first constructing a rectangle in the feature space, then reducing its size until it covers instances from positive bags only.

After this framework and algorithm were presented, various approaches were proposed. Some of them extended the existing supervised learning algorithm. Wang and Zucker applied k-NN algorithm for multiple-instance problem [3]. Chevaleyre and Zucker proposed generic framework for extending propositional rule learner to handle multiple-instance data [4]. They implemented the extension of RIPPER. Gärtner et al. proposed a new kernel function for multiple-instance learning [5]. Maron et al. proposed the original approach for multiple-instance learning using Diverse Density (DD) [6]. This approach is applied in the proposed system. We then explain this approach in detail.

Diverse Density. Diverse Density (DD) algorithm aims to measure a point in an n-dimensional feature space to be a positive instance. DD value at point p in the feature space shows both how many *different* positive bags have an instance near p, and how *far* the negative instances are from p. Thus, DD is high in the area where instances from various positive bags are located together. It is originally defined as follows.

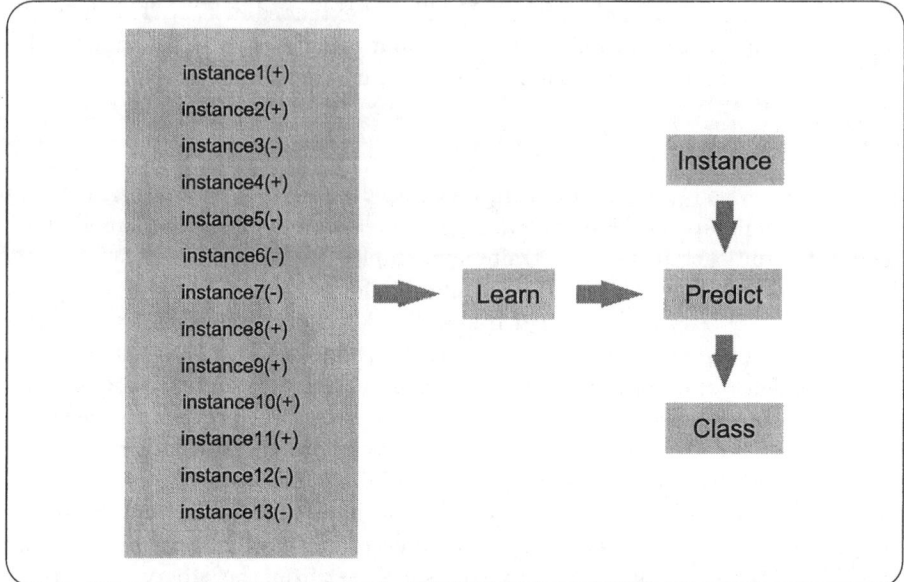

Fig. 1. Supervised learning framework

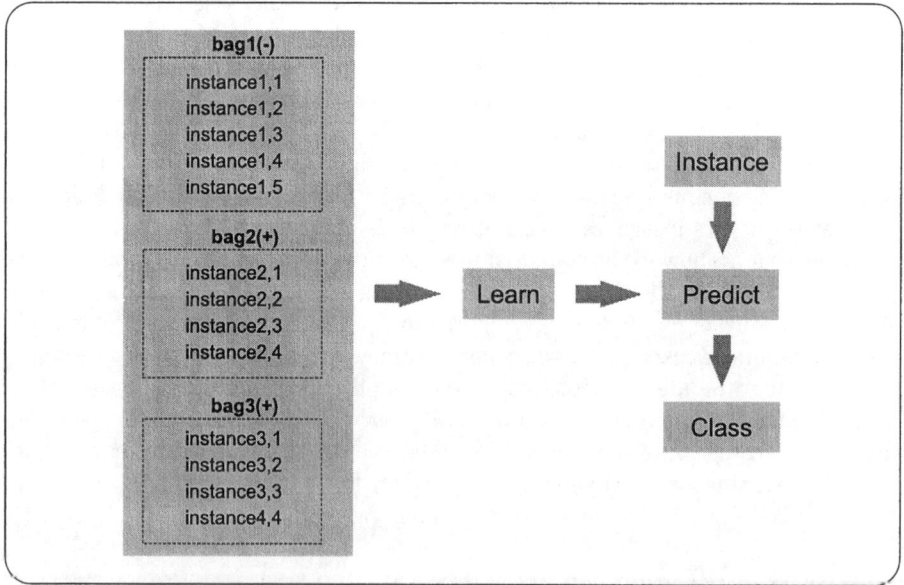

Fig. 2. Multiple-instance learning framework

Let B_i^+ denote a positive bag, B_{ij}^+ denote the jth instance in B_i^+, and B_{ijk}^+ represents the kth feature of that instance. In the same way, B_{ij}^- represents a

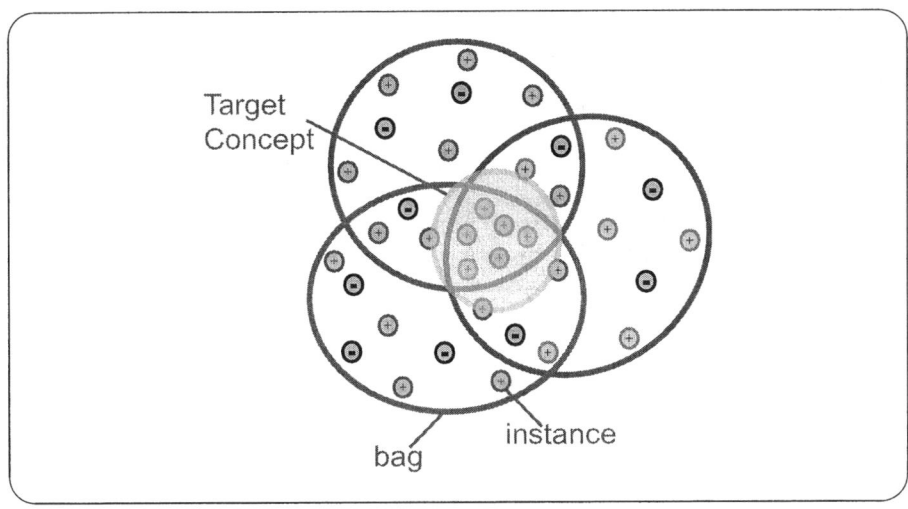

Fig. 3. Feature space in multiple-instance learning framework

negative instance. Assuming that the target concept is a single point t. The Diverse Density is defined as:

$$DD(t) = Pr(x = t | B_1^+, B_2^+, \ldots, B_n^+, B_1^-, B_2^-, \ldots, B_m^-)$$

Using Bayes' rule,

$$DD(t) = \frac{Pr(B_1^+, B_2^+, \ldots, B_n^+, B_1^-, B_2^-, \ldots, B_m^- | x = t) Pr(x = t)}{Pr(B_1^+, B_2^+, \ldots, B_n^+, B_1^-, B_2^-, \ldots, B_m^-)}$$

However, $Pr(x = t)$ is constant because of assuming a uniform prior over concept location and $Pr(B_1^+, B_2^+, \ldots, B_n^+, B_1^-, B_2^-, \ldots, B_m^-)$ is also constant with respect to t. Then, $DD(t)$ is estimated from

$$Pr(B_1^+, B_2^+, \ldots, B_n^+, B_1^-, B_2^-, \ldots, B_m^- | x = t)$$

Using Bayes's rule and assuming a uniform prior over concept location again, this is equivalent to

$$\prod_i Pr(x = t | B_i^+) \prod_i (x = t | B_i^-)$$

This probability is estimated by using noisy-or model from Bayesian Networks. Then,

$$Pr(x = t | B_i^+) = 1 - \prod_j (1 - Pr(x = t | B_{ij}^+))$$

$$Pr(x = t | B_i^-) = \prod_j (1 - Pr(x = t | B_{ij}^-))$$

Intuitively, $Pr(x = t|B_i^+)$ is high if x is closed to one of the instances in a positive bag. This is opposite for $Pr(x = t|B_i^-)$ that is related to negative bags. Then, the probability of an individual instance on the target point ($Pr(x = t|B_{ij})$) is defined based on the distance between them.

$$Pr(x = t|B_{ij}) = exp(-\|B_{ij} - x\|^2)$$

Euclidean distance is used, then $\|B_{ij} - x\|^2 = \sum_k s_k^2 (B_{ijk} - x_k)^2$ where s_k is the scaling factor of the kth feature. Likewise, if an instance is closed to x, this probability will be high. Finally, the DD is approximated from the formula below.

$$DD(x) = \prod_i (1 - \prod_j (1 - exp(-\|B_{ij}^+ - x\|^2))) \cdot$$
$$\prod_i \prod_j (1 - exp(-\|B_{ij}^- - x\|^2)) \qquad (4)$$

where x is a point in the feature space and B_{ij} represents the jth instance of the ith bag in training examples. For the distance, the Euclidean distance is adopted then

$$\|B_{ij} - x\|^2 = \sum_k (B_{ijk} - x_k)^2 \qquad (5)$$

In the previous approaches, several searching techniques are proposed for determining the value of features or the area in the feature space maximizing DD.

3   Proposed Method

We present top-down ILP system that is able to learn more efficiently hypotheses from set of examples, each consisting of several small parts, or when trying to predict class of data from the common substructure. The proposed system incorporates existing top-down ILP system (FOIL) and applies multiple-instance based measure to find common characteristics among parts of positive examples. This measure is then used as a weight attached to each part of the example and the common parts among positive examples are attached with high-valued weights. With these weights and heuristic function based on example coverage, the system generates more precise and higher coverage hypotheses from training examples. Next, we define multiple-part data, and then, explain modified heuristics.

3.1   Multiple-Part Data

In this section, we define multiple-part data and multiple-part learning problem.
    Multiple-part data consists of at least one component with part-of relations between each component and the whole data as well as relations among parts. Because of flexibility of the first-order logic, there are many ways to denote multiple-part data. We set a common way for data representation to make preprocessing easier. A part is denoted using only one predicate. The first two

parameters denote the identification of data and part. The rest parameters are used for attributes. For denoting a relation between parts, we use one predicate for one relation in similar manner to a part. The predicate is written as

- *part(Data-ID, Part-ID, Attr-1, Attr-2, ...)*.
- *relation(Data-ID, Part-ID$_1$, Part-ID$_2$, ...)*.

For better understanding, we explain the multiple-part data using chemical compound structure data as shown in Fig. 4. The predicate **atom** denotes a part of multiple-part data, while **bond** shows a relation between two parts (atoms). Using the first-order representation, each compound can be denoted by using two predicates:

- *atom(Compound-ID, Atom-ID, Element, Charge)* for an atom.
- *bond(Compound-ID, Atom-ID$_1$, Atom-ID$_2$, Bond-Type)* for a bond.

We use *Compound-ID* and *Atom-ID* to identify each compound and each atom. A bond is a relation consisting of two atoms (*Atom-ID$_1$* and *Atom-ID$_2$*). Moreover, we also include features to characterize atoms and bonds, which are *Element*, *Charge*, and *Bond-Type*. These features are useful for categorizing the atoms and bonds. which will be used in the experiments. From the chemical structure, each chemical compound or molecule represents the whole multiple-part data. It consists of several atoms as parts as well as bonds which are relations between two atoms.

Given a training example $\mathbb{E} = \{(x_1, y_1), (x_2, y_2), \ldots, (x_n, y_n)\}$ where x_i is a multiple-part data composing of $P_i \subseteq \mathbb{P}$ and $R_i \subseteq \mathbb{P} \times \mathbb{P}$ where $\mathbb{P}$ is a set of part, $\mathbb{R}$ is a set of relation between parts and y_i is a class (simply positive or negative). Multiple-part learning problem aims to approximate a function $f(P, R) = y$ where $P \subseteq \mathbb{P}$ and $R \subseteq \mathbb{R}$. This learning problem is considered a special case of supervised learning since it aims to find the class of data from substructure or subset of parts and relations. For example, in case of chemical compound data, we want to find substructures that are common among compounds with the same label or class, such as a group of atoms and bonds including their features. This problem is different from the traditional supervised learning that aims to predict class from the whole characteristics of data like predicting class of compound from its weight, or some special value computed.

3.2 Modified Heuristic Function

Heuristic function is used to control the way algorithm explores hypothesis space. FOIL (equation 1 and 3) adapts this function based on information theory that counts the number of positive and negative examples covered by partially developed clause. With this, FOIL selects the literal that covers many positive tuples but few negative tuples. In order to help heuristics select better literals, we apply DD value to each tuple, and we have to adapt heuristic function and the parts with high DD values are selected first, making the hypothesis cover common characteristics among parts from positive examples.

From equation 1, T_i^+ and T_i^- denote the set of positive and negative tuples respectively, as DD value can be used to show the importance of the part of data by representing each instance of multiple-part data as a bag and each part as an instance in the bag. The distance between two parts is calculated by first constructing a vector p for each part where p_i denotes *Attr-i* in the *part* predicate explained in the previous section. Then, equation 5 is used to calculate distance between two attribute vectors. From Fig. 4, distance between `atom(c1,a1,c,-1.2)` and `atom(c1,a2,o,1.3)` is computed by constructing two vectors $[c, -1.2]$ and $[o, 1.3]$ and using equation 5. To compute DD value of each atom, distances between all atom pairs are calculated first. Then, x in equation 4 is assigned to the vector of atom being considered. $||B_{ij}^+ - x||^2$ and $||B_{ij}^- - x||^2$ are obtained from the computed distances.

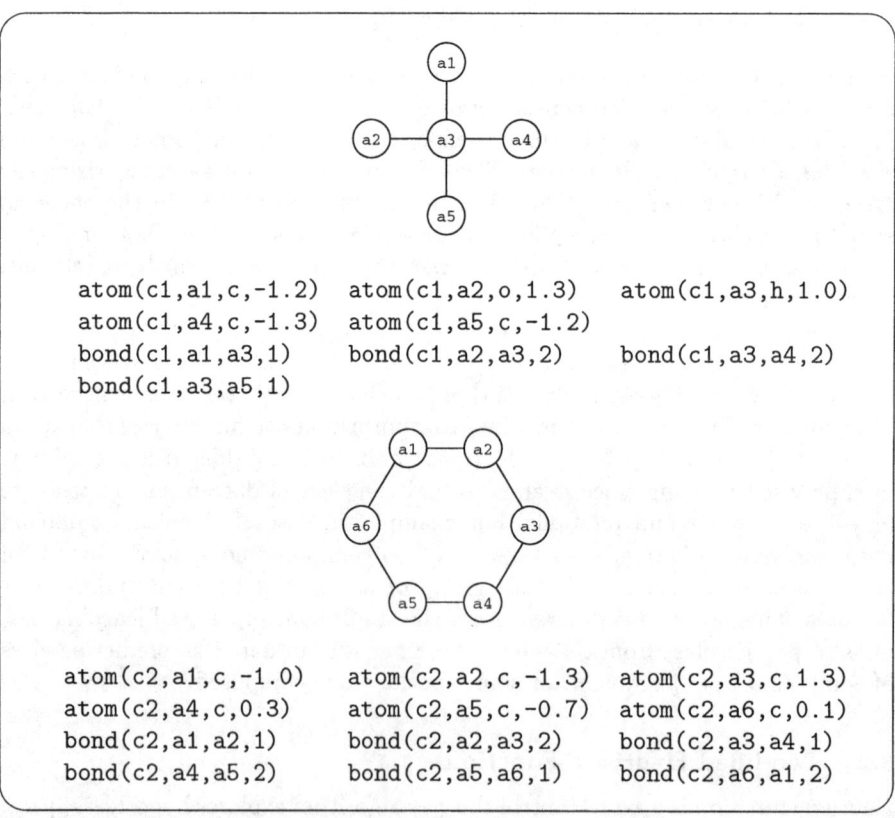

```
atom(c1,a1,c,-1.2)   atom(c1,a2,o,1.3)    atom(c1,a3,h,1.0)
atom(c1,a4,c,-1.3)   atom(c1,a5,c,-1.2)
bond(c1,a1,a3,1)     bond(c1,a2,a3,2)     bond(c1,a3,a4,2)
bond(c1,a3,a5,1)
```

```
atom(c2,a1,c,-1.0)   atom(c2,a2,c,-1.3)   atom(c2,a3,c,1.3)
atom(c2,a4,c,0.3)    atom(c2,a5,c,-0.7)   atom(c2,a6,c,0.1)
bond(c2,a1,a2,1)     bond(c2,a2,a3,2)     bond(c2,a3,a4,1)
bond(c2,a4,a5,2)     bond(c2,a5,a6,1)     bond(c2,a6,a1,2)
```

Fig. 4. Examples of multiple-part data

We incorporate DD values to heuristic function by altering $|T_i^+|$ to be the sum of tuple DD values. If this sum is high, it means that the literal can cover more common parts among positive examples. Thus, the heuristic function is adapted as follows:

$$DD(t) = \frac{\sum_k(t_k)}{m}, t = < t_1, t_2, \ldots, t_m > \tag{6}$$

$$DD_s(T) = \sum_{t_i \in T} DD(t_i) \tag{7}$$

$$I(T_i) = -\log_2 \frac{DD_s(T_i^+)}{DD_s(T_i^+) + |T_i^-|} \tag{8}$$

$$Gain(L_i) = DD_s(T_i^{++}) \times (I(T_i) - I(T_{i+1})) \tag{9}$$

This function weighs each part with DD value and uses the sum of these weights to select the literal, while the original heuristic function weighs all parts with the same value as 1. Nevertheless, we still use the number of negative tuples $|T_i^-|$ in the same way as the original heuristics, because we know that all parts of negative examples show the same strength. Therefore, it weighs all negative parts with value 1.

From the above function, one problem is left to be considered. Each tuple may consist of more than one part. The algorithm has to calculate DD value of a relation among parts, e.g. a bond makes each tuple contains two atoms. We then have to select the weight to represent each tuple from DD value of the parts. We solve this problem by simply selecting average DD value in the tuple as the weight of tuple (equation 6).

3.3   Algorithm

From this modified function, we implement the prototype system called FOILMP (**FOIL** for **M**ultiple-**P**art data). This system basically uses the same algorithm as proposed in [1]. Nevertheless, in order to construct accurate hypotheses, beam search is applied so that the algorithm maintains a set of good candidates instead of selecting the best candidate at that time. This searching method enables the algorithm to backtrack to the right direction and finally get to the goal. Moreover, in order to obtain rules with high coverage, we define coverage ratio, and the algorithm is set to select only the rules covering positive examples higher than the coverage ratio. Fig. 5 shows the main algorithm used in the proposed

---

FOILmp

- $Theory \leftarrow \emptyset$
- $Remaining \leftarrow Positive(Examples)$
- While not $StopCriterion(Examples, Remaining)$
    - $Rule \leftarrow$ **FindBestRule**$(Examples, Remaining)$
    - $Theory \leftarrow Theory \cup Rule$
    - $Covered \leftarrow Cover(Remaining, Rule)$
    - $Remaining \leftarrow Remaining - Covered$

Fig. 5. The main algorithm

FindBestRule(Examples, Remaining)

- Initialize *Beam* and add a rule with empty body.
- Do
    - *NewBeam* ← {}
    - For each clause *C* in *Beam*
        * Generate *Candidates* by selecting a possible literal and adding to *C*.
        * For each new clause *nC* in *Candidates*
            · Calculate *heuristic* of *nC* using DD values.
            · Append *nC* to *NewBeam*.
    - *Beam* ← Best *BeamWidth* clauses in *NewBeam*
    - *R* ← Best clause in *Beam*
- Until (Accuracy(R) > ε and PositiveCoverage(R) > γ) or (Gain(R) ≤ 0)
- Return R

Fig. 6. Algorithm for finding the best rule from the remaining positive examples

system. This algorithm starts by initialising the set *Theory* to null, and the set *Remaining* to the set of positive examples. The algorithm loops to find rules and add each rule found to *Theory* until all positive examples are covered. The modified subroutine for selecting rules is shown in Fig. 6. There are two user-defined parameters: ε for the minimum accuracy and γ for the minimum positive example coverage.

4   Experiments

We conducted experiments on two datasets for SAR: Mutagenicity and Dopamine antagonist data. To evaluate performance of the proposed system, these experiments are conducted in ten-fold cross validation manner and we compare the results to the existing approaches.

4.1   Dataset

In this research, we aim to discover rules describing the activities of chemical compounds from their structures. Two kinds of SAR data were studied: mutagenesis dataset [7] and dopamine antagonist dataset.

Mutagenesis Dataset. aims to test mutagenicity in nitroaromatic compounds which are often known to be carcinogenic and cause damage to DNA. These compounds are found in automobile exhaust fumes and are common intermediates used in chemical industry. In this dataset, 230 compounds were obtained from the standard molecular modeling package QUANTA. Two predicates (atm and bond) are used to denote each compound:

– *atm(comp, atom, element, type, charge)*, stating that there is the atom *atom* in the compound *comp* that has element *element* of *type* and partial charge *charge*.
– *bond(comp, atom1, atom2, type)*, describing that there is a bond of *type* between the atoms *atom1* and *atom2* in the compound *comp*.

The background knowledge in this dataset is already formalized in the form of multiple-part data, and thus, no preprocessing is necessary.

Dopamine Antagonist Dataset. describes each compound as atoms and bonds when a compound is plotted in the 3-dimensional area. Each atom is represented by element type and its position in the 3-dimensional area. Each bond is represented by two atoms and bond type. From this information, it can be seen that the position of atom has no meaning, since a compound can be plotted in many different ways. Therefore, the positions are not used directly but are used for computing length of bond between atoms. Hence, after preprocessing, the background knowledge consists of two kinds of predicate.

– *atom* – element type (such as, C for Carbon, N for Nitrogen, O for Oxygen), position when it is plotted in 3D space (X, Y, and Z).
– *bond* – two atoms that are linked by the bond, bond type which can be 1 for a single bond, or 2 for a double bond.

To convert information above into predicates, we first found that the position (X, Y, and Z) in 3D space has no meaning, since we can rotate and re-plot the compound and it makes the position of atoms changed to other values. We then used the position of atom to compute length of bond which is a fixed feature not related to moving or rotating. Two predicates were generated:

– *atm(compound, atom, element)* – stating an atom *atom* in compound *compound* with element *element*.
– *bond(compound, atom1, atom2, bondtype, length)* – describing a bond *bond* in compound *compound*. This bond links atom *atom1* and atom *atom2* together with type *bondtype* and length *length*.

However, after discussion with the domain expert, we found that excepting bond, there are as well other kinds of link whose energy is not so strong as bond but it is frequently important to identify the compound structure. Therefore, we add another predicate in order to show this kind of information and call it *link* as below.

– *link(compound, atom1, atom2, length)* – describing a relation *link* in compound *compound*. It links atom *atom1* and atom *atom2* with length *length*.

Finally, three kinds of predicate are used in the background knowledge. Nevertheless, there is only one feature to characterize each atom, that is, element type. This would not be enough to compute DD value if we use element type only. It means that we can separate dopamine antagonist compound by checking only elements included in that compound. Therefore, we need to add other features to characterize each atom. After discussing with the domain expert, the other features based on basic knowledge in chemistry are added: number of bonds linked to an atom, average length of bonds linked to an atom, connection to oxygen atom, minimum distance to oxygen and nitrogen.

Most of features are related to oxygen and nitrogen because the expert said that the position of oxygen and nitrogen has an effect to the activity of dopamine antagonist. Hence, the predicate *atm* is modified to *atm(compound, atom, element, number-bond, avg-bond-len, o-connect, o-min-len, n-min-len)*.

Although, the proposed method can handle only two-class data (only positive or negative), there are four classes for the dopamine antagonist compounds, however. Then, hypotheses for each class are learned by the one-against-the-rest

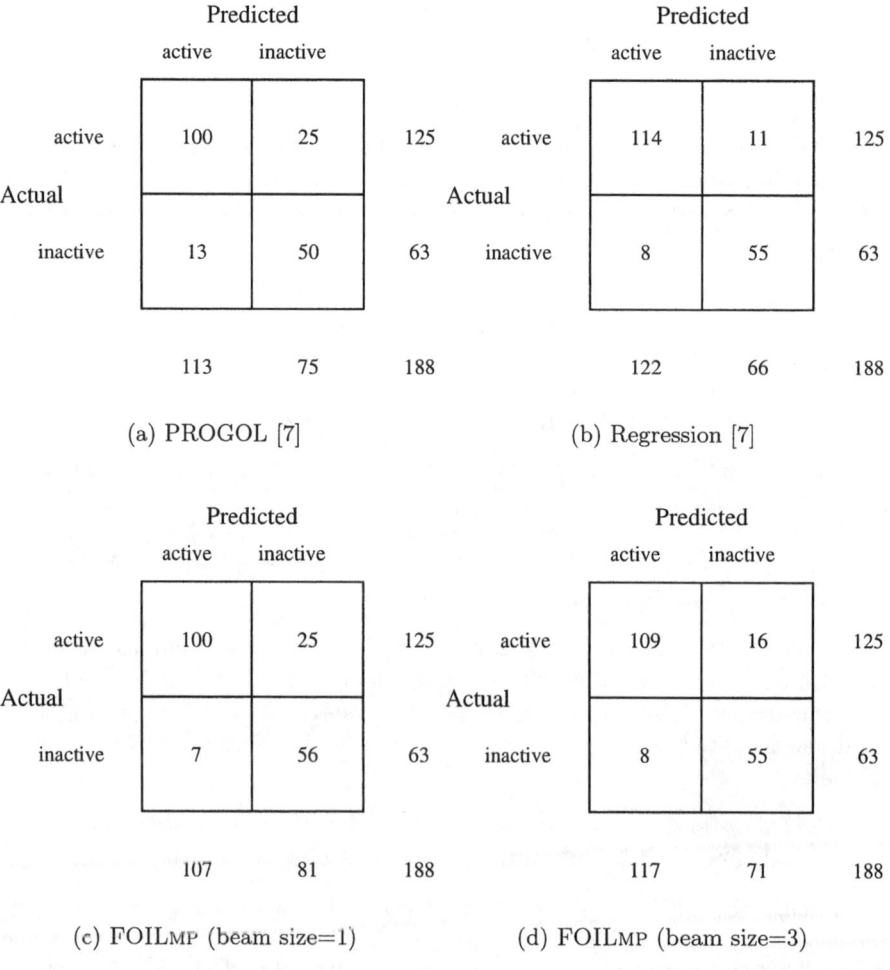

Fig. 7. Performance tables for Mutagenicity Data comparing FOILMP to PROGOL and the regression technique

technique, for instance, learning class D1 by using D1 as positive examples and D2, D3, D4 as negative examples.

4.2 Experimental Results and Discussion

We first compare performance of FOILMP using all data which consist of 125 compounds for positive class and 63 compounds for negative class. In this experiment, beam search is applied in FOILMP by setting the beam size = 1 (hill-climbing search) and 3 subsequently. The results are compared to the existing results described in [7]. Fig. 7 shows performance tables.

From the performance tables, it can be seen that even FOILMP with hill-climbing search strategy can learn from this dataset better than PROGOL with accuracy 83.0% for FOILMP and 79.8% for PROGOL. When compared to the regression technique based on the model called *logM* [7], FOILMP with the beam size = 3 still performs worse than the regression model that can predict at 89.9% whereas FOILMP can predict at only 87.2%. However, these experimental results show the advantage of FOILMP as follows: to use the regression model, a human expert is required to choose useful features to construct the model and the results are based on features difficult to be comprehended by other chemists.

Rule1:

```
active(A) :- atm(A,B,C,D,E), D=27, atm(A,F,G,H,I), H=27, neq(E,I).
```

Accuracy = 92.5% Coverage = 49.6%

This rule shows that the molecule contains two atoms of Type 27 which means a carbon atom that merges two six-numbered aromatic rings. However, these two atoms has different charge.

Rule2:

```
active(A) :- atm(A,B,C,D,E), E>0.81, atm(A,F,G,H,I), H=29.
```

Accuracy = 90.9% Coverage = 16.0%

This rule is similar to Rule1 but the first atom has charge greater than 0.81 and the second atom is of Type 29.

Rule3:

```
active(A) :- atm(A,B,C,D,E), D=32, atm(A,F,G,H,I), I<-0.4,
             bond(A,F,J,K), neq(B,F), eq(C,G), eq(D,H).
```

Accuracy = 77.8% Coverage = 5.0%

This rule shows that there are two atoms of Type 32 which occurs in an amide group. But the second atom has charge less than 0.4 and there is also a bond from this atom to another atom.

Fig. 8. Examples of rules obtained by FOILMP

Table 1. Ten-fold cross validation test comparing the accuracy on Mutagenesis data

Approach	Accuracy
The proposed method	0.82
PROGOL	0.76
FOIL	0.61

Fig. 8 shows example of rules obtained from FOILMP. We found that FOILMP obtains rules with high coverage, such as, the first rule can cover around 50% of the all positive examples.

Table 1 shows experimental results on Mutagenicity data. Prediction accuracy on test examples using ten-fold cross validation is compared to the existing approaches (FOIL and PROGOL). It shows that the proposed method can predict more accurately than the existing approaches.

Actual \ Predicted	positive	negative	
positive	126	19	145
negative	7	1085	1092
	133	1104	1237

(a) FOILMP

Actual \ Predicted	positive	negative	
positive	124	21	145
negative	11	1081	1092
	136	1102	1237

(b) Aleph

Fig. 9. Performance table for fold 1 comparing FOILMP and Aleph

Table 2. Ten-fold cross-validation test comparing the accuracy on dopamine antagonist data; Superscripts denote confidence levels for the difference in accuracy between FOILMP and Aleph, using a one-paired t-test: * is 95.0%, ** is 99.0%; no superscripts denote confidence levels below 95%

Activity	FOILMP Accuracy(%) (overall)	FOILMP Accuracy(%) (only positive)	Aleph Accuracy(%) (overall)	Aleph Accuracy(%) (only positive)
D1	97.0	85.5	96.0*	78.6**
D2	88.1	79.1	86.4*	70.5*
D3	93.4	78.4	93.1	75.1*
D4	88.4	85.1	87.6*	83.2*

Rule 1

```
d1(A) :- atm(A,B,C,D,E,F), E>=3.7, F=3.3, bond(A,L,B,H,M,N),
    bond(A,G,H,I,J,K), K=1.5, bond(A,O,B,P,Q,R),
        not_equal(H,P).
```

Accuracy = 93.2% Coverage = 47.6%

This rule shows a molecule contains an atom B with the minimum distance to oxygen is greater or equal to $3.7\mathring{A}$, and the minimum distance to nitrogen is $3.3\mathring{A}$. From B, there are two bonds to two different atoms (H and P). Moreover, there is another bond from H to I with bond length is equal to $1.5\mathring{A}$.

Rule 2

```
d1(A) :- atm(A,B,C,D,E,F), F=3.0, E>=3.9, bond(A,G,B,H,I,J),
    J<1.4.
```

Accuracy = 93.8% Coverage = 10.3%

This rule is similar to Rule 1 that there is one atom with specified minimum distance to oxygen and nitrogen. But there is only one bond with length less than $1.4\mathring{A}$.

Fig. 10. Rules obtained by FOILMP using data for D1 activity

Rule 1

```
d1(A) :- link(A,B,C,D), bond(A,E,F,C,G,H), D=6.9, H=1.4,
         bond(A,I,J,F,K,H), bond(A,L,M,J,G,H), bond(A,N,B,O,G,P).
```

Accuracy = 91.3% Coverage = 36.5%

This rule shows a molecule contains a link between atom B and C with length $6.9\mathring{A}$. There is a bond from atom F to C with length $1.4\mathring{A}$ and there are bonds from J to F, M to J and B to O.

Rule 2

```
d1(A) :- link(A,B,C,D), D=2.7, bond(A,E,C,F,G,H), H=1.5,
         bond(A,I,J,B,G,K), atm(A,L,M,N,O,P), O=<2.9.
```

Accuracy = 81.0% Coverage = 11.7%

This rule shows a molecule contains a link between atom B and C with length $2.7\mathring{A}$. There is a bond from atom C to F with length $1.5\mathring{A}$ and there is a bond from atom B to J. The molecule contains an atom L with the minimun distance to oxygen is less than or equal to $2.9\mathring{A}$.

Fig. 11. Rules obtained by Aleph using data for D1 activity

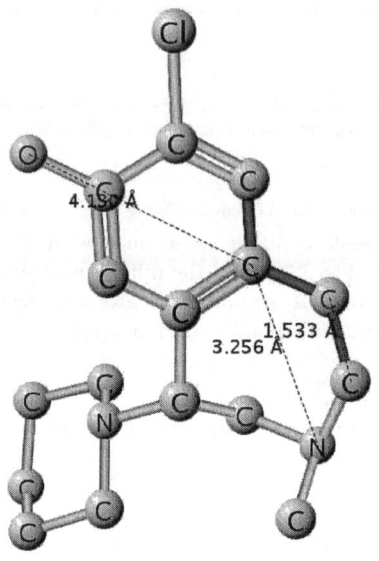

(a) FOILMP

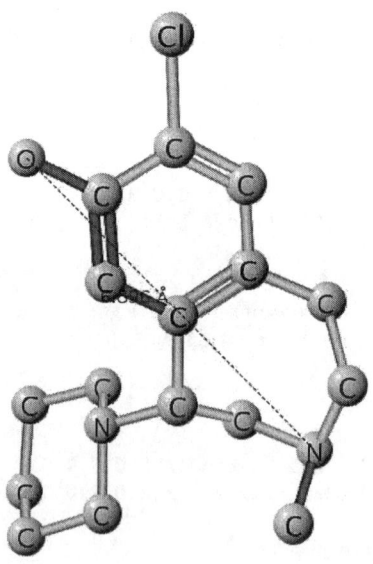

(b) Aleph

Fig. 12. Visualization of a molecule described by Rule 1 from FOILMP and Aleph

For Dopamine Antagonist data, we conducted ten-fold cross validation to predict D1, D2, D3, and D4 activities. However, we compared the experimental results with Aleph [8], since PROGOL cannot generate accurate rules from this dataset in reasonable time. Aleph is an ILP system based on inverse entailment and similar algorithm with PROGOL. However, Aleph has adopted several search strategies, such as randomized search which helps improve the performance of the system. In this experiment, we set Aleph to use GSAT [9], which is one of the randomized search algorithms where the best results can be generated.

Fig. 9 shows the performance table comparing the experimental results in the first fold. Table 2 shows the prediction accuracy computed for both positive and negative examples, and then, for only the positive examples. The table also shows the results of significance test using a one-paired t-test. The experiment results show that FOILMP predicts more accurately than Aleph in both accuracy computation methods. The significance tests also show the confidence level in the difference between accuracy. Fig. 10 and 11 show details of rules obtained by FOILMP and Aleph respectively. We also found that FOILMP generates rule with higher coverage than Aleph where the rule covers 36.5% of positive examples.

5   Related Work

In recent years, many researches were made to learn from chemical compound structure data because learning results can be applied directly to produce new drugs for curing some difficult diseases. Muggleton, Srinivasan and King [7, 10, 11] proposed the approach that applies PROGOL to predict several datasets including mutagenicity of chemical compounds used in our experiments.

King et al. also discussed whether propositional learner or ILP is better for learning from chemical structure [10]. Actually, the first-order representation can denote chemical structure without losing any information. Since denoting the relational data using propositional logic is beyond its limit, some special techniques are required, e.g., for relations among parts, we may use only average value of features or use domain-related knowledge to calculate a new feature for categorization. However, a propositional learner can perform better than a learner using first-order representation because ILP learners have some restrictions from the logic theory. However, comparing only accuracy may not be good assessment because chemist's natural inclination is related to chemical structure and the learning results from ILP is comprehensible to chemists.

However, King et al. [10] reviewed four case studies related to SAR studies: inhibition of dihydrofolate reductase by pyrimidines, inhibition of dihydrofolate reductase by triazines, design of tacrine analogues, and mutagenicity of nitroaromatic and heteroaromatic compounds. The experimental results are compared with two propositional learner: *Regression*, a linear regression technique and *CART*, a decision tree learner. They found that with these chemical structure data, propositional learners with limited number of features in one instance are sufficient to all problems. However, when more complex chemical structures and background knowledge are added, propositional representations become unmanageable. Therefore, first-order representations would provide more possibility with more comprehensible results.

From multiple-instance learning problem, Wiedmann et al. [12] proposed an extension of the process for determining labels of a bag. This is a generalization of the assumption used in multiple-instance learning where a bag is labeled as positive if there exists at least one positive instance. The author proposed the idea of two-level classification for handling generalized multiple-instance problem. However, the research focuses on learning from propositional data representation.

McGovern and Jensen [13] proposed extension of diverse density and chi-squared measure to relational data using the metric based on the found maximal common subgraph. This work is similar to the proposed approach that also aims to handle ambiguous relational data. Because each bag is represented in form of graph, relations between bags cannot be denoted. Nevertheless, the proposed metric is interesting enough to apply modified version of the metric to our proposed method.

Zucker et al. [14, 15] applied multiple-instance learning on Mutagenesis data and proposed the extension of decision tree and propositional rule learner for multiple-instance learning. The molecular property, such as $logP$ and $lumo$, are applied in the experiments, but comparison to the proposed method is difficult to make. However, the dataset is transformed into propositional representation due to the user-defined setting. It limits usage of relations in the hypotheses.

6   Conclusion and Future Works

We presented extension of FOIL for handling multiple-part data more efficiently by using Diverse Density from multiple-instance learning to evaluate parts and parts with common characteristics among positive examples have high-valued weight and help enable the searching process to generate better results. We conducted experiments on chemical compound data for structure-activity relationship studies. The experimental results showed that the proposed method can predict test examples more accurately than the previous ILP approaches.

For future works, scaling factor of the feature should be considered in heuristic value calculation in order to produce more suitable heuristics. Because the proposed approach works only in the top-down ILP system such as FOIL, it is better to adopt this approach to other kinds of system such as the one with bottom-up approach. We plan to evaluate the proposed system to other domains. Moreover, as the proposed approach mainly focuses on a part, it is difficult to incorporate relational information into the heuristic function. We plan to overcome this limitation in our future works.

References

1. Quinlan, J.R.: Learning logical definitions from relations. Machine Learning **5** (1990) 239–266
2. Dietterich, T.G., Lathrop, R.H., Lozano-Perez, T.: Solving the multiple instance problem with axis-parallel rectangles. Artificial Intelligence **89** (1997) 31–71

3. Wang, J., Zucker, J.D.: Solving the multiple-instance problem: A lazy learning approach. In: Proc. 17th International Conf. on Machine Learning, Morgan Kaufmann, San Francisco, CA (2000) 1119–1125
4. Chevaleyre, Y., Zucker, J.D.: A framework for learning rules from multiple instance data. In: Proc. 12th European Conf. on Machine Learning. Volume 2167 of LNCS., Springer (2001) 49–60
5. Gärtner, T., Flach, P.A., Kowalczyk, A., Smola, A.J.: Multi-instance kernels. In: Proc. 19th International Conf. on Machine Learning, Morgan Kaufmann (2002) 179–186
6. Maron, O., Lozano-Pérez, T.: A framework for multiple-instance learning. In Jordan, M.I., Kearns, M.J., Solla, S.A., eds.: Advances in Neural Information Processing Systems. Volume 10., The MIT Press (1998)
7. Srinivasan, A., Muggleton, S., King, R., Sternberg, M.: Mutagenesis: ILP experiments in a non-determinate biological domain. In Wrobel, S., ed.: Proc. 4th International Workshop on Inductive Logic Programming. Volume 237., Gesellschaft für Mathematik und Datenverarbeitung MBH (1994) 217–232
8. Srinivasan, A.: The Aleph manual (2001) http://web.comlab.ox.ac.uk/oucl/-research/areas/machlearn/Aleph/.
9. Selman, B., Levesque, H.J., Mitchell, D.: A new method for solving hard satisfiability problems. In: Proceedings 10th National Conference on Artificial Intelligence. (1992) 440–446
10. King, R.D., Sternberg, M.J.E., Srinivasan, A.: Relating chemical activity to structure: An examination of ILP successes. New Generation Computing 13 (1995) 411–433
11. Srinivasan, A., Muggleton, S., Sternberg, M.J.E., King, R.D.: Theories for mutagenicity: A study in first-order and feature-based induction. Artificial Intelligence 85 (1996) 277–299
12. Weidmann, N., Frank, E., Pfahringer, B.: A two-level learning method for generalized multi-instance problems. In: Proceedings of the European Conference on Machine Learning (ECML-2003). (2003) 468–479
13. McGovern, A., Jensen, D.: Identifying predictive structures in relational data using multiple instance learning. In: Proceedings of the 20th International Conference on Machine Learning (ICML-2003). (2003)
14. Chevaleyre, Y., Zucker, J.D.: Solving multiple-instance and multiple-part learning problems with decision trees and decision rules: Application to the mutagenesis problem. Technical report, LIP6-CNRS, University Paris VI (2000)
15. Zucker, J.D.: Solving multiple-instance and multiple-part learning problems with decision trees and rule sets. application to the mutagenesis problem. In: Proceedings of Canadian Conference on AI 2001. (2001) 204–214

First-Order Rule Mining by Using Graphs Created from Temporal Medical Data

Ryutaro Ichise[1] and Masayuki Numao[2]

[1] Intelligent Systems Research Division,
National Institute of Informatics,
2-1-2 Hitotsubashi, Chiyoda, Tokyo 101-8430, Japan
ichise@nii.ac.jp
[2] The Institute of Scientific and Industrial Research,
Osaka University,
8-1 Mihogaoka, Ibaraki, Osaka 567-0047, Japan
numao@ai.sanken.osaka-u.ac.jp

Abstract. In managing medical data, handling time-series data, which contain irregularities, presents the greatest difficulty. In the present paper, we propose a first-order rule discovery method for handling such data. The present method is an attempt to use graph structure to represent time-series data and reduce the graph using specified rules for inducing hypothesis. In order to evaluate the proposed method, we conducted experiments using real-world medical data.

1   Introduction

Hospital information systems that store medical data are very popular, especially in large hospitals. Such systems hold patient medical records, laboratory data, and other types of information, and the knowledge extracted from such medical data can assist physicians in formulating treatment strategies. However, the volume of data is too large to allow efficient manual extraction of data. Therefore, physicians must rely on computers to extract relevant knowledge.

Medical data has three notable features [14]; namely, the number of records increases each time a patient visits a hospital; values are often missing, usually because patients do not always undergo all examinations; and the data include time-series attributes with irregular time intervals. To handle medical data, a mining system must have functions that accommodate these features. Methods for mining data include K-NN, decision trees, neural nets, association rules, and genetic algorithms [1]. However, these methods are unsuitable for medical data, in view of the inclusion of multiple relationships and time relationships with irregular intervals.

Inductive Logic Programming (ILP) [4] is an effective method for handling multiple relationships, because it uses horn clauses that constitute a subset of first order logic. However, ILP is difficult to apply to data of large volume, in view of computational cost. We propose a new graph-based algorithm for inducing

S. Tsumoto et al. (Eds.): AM 2003, LNAI 3430, pp. 112–125, 2005.

Table 1. Example medical data

ID	Examination Date	GOT	GPT	WBC	RNP	SM
14872	19831212	30	18			
14872	19840123	30	16			
14872	19840319	27	17	4.9		
14872	19840417	29	19	18.1		
14872	...					
5482128	19960516	18	11	9.1	-	-
5482128	19960703	25	23	9.6		
5482779	19980526	52	59	3.6	4	-
5482779	19980811			4		
5482779	...					

horn clauses for representing temporal relations from data in the manner of ILP systems. The method can reduce computational cost of exploring in hypothesis space. We apply this system to a medical data mining task and demonstrate the performance in identifying temporal knowledge in the data.

This paper is organized as follows. Section 2 characterizes the medical data with some examples. Section 3 describes related work in time-series data and medical data. Section 4 presents new temporal relationship mining algorithms and mechanisms. Section 5 applies the algorithms to real-world medical data to demonstrate our algorithm's performance, and Section 6 discusses our experimental result and methods. Finally, in Section 7 we present our conclusions.

2 Medical Data

As described above, the sample medical data shown here have three notable features. Table 1 shows an example laboratory examination data set including seven attributes. The first attribute, ID, means personal identification. The second is Examination Date, which is the date the patient consults a physician. The remaining attributes designate results of laboratory tests.

The first feature shows that the data contain a large number of records. The volume of data in this table increases quickly, because new records having numerous attributes are added every time a patient undergoes an examination.

The second feature is that many values are missing from the data. Table 1 shows that many values are absent from the attributes that indicate the results of laboratory examinations. Since this table is an extract from medical data, the number of missing values is quite low. However, in the actual data set this number is far higher. That is, most of the data are missing values, because each patient undergoes only some tests during the course of one examination. In addition, Table 1 does not contain data when laboratory tests have not been conducted. This means that the data during the period 1983/12/13 to 1984/01/22 for patient ID 14872 can also be considered missing values.

The other notable feature of the medical data is that it contains time-series attributes. When a table does not have these attributes, then the data contain only a relationship between ID and examination results. Under these circumstances, the data can be subjected to decision tree learning or any other propositional learning method. However, relationships between examination test dates are also included; that is, multiple relationships.

3   Related Work

These kinds of data can be handled by any of numerous approaches. We summarize related work for treating such data from two points of view: time-series data and medical data.

3.1   Time-Series Data

One approach is to treat the data described in Section 2 as time-series data. When we plot each data point, we can obtain a graph similar to stock market chart, and can apply a mining method to such data. Mining methods include the window sliding approach [3] and dynamic time warping [7]. Those methods can identify similar graphs. However, when there are missing data in the time series, or when the time series data can not be obtained continuously, can methods based on the similarity of graphs be assumed to work well? Let us consider the data listed in Table 2. Each row represents one set of time series data, and each set consists of four data, collected at four different points in time. First, we will examine the problem in which conventional mining methods, which are based on graph similarity, can not find a feature among the data. Assume that we have time series ID1 and ID2, given in Table 2. As shown in the upper left-hand graph in Figure 1, the two example time series look very different. However, if we exclude the datum at time 2 for ID1 and that at time 3 for ID2, we obtain the upper right-hand graph in Figure 1. The shapes of the graphs are now identical. Thus, the graph similarity approach can not find a feature common to ID1 and ID2. This type of problem may also occur under different circumstances. Looking at the ID1 time series, we first suppose the datum at time 1 is missing. We will call this time series ID1'. Now suppose that for the same original time series (ID1), the datum at time 2 is missing. Let us call this time series ID1". These time series are given in Table 2 and are graphed in the lower left-hand and lower right-hand graphs, respectively, in Figure 1. Even when generated from the same actual time series, the graph shape may differ greatly when data are missing. From the above discussion, this type of method is not robust for missing values and is not directly applicable to the medical data described in Section 2.

3.2   Medical Data

Many systems for finding useful knowledge from medical data have been developed [8]. However, not many systems for treating temporal medical data have been developed. Active mining projects [9] progressing in Japan are now being

Table 2. Example time series

Data	1	2	3	4
ID1	50	100	50	50
ID2	50	50	0	50
ID1'	-	100	50	50
ID1"	50	-	50	50

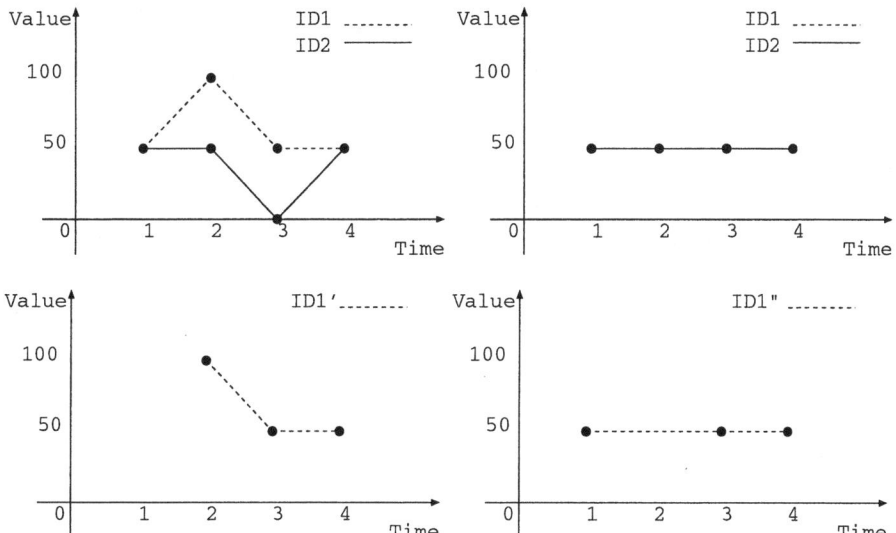

Fig. 1. Graphs of the example time series of Table 2

developed in order to obtain knowledge from such data. The temporal description
is usually converted into attribute features by some special function or dynamic
time warping method. Subsequently, the attribute feature in a standard machine
learning method such as decision tree [15] or clustering [2] is used. Since these
methods do not treat the data directly, the obtained data can be biased by
summarization of the temporal data.

Another approach incorporates InfoZoom [13], which is a tool for visualization
of medical data in which the temporal data are shown to a physician, and the
physician tries to find knowledge from medical data interactively. This tool lends
useful support for the physician, but does not induce knowledge by itself.

4   Temporal Relationship Mining

4.1   Approach

An important consideration for obtaining knowledge from medical data is to
have a knowledge representation scheme that can handle the features described

in Section 2. One such scheme is Inductive Logic Programming (ILP)[4], because it uses horn clauses, which can represent such complicated and multi-relationship data [6]. Since ILP framework is based on the proof of logic, only observed data are processed for finding features. This means not adding false data when actual data cannot be obtained. Therefore, ILP constitutes one solution for the second problem inherent to medical data described in Section 2. Horn clause representation permits multiple relations, such as time-series relation and attributes relations. It can also be a solution to the third problem inherent to medical data. However, the ILP system does not provide a good solution to the first problem, because its computational cost is much higher than that of other machine learning methods. In this section, we propose a new algorithm for solving the problem by using graphs.

4.2   Temporal Predicate

Data mining of medical data requires a temporal predicate, which can represent irregular intervals for the treatment of temporal knowledge. We employ a predicate similar to one proposed by Rodríguez et al. [12]. The predicate has five arguments and is represented as follows:

$$blood\_test(ID, Test, Value, BeginningDate, EndingDate)$$

The arguments denote the patient ID, kind of laboratory test, value of the test, beginning date of the period being considered, and ending date of the period being considered, respectively. This predicate returns true if all tests conducted within the period have a designated value. For example, the following predicate is true if patient ID 618 had at least one GOT test from Oct. 10th 1982 to Nov. 5th 1983, and all tests during this period yield very high values.

$$blood\_test(618, got, veryhigh, 19821010, 19831105)$$

This predicate is a good example for representing temporal knowledge in medical data, because it can represent the predisposition within a certain period, regardless of test intervals. Moreover, it can handle missing values without affecting the truth value. This naturally implies that our approach is a good solution for two of the problems inherent to medical data (e.g., multiple relationships and time relationships with irregular intervals) described in Section 2.

4.3   Rule Induction Algorithm

In this paper, we utilize a top-down ILP algorithm similar to FOIL[11]. We can divide this algorithm into two parts. One part is an external loop for covering algorithm[10]. This algorithm is used for deleting from a positive example set examples that are covered by a generated hypothesis, and is shown in Table 3. The second part of the algorithm is an internal loop for generating a hypothesis. The algorithm is shown in Table 4. Initially, the algorithm creates the most general

Table 3. The external loop algorithm

E^+ is a set of positive examples, R is a set of discovered rules.

1. If $E^+ = \phi$, return R
2. Construct clause H by using the internal loop algorithm
3. Let $R = R \cup H$
4. Goto 1

Table 4. The internal loop algorithm

H is a hypothesis.

1. Generate H, which contains only head
2. Use refinement operator to generate literal candidate
3. Select the best literal L according to MDL criteria
4. Add L as a body of literal H
5. If H qualified criteria, return H, otherwise goto 2

---

hypothesis. Subsequently, it generates literal candidates by using a refinement operator discussed in the following section. Next, the algorithm chooses the most promising literal according to MDL criteria, and adds it to the body of the hypothesis. If the MDL cannot be decreased by adding a literal, the algorithm returns the hypothesis.

4.4   Refinement

In our method, the search space for the hypothesis is constructed by combinations of predicates described in Section 4.2. Suppose that the number of the kinds of tests is N_a, the number of test domains is N_v, and the number of date possibilities is N_d. Then, the number of candidate literals is $N_a \times N_v \times N_d^2/2$. As we described in Section 2, because medical data consist of a great number of records, the computational cost for handling medical data is also great. However, medical data have many missing values and consequently, often consist of sparse data. When we make use of this fact, we can reduce the search space and computational cost.

To create candidate literals which are used for refinement, we propose employing graphs created from temporal medical data. The purpose of this literal creation is to find literals which cover many positive examples. In order to find them, a graph is created from positive examples. The nodes in the graph are defined by each medical data record and the node has four labels; i.e. patient ID, laboratory test name, laboratory test value, and date test conducted. Arcs are created for each node. Suppose that two nodes represented by $n(Id_0, Att_0, Val_0, Dat_0)$ and $n(Id_1, Att_1, Val_1, Dat_1)$ exist. The arc is created if all the following conditions hold:

Table 5. Example data

Id	Attribute	Value	Date
23	got	vh	80
31	got	vh	72
31	got	vh	84
35	got	vh	74

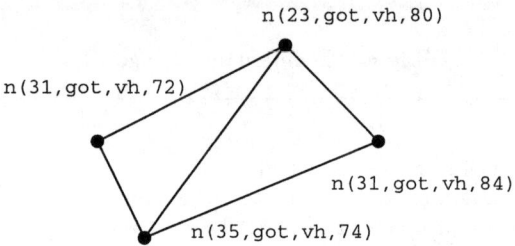

Fig. 2. Example graph

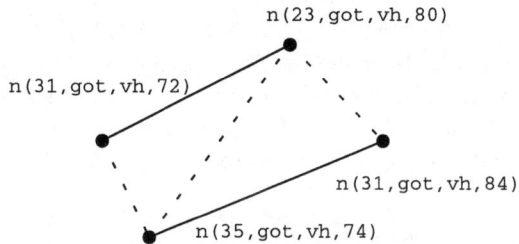

Fig. 3. Graph after deletion

- $Id_0 \neq Id_1$
- $Att_0 = Att_1$
- $Val_0 = Val_1$
- For all $D\{D \geq Dat_0 \wedge D \leq Dat_1\}$,
  if $n(Id_0, Att_0, Val, D)$ exists, $Val = Val_0$
  and
  if $n(Id_1, Att_1, Val, D)$ exists, $Val = Val_1$

For example, supposing that we have data shown in Table 5, we can obtain the graph shown in Figure 2.

After constructing the graph, the arcs are deleted by the following reduction rules:

- The arc $n_0 - n_1$ is deleted if a node n_2 which is connected to both n_0 and n_1 exists, and
  - Dat_2 for n_2 is greater than both Dat_0 and Dat_1 or
  - Dat_2 for n_2 is smaller than both Dat_0 and Dat_1

After deleting all arcs for which the above conditions hold, we can obtain the maximum period which contains positive examples. Then we pick up the remaining arcs and set the node date as *BeginingDate* and *EndingDate*. After applying the deletion rules for the graph shown in Figure 2, we obtain the graph shown in Figure 3. Then the final literal candidate for refinement is $blood\_test(Id, got, veryhigh, 72, 80)$ and $blood\_test(Id, got, veryhigh, 74, 84)$, which in this case covers all three patients.

5   Experiment

5.1   Experimental Settings

In order to evaluate the proposed algorithm, we conducted experiments on real medical data donated from Chiba University Hospital. These medical data contains data of hepatitis patients, and the physician requires us to find an effective timing for starting interferon therapy. Interferon is a kind of medicine for reducing the hepatitis virus. It has great effect for some patients; however, some patients exhibit no effect, and some patients exhibit deteriorated condition. Further, the medicine is expensive and has side effects. Therefore, physicians wants to know the effectiveness of Interferon before starting the therapy. According to our consulting physician, the effectiveness of the therapy could be changed by the patient's condition and could be affected by the timing for starting it.

We input the data of patients whose response is complete as positive examples, and the data of the remaining patients as negative examples. Complete response is judged by virus tests and under advice from our consulting physician. The number of positive and negative examples are 57 and 86, respectively. GOT, GPT, TTT, ZTT, T-BIL, ALB, CHE, TP, T-CHO, WBC, and PLT, which are attributes of the blood test, were used in this experiment. Each attribute value was discretized by the criteria suggested by the physician. We treat the starting date for interferon therapy as base date, in order to align data from different patients. According to the physician, small changes in blood test results can be ignored. Therefore, we consider the predicate blood_test to be true if the percentage p, which is set by parameter, of the blood tests in the time period show the specified value.

5.2   Result

Since not all results can be explained, we introduce only five of the rules obtained by our system.

```
inf_effect(Id):-
        blood_test(Id,wbc,low,149,210). (1)
```

This rule is obtained when the percentage parameter p is set at 1.0. Among the 143 patients, 13 satisfied the antecedent of this rule, and interferon therapy was effective in 11 of these. The rule held for 19.3 percent of the effective patients and had 84.6 percent accuracy. The blood

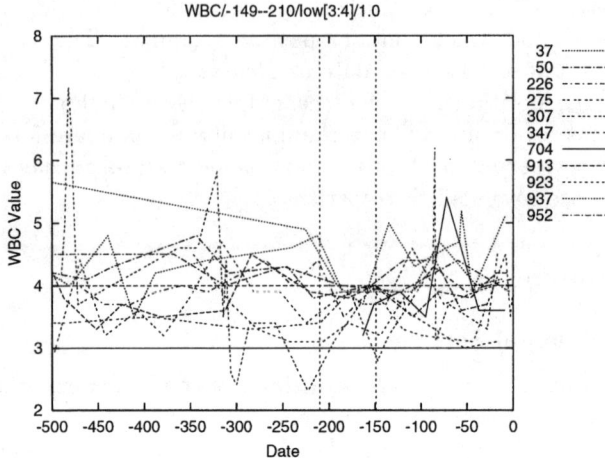

Fig. 4. Blood test graph for rule (1)

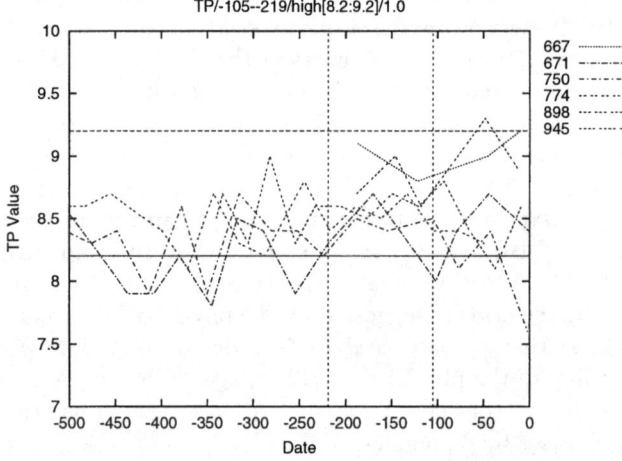

Fig. 5. Blood test graph for rule (2)

test data for effective patients are shown in Figure 4. The number of the graph line represents patient ID, and the title of the graph represents test-name/period/value[low:high]/parameter p, respectively.

```
inf_effect(Id):-
        blood_test(Id,tp,high,105,219).  (2)
```

This rule is obtained when the percentage parameter p is set at 1.0. Among the 143 patients, 7 satisfied the antecedent of this rule, and interferon therapy was effective for 6 of these. The rule held for 10.5 percent of the effective patients and had 85.7 percent accuracy. The blood test data for effective patients are shown in Figure 5.

```
inf_effect(Id):-
        blood_test(Id,wbc,normal,85,133),
        blood_test(Id,tbil,veryhigh,43,98). (3)
```

This rule is obtained when the percentage parameter p is set at 0.8. Among the 143 patients, 5 satisfied the antecedent of this rule, and interferon therapy was effective in all of these. The rule held for 8.8 percent of the effective patients and had 100 percent accuracy. The blood

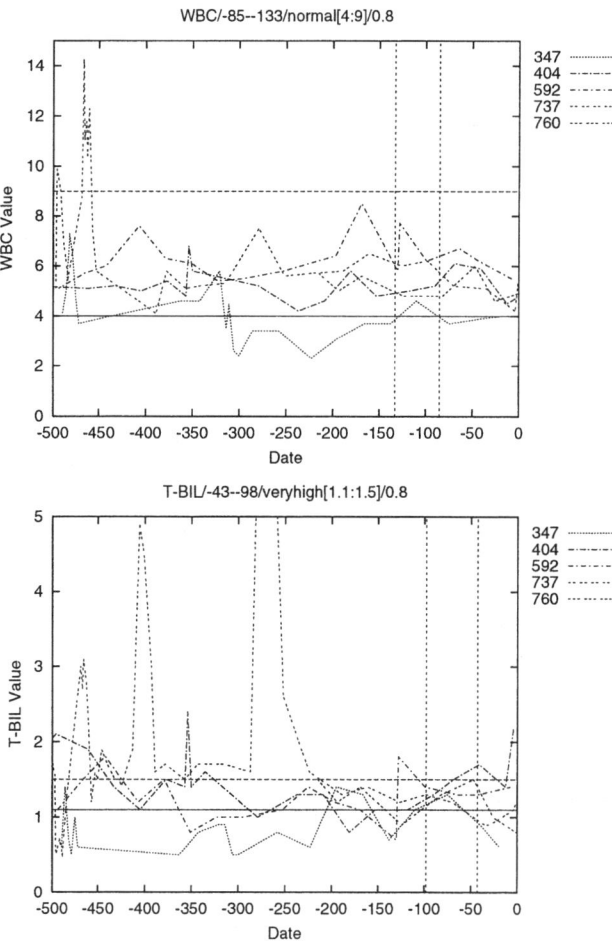

Fig. 6. Blood test graph for rule (3)

test data for effective patients are shown in Figure 6. The patients who
satisfied both test in rule (3) are positive patients. This means that we
have to view both graphs in Figure 6 simultaneously.

```
inf_effect(Id):-
        blood_test(Id,tbil,medium,399,499). (4)
```

This rule is obtained when the percentage parameter p is set at 0.8.
Among the 143 patients, 6 satisfied the antecedent of this rule, and
interferon therapy was effective in 5 of these. The rule held for 8.8 percent

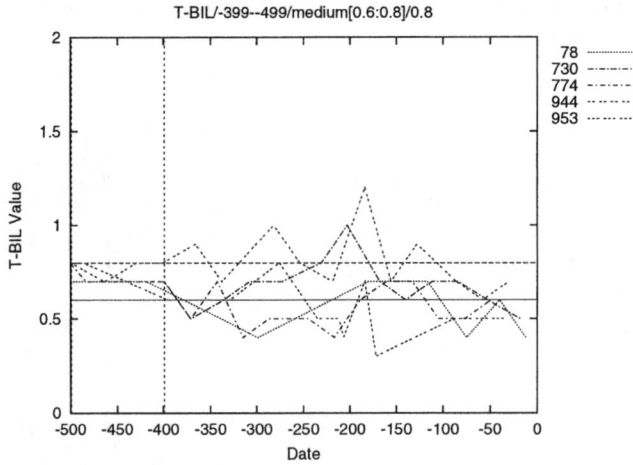

Fig. 7. Blood test graph for rule (4)

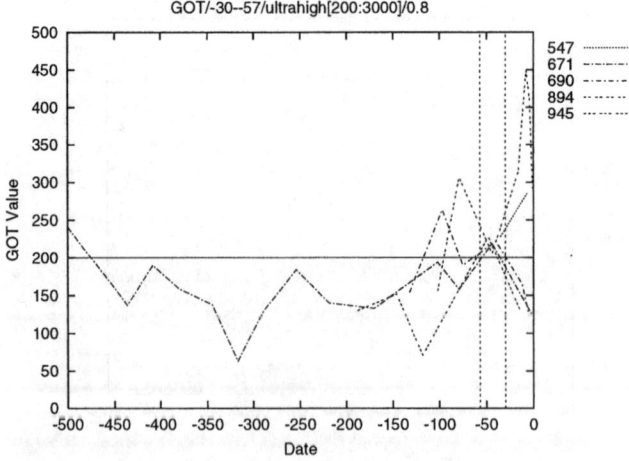

Fig. 8. Blood test graph for rule (5)

of the effective patients and had 83.3 percent accuracy. The blood test data for effective patients are shown in Figure 7.

```
inf_effect(Id):-
          blood_test(Id,got,ultrahigh,30,57). (5)
```

This rule is obtained when the percentage parameter p is set at 0.8. Among the 143 patients, 6 satisfied the antecedent of this rule, and interferon therapy was effective in 5 of these. The rule held for 8.8 percent of the effective patients and had 83.3 percent accuracy. The blood test data for effective patients are shown in Figure 8.

6   Discussion

The results of our experiment demonstrate that our method successfully induces rules with temporal relationships in positive examples. For example, in Figure 4, the value range of WBC for the patients is wide except for the period between 149 and 210, but during that period, patients exhibiting interferon effect have the same value. This implies that our system can discover temporal knowledge within the positive examples.

We showed these results to our consulting physician. He stated that if the rule specified about half a year before therapy starting day, causality between the phenomena and the result would be hard to imagine. It was necessary to find a connection between them during the period. In relation to the third rule, he also commented that the hypothesis implies that temporary deterioration in a patient's condition would indicate the desirability to start interferon therapy with complete response.

The current system utilizes a cover set algorithm to induce knowledge. This method starts from finding the largest group in positive examples, then progresses to find smaller groups. According to our consulting physician, the patients could be divided into groups, even within the interferon effective patients. One method for identifying such groups is the subgroups discovery method [5], which uses a covering algorithm involving example weighting for rule set construction. When it is used in place of the cover set algorithm, this method could assist the physician.

In its present form, our method uses only the predicate defined in Section 4.2. When we use this predicate with the same rule and different time periods, we can represent movement of blood test values. However, this induction is somewhat difficult for our system, because each literal is treated in each refinement step separately. This means that the possibility to obtain rules including movement of blood test is very small. This is a current limitation for representing the movement of blood tests. Rodrígues et al. [12] also propose other types of temporal literals. As we mentioned previously, the hypothesis space constructed by the temporal literal requires a high computational cost for searching, and only a limited hypothesis space is explored. In this paper, we propose inducing the literals efficiently by using graph representation of hypothesis space. We believe that we can extend this approach to other types of temporal literals.

7   Conclusion

In this paper, we propose a new data mining algorithm. The performance of the algorithm was tested experimentally by use of real-world medical data. The experimental results show that this algorithm can induce knowledge about temporal relationships from medical data. The temporal knowledge is hard to obtain by existing methods, such as a decision tree. Furthermore, physicians have shown interest in the rules induced by our algorithm.

Although our results are encouraging, several areas of research remain to be explored. As shown in Section 5.2, our system induces hypothesis regardless of the causality. We must bias the induction date period to suit the knowledge of our consulting physicians. In addition, our algorithm must be subjected to experiments with different settings. We plan to apply this algorithm to other domains of medical data and also apply it to non-medical, temporal data. Extensions to treating numerical values also must be investigated. Our current method require attributes in discrete values. We plan to investigate these points in our future work.

Acknowledgments

We are grateful to Hideto Yokoi for fruitful discussions.

References

1. Adriaans, P., & Zantinge, D. (1996). *Data Mining*. London: Addison Wesley.
2. Baxter, R., Williams, G., & He, H. (2001). Feature Selection for Temporal Health Records. *Lecture Notes in Computer Science*. 2035, 198–209.
3. Das, D., Lin, K., Mannila, H., Renganathan, G. & Smyth, P. (1998). Rule Discovery from Time Series. *In Proceedings of the Fourth International Conference on Knowledge Discovery and Data Mining* (pp. 16–22).
4. Džeroski, S. & Lavrač, N. (2001). *Relational Data Mining*. Berlin: Springer.
5. Gamberger, D., Lavrač, N., & Krstačić, G. (2003). Active subgroup mining: a case study in coronary heart disease risk group detection, *Artificial Intelligence in Medicine*, 28, 27–57.
6. Ichise, R., & Numao, M. (2001). Learning first-order rules to handle medical data. *NII Journal*, 2, 9–14.
7. Keogh, E., & Pazzani, M. (2000). Scaling up Dynamic Time Warping for Datamining Applications, *In the Proceedings of the Sixth International Conference on Knowledge Discovery and Data Mining* (pp. 285–289)
8. Kononenko, I. (2001). Machine learning for medical diagnosis: history, state of the art and perspective, *Artificial Intelligence in Medicine*, 23, 89–109.
9. Motoda, H. editor. (2002) Active mining: new directions of data mining. In: Frontiers in artificial intelligence and applications, 79. IOS Press.
10. Muggleton, S., & Firth, J. (2001). Relational rule induction with CPROGOL4.4: a tutorial introduction, *Relational Data Mining* (pp. 160–188).
11. Quinlan, J. R. (1990). Learning logical definitions from relation. *Machine Learning*, 5, 3, 239–266.

12. Rodríguez, J. J., Alonso, C. J., & Boström, H. (2000). Learning First Order Logic Time Series Classifiers: Rules and Boosting. *Proceedings of the Fourth European Conference on Principles and Practice of Knowledge Discovery in Databases* (pp. 299–308).
13. Spenke, M. (2001). Visualization and interactive analysis of blood parameters with InfoZoom. *Artificial Intelligence in Medicine*, 22, 159–172.
14. Tsumoto, S. (1999). Rule Discovery in Large Time-Series Medical Databases. *Proceedings of Principles of Data Mining and Knowledge Discovery: Third European Conference* (pp. 23–31).
15. Yamada, Y., Suzuki, E., Yokoi, H., & Takabayashi, K. (2003) Classification by Time-series Decision Tree, *Proceedings of the 17th Annual Conference of the Japanese Society for Artificial Intelligence*, in Japanese, 1F5-06.

Extracting Diagnostic Knowledge from Hepatitis Dataset by Decision Tree Graph-Based Induction

Warodom Geamsakul[1], Tetsuya Yoshida[1],
Kouzou Ohara[1], Hiroshi Motoda[1], Takashi Washio[1],
Hideto Yokoi[2], and Katsuhiko Takabayashi[2]

[1] Institute of Scientific and Industrial Research, Osaka University, Japan
{warodom, yoshida, ohara, motoda, washio}@ar.sanken.osaka-u.ac.jp
[2] Division for Medical Informatics, Chiba University Hospital, Japan
yokoi@telemed.ho.chiba-u.ac.jp takaba@ho.chiba-u.ac.jp

Abstract. We have proposed a method called Decision Tree Graph-Based Induction (DT-GBI), which constructs a classifier (decision tree) for graph-structured data while simultaneously constructing attributes for classification. Graph-Based Induction (GBI) is utilized in DT-GBI for efficiently extracting typical patterns from graph-structured data by stepwise pair expansion (pairwise chunking). Attributes, i.e., substructures useful for classification task, are constructed by GBI on the fly while constructing a decision tree in DT-GBI. We applied DT-GBI to four classification tasks of hepatitis data using only the time-series data of blood inspection and urinalysis, which was provided by Chiba University Hospital. In the first and second experiments, the stages of fibrosis were used as classes and a decision tree was constructed for discriminating patients with F4 (cirrhosis) from patients with the other stages. In the third experiment, the types of hepatitis (B and C) were used as classes, and in the fourth experiment the effectiveness of interferon therapy was used as class label. The preliminary results of experiments, both constructed decision trees and their predictive accuracies, are reported in this paper. The validity of extracted patterns is now being evaluated by the domain experts (medical doctors). Some of the patterns match experts' experience and the overall results are encouraging.

1 Introduction

Viral hepatitis is a very critical illness. If it is left without undergoing a suitable medical treatment, a patient may suffer from cirrhosis and fatal liver cancer. The progress speed of the condition is slow and subjective symptoms are not noticed easily. Hence, in many cases, it has already become very severe when subjective symptoms are noticed. Although periodic inspection and proper treatment are important in order to prevent this situation, there are problems of expensive cost and physical burden on a patient. There is an alternative much cheaper method of inspection such as blood test and urinalysis. However, the amount of data becomes enormous since the progress speed of the condition is slow.

S. Tsumoto et al. (Eds.): AM 2003, LNAI 3430, pp. 126–151, 2005.

We have proposed a method called Decision Tree Graph-Based Induction (DT-GBI), which constructs a classifier (decision tree) for graph-structured data while simultaneously constructing attributes for classification using GBI [10, 11]. A pair extracted by Graph-based Induction (GBI) [13, 4], which consists of nodes and the edges between them, is treated as an attribute and the existence/non-existence of the pair in a graph is treated as its value for the graph. Thus, attributes (pairs) that divide data effectively are extracted by GBI while a decision tree is being constructed. To classify graph-structured data after the construction of a decision tree, attributes are produced from data before the classification. We applied DT-GBI for the hepatitis data which was provided by Chiba University Hospital as a part of evidence-based medicine. In our analysis temporal records in the provided dataset was converted into graph structured data with respect to time correlation so that both intra-correlation of individual inspection at one time and inter-correlation among inspections at different time are represented in graph-structured data. The decision trees were constructed by DT-GBI to discriminate between two groups of patients without using any biopsy results but using only the time sequence data of blood inspection and urinalysis. The stages of fibrosis were used as classes in the first and second experiments and a decision tree was constructed for discriminating patients with F4 (cirrhosis) from patients with the other stages. The types of hepatitis (B and C) were used as classes in the third experiment, and the effectiveness of interferon therapy was used as class label in the fourth experiment. The results of experiments are reported and discussed in this paper.

There are some other analyses already conducted and reported on this dataset. [12] analyzed the data by constructing decision trees from time-series data without discretizing numeric values. [3] proposed a method of temporal abstraction to handle time-series data, converted time phenomena to symbols and used a standard classifier. [9] used multi-scale matching to compare time-series data and clustered them using rough set theory. [5] also clustered the time-series data of a certain time interval into several categories and used a standard classifier. These analyses examine the temporal correlation of each inspection separately and do not explicitly consider the relations among inspections. Thus, these approaches do not correspond to the structured data analysis.

Section 2 briefly describes the framework of GBI. Section 3 explains our method called DT-GBI for constructing a classifier with GBI for graph-structured data and illustrates how decision tree is constructed with a simple example. Section 4 describes the details of how we applied DT-GBI for the hepatitis dataset and reports the results of experiments, both constructed decision trees and their predictive accuracies. Section 5 concludes the paper with a summary of the results and the planned future work.

2   Graph-Based Induction (GBI)

2.1   Principle of GBI

GBI employs the idea of extracting typical patterns by stepwise pair expansion as shown in Figure 1. In the original GBI an assumption is made that typical pat-

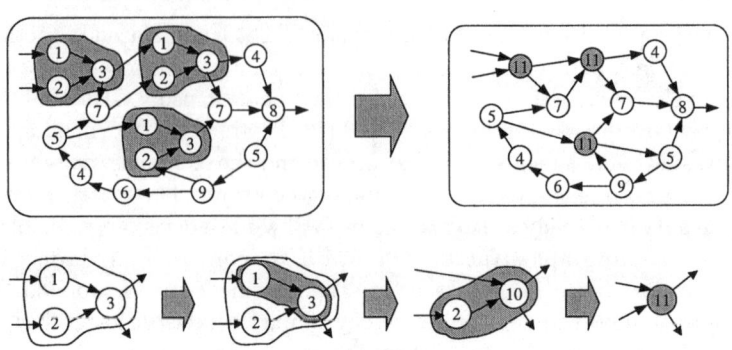

Fig. 1. The basic idea of the GBI method

GBI(G)
Enumerate all the pairs P_{all} in G
Select a subset P of pairs from P_{all} (all the pairs in G)
based on typicality criterion
Select a pair from P_{all} based on chunking criterion
Chunk the selected pair into one node c
G_c := contracted graph of G
while termination condition not reached
$P := P \cup \text{GBI}(G_c)$
return P

Fig. 2. Algorithm of GBI

terns represent some concepts/substructures and "typicality" is characterized by the pattern's frequency or the value of some evaluation function of its frequency. We can use statistical indexes as an evaluation function, such as frequency itself, Information Gain [6], Gain Ratio [7] and Gini Index [1], all of which are based on frequency. In Figure 1 the shaded pattern consisting of nodes 1, 2, and 3 is thought typical because it occurs three times in the graph. GBI first finds the 1→3 pairs based on its frequency, chunks them into a new node 10, then in the next iteration finds the 2→10 pairs, chunks them into a new node 11. The resulting node represents the shaded pattern.

It is possible to extract typical patterns of various sizes by repeating the above three steps. Note that the search is greedy. No backtracking is made. This means that in enumerating pairs no pattern which has been chunked into one node is restored to the original pattern. Because of this, all the "typical patterns" that exist in the input graph are not necessarily extracted. The problem of extracting all the isomorphic subgraphs is known to be NP-complete. Thus, GBI aims at extracting only meaningful typical patterns of a certain size. Its objective is not finding all the typical patterns nor finding all the frequent patterns.

As described earlier, GBI can use any criterion that is based on the frequency of paired nodes. However, for finding a pattern that is of interest any of its subpatterns must be of interest because of the nature of repeated chunking.

In Figure 1 the pattern 1→3 must be typical for the pattern 2→10 to be typical. Said differently, unless pattern 1→3 is chunked, there is no way of finding the pattern 2→10. The frequency measure satisfies this monotonicity. However, if the criterion chosen does not satisfy this monotonicity, repeated chunking may not find good patterns even though the best pair based on the criterion is selected at each iteration. To resolve this issue GBI was improved to use two criteria, one for frequency measure for chunking and the other for finding discriminative patterns after chunking. The latter criterion does not necessarily hold monotonicity property. Any function that is discriminative can be used, such as Information Gain [6], Gain Ratio [7] and Gini Index [1], and some others.

The improved stepwise pair expansion algorithm is summarized in Figure 2. It repeats the following four steps until the chunking threshold is reached (normally minimum support value is used as the stopping criterion).

Step 1. Extract all the pairs consisting of connected two nodes in the graph.

Step 2a. Select all the typical pairs based on the typicality criterion from among the pairs extracted in Step 1, rank them according to the criterion and register them as typical patterns. If either or both nodes of the selected pairs have already been rewritten (chunked), they are restored to the original patterns before registration.

Step 2b. Select the most frequent pair from among the pairs extracted in Step 1 and register it as the pattern to chunk. If either or both nodes of the selected pair have already been rewritten (chunked), they are restored to the original patterns before registration. Stop when there is no more pattern to chunk.

Step 3. Replace the selected pair in Step 2b with one node and assign a new label to it. Rewrite the graph by replacing all the occurrence of the selected pair with a node with the newly assigned label. Go back to Step 1.

The output of the improved GBI is a set of ranked typical patterns extracted at Step 2a. These patterns are typical in the sense that they are more discriminative than non-selected patterns in terms of the criterion used.

2.2   Beam-Wise Graph-Based Induction (B-GBI)

Since the search in GBI is greedy and no backtracking is made, which patterns are extracted by GBI depends on which pair is selected for chunking. There can be many patterns which are not extracted by GBI. A beam search is incorporated to GBI, still, within the framework of greedy search [4] in order to relax this problem, increase the search space, and extract more discriminative patterns while still keeping the computational complexity within a tolerant level. A certain fixed number of pairs ranked from the top are selected to be chunked individually in parallel. To prevent each branch growing exponentially, the total number of pairs to chunk (the beam width) is fixed at every time of chunking. Thus, at any iteration step, there is always a fixed number of chunking that is performed in parallel.

Figure 3 shows how search is conducted in B-GBI when beam width is
set to five. First, five frequent pairs are
selected from the graphs at the starting state in search (cs in Figure 3).
Graphs in cs are then copied into the
five states (c11 ~ c15), and each of five
pairs is chunked in the copied graphs
at the respective state. At the second
cycle in search, pairs in graphs are enumerated in each state and five frequent
pairs are selected from all the states.
In this example, two pairs are selected
from c11, one pair from c13, and two
pairs from c14. At the third cycle in
search, graphs in c11 are copied into
c21 and c22, graphs in c13 are copied
into c23, and graphs in c24 are copied

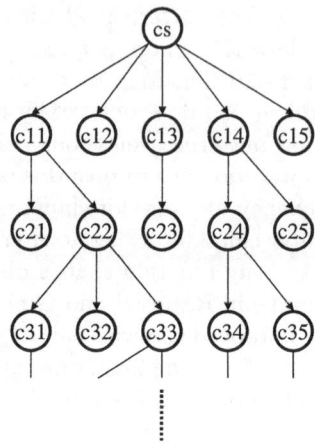

Fig. 3. Beam search in B-GBI (beam
width = 5)

into c24 and c25. As in the second cycle, the selected pairs are chunked in the
copied graphs. The states without the selected pairs (in this example c12 and
c15) are discarded.

2.3 Canonical Labelling

GBI assigns a new label for each newly chunked pair. Because it recursively
chunks pairs, it happens that the new pairs that have different labels because of
different chunking history happen to be the same pattern (subgraph).

To identify whether the two pairs represent the same pattern or not, each
pair is represented by its canonical label[8, 2] and only when the label is the
same, they are regarded as identical. The basic procedure of canonical labelling
is as follows. Nodes in the graph are grouped according to their labels (node
colors) and the degrees of node (number of links attached to the node) and
ordered lexicographically. Then an adjacency matrix is created using this node
ordering. When the graph is undirected, the adjacency matrix is symmetric, and
the upper triangular elements are concatenated scanning either horizontally or
vertically to codify the graph. When the graph is directed, the adjacency matrix
is asymmetric, and all the elements in both triangles are used to codify the graph
in a similar way. If there are more than one node that have identical node label
and identical degrees of node, the ordering which results in the maximum (or
minimum) value of the code is searched. The corresponding code is the canonical
label. Let M be the number of nodes in a graph, N be the number of groups
of the nodes, and $p_i (i = 1, 2, \ldots, N)$ be the number of the nodes within group
i. The search space can be reduced to $\prod_{i=1}^{N} (p_i!)$ from $M!$ by this grouping and
lexicographical ordering. The code of an adjacency matrix for the case in which
elements in the upper triangle are vertically concatenated is defined as

$$A = \begin{pmatrix} a_{11} \; a_{12} \; \cdots \; a_{1n} \\ \quad a_{22} \; \cdots \; a_{2n} \\ \qquad \ddots \quad \vdots \\ \qquad \qquad a_{nn} \end{pmatrix} \quad \begin{aligned} code(A) &= a_{11}a_{12}a_{22}a_{13}a_{23} \ldots a_{nn} \qquad\qquad (1) \\ &= \sum_{j=1}^{n}\sum_{i=1}^{j}\left((L+1)^{\{(\sum_{k=j+1}^{n} k)+j-i\}}a_{ij}\right). \ (2) \end{aligned}$$

Here L is the number of different link labels. It is possible to further prune the search space. We choose the option of vertical concatenation. Elements of the adjacency matrix of higher ranked nodes form higher elements (digits) of the code. Thus, once the locations of higher ranked nodes in the adjacency matrix are fixed, corresponding higher elements of the code are also fixed and are not affected by the order of elements of lower ranks. This reduces the search space of $\prod_{i=1}^{N}(p_i!)$ to $\sum_{i=1}^{N}(p_i!)$.

However, there is still a problem of combinatorial explosion for a case where there are many nodes of the same labels and the same degrees of node such as the case of chemical compounds because the value of p_i becomes large. What we can do is to make the best of already determined nodes of higher ranks. Assume that the order of the nodes $v_i \in V(G)(i = 1, 2, \ldots, N)$ is already determined in a graph G. Consider finding the order of the nodes $u_i \in V(G)(i = 1, 2, \ldots, k)$ of the same group that gives the maximum code value. The node that comes to v_{N+1} is the one in $u_i(i = 1, \ldots, k)$ that has a link to the node v_1 because the highest element that v_{N+1} can make is a_{1N+1} and the node that makes this element non-zero, that is, the node that is linked to v_1 gives the maximum code. If there are more than one node or no node at all that has a link to v_{N+1}, the one that has a link to v_2 comes to v_{N+1}. Repeating this process determines which node comes to v_{N+1}. If no node can be determined after the last comparison at v_N, permutation within the group is needed. Thus, the computational complexity in the worst case is still exponential. Our past experience indicates that computation required for canonical labeling is less than 10% of the total computation time in GBI.

3   Decision Tree Graph-Based Induction (DT-GBI)

3.1   Decision Tree for Graph-Structured Data

We formulate the construction of decision tree for graph-structured data by defining attributes and attribute-values as follows:

- attribute: a pattern/subgraph in graph-structured data
- value for an attribute: existence/non-existence of the pattern in a graph

Since the value for an attribute is yes (the classifying pattern exists) and no (the classifying pattern does not exist), the constructed decision tree is represented as a binary tree. Data (graphs) are divided into two groups, namely, the one with the pattern and the other without the pattern. The above process is summarized in Figure 4. One remaining question is how to determine classifying patterns which are used as attributes for graph-structured data. Our approach is described in the next subsection.

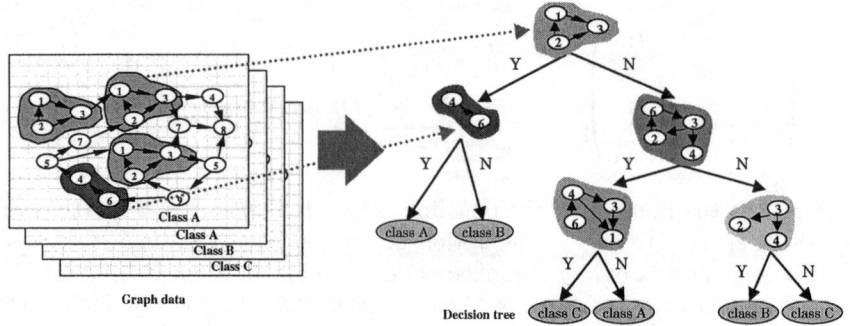

Fig. 4. Decision tree for classifying graph-structured data

DT-GBI(D)
Create a node DT for D
if termination condition reached
return DT
else
$P :=$ GBI(D) (with the number of chunking specified)
Select a pair p from P
Divide D into D_y (with p) and D_n (without p)
Chunk the pair p into one node c
$D_{yc} :=$ contracted data of D_y
for $D_i := D_{yc}, D_n$
$DT_i :=$ DT-GBI(D_i)
Augment DT by attaching DT_i as its child along yes(no) branch
return DT

Fig. 5. Algorithm of DT-GBI

3.2   Feature Construction by GBI

In our Decision Tree Graph-Based Induction (DT-GBI) method, typical patterns
are extracted using B-GBI and used as attributes for classifying graph-structured
data. When constructing a decision tree, all the pairs in data are enumerated
and one pair is selected. The data (graphs) are divided into two groups, namely,
the one with the pair and the other without the pair. The selected pair is then
chunked in the former graphs and these graphs are rewritten by replacing all
the occurrences of the selected pair with a new node. This process is recursively
applied at each node of a decision tree and a decision tree is constructed while
attributes (pairs) for classification task are created on the fly. The algorithm
of DT-GBI is summarized in Figure 5. As shown in Figure 5, the number of
chunking applied at one node is specified as a parameter. For instance, when it
is set to 10, chunking is applied for 10 times to construct a set of pairs P, which
consists of all the pairs by applying chunking $1 \sim 10$ times. Note that the pair p
selected from P is not necessarily constructed by applying chunking at depth 10.

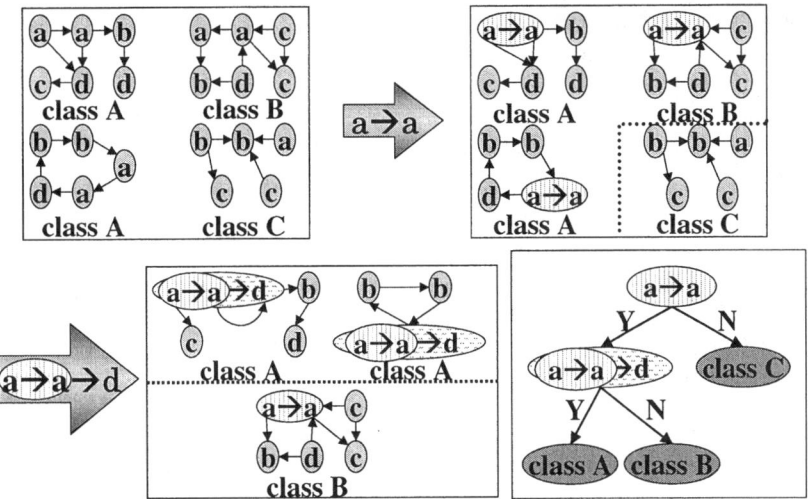

Fig. 6. Example of decision tree construction by DT-GBI

Each time when an attribute (pair) is selected to divide the data, the pair is chunked into a larger node in size. Thus, although initial pairs consist of two nodes and the edge between them, attributes useful for classification task are gradually grown up into larger pair (subgraphs) by applying chunking recursively. In this sense the proposed DT-GBI method can be conceived as a method for feature construction, since features, namely attributes (pairs) useful for classification task, are constructed during the application of DT-GBI.

Note that the criterion for chunking and the criterion for selecting a classifying pair can be different. In the following experiments, frequency is used as the evaluation function for chunking, and information gain is used as the evaluation function for selecting a classifying pair[3].

3.3 Working Example of DT-GBI

Suppose DT-GBI receives a set of 4 graphs in the upper left-hand side of Figure 6. The number of chunking applied at each node is set to 1 to simplify the working of DT-GBI in this example. By enumerating all the pairs in these graphs, 13 kinds of pair are extracted from the data. These pairs are: a→a, a→b, a→c, a→d, b→a, b→b, b→c, b→d, c→b, c→c, d→a, d→b, d→c. The existence/non-existence of the pairs in each graph is converted into the ordinary table representation of attribute-value pairs, as shown in Figure 7. For instance, for the pair a→a, graph 1, graph 2 and graph 3 have the pair but graph 4 does not have it. This is shown in the first column in Figure 7.

Next, the pair with the highest evaluation for classification (i.e., information gain) is selected and used to divide the data into two groups at the root node.

---

[3] We did not use information gain ratio because DT-GBI constructs a binary tree.

Graph	a→a	a→b	a→c	a→d	b→a	b→b	b→c	b→d	c→b	c→c	d→a	d→b	d→c
1 (class A)	1	1	0	1	0	0	0	1	0	0	0	0	1
2 (class B)	1	1	1	0	0	0	0	0	0	1	1	1	0
3 (class A)	1	0	0	1	1	1	0	0	0	0	0	1	0
4 (class C)	0	1	0	0	0	1	1	0	1	0	0	0	0

Fig. 7. Attribute-value pairs at the first step

Graph	a→a→b	a→a→c	a→a→d	b→a→a	b→a	⋯	d→c
1 (class A)	1	0	1	0	0	⋯	1
2 (class B)	1	1	0	0	0	⋯	0
3 (class A)	0	0	1	1	1	⋯	0

Fig. 8. Attribute-value pairs at the second step

In this example, the pair "a→a" is selected. The selected pair is then chunked in graph 1, graph 2 and graph 3 and these graphs are rewritten. On the other hand, graph 4 is left as it is.

The above process is applied recursively at each node to grow up the decision tree while constructing the attributes (pairs) useful for classification task at the same time. Pairs in graph 1, graph 2 and graph 3 are enumerated and the attribute-value tables are constructed as shown in Figure 8. After selecting the pair "(a→a)→d", the graphs are separated into two partitions, each of which contains graphs of a single class. The constructed decision tree is shown in the lower right-hand side of Figure 6.

3.4 Pruning Decision Tree

Recursive partitioning of data until each subset in the partition contains data of a single class often results in overfitting to the training data and thus degrades the predictive accuracy of decision trees. To avoid overfitting, in our previous approach [10] a very naive *prepruning* method was used by setting the termination condition in DT-GBI in Figure 5 to whether the number of graphs in D is equal to or less than 10. A more sophisticated *postpruning* method, is used in C4.5 [7] (which is called "pessimistic pruning") by growing an overfitted tree first and then pruning it to improve predictive accuracy based on the confidence interval for binomial distribution. To improve predictive accuracy, pessimistic pruning used in C4.5 is incorporated into the DT-GBI by adding a step for postpruning in Figure 5.

4   Data Preprocessing

The dataset contains long time-series data (from 1982 to 2001) on laboratory examination of 771 patients of hepatitis B and C. The data can be split into

MID	Date of examination	Object to examine	Name of examination	...	Result value	Unit	Judge result	Comment	...
1	19850711	1	CA19-9		8	U/ML			...
1	19870114	1	CMV.IGG(ELISA)		0.729		(2+)		...
1	19870114	1	CMV.IGM(ELISA)		0.214		(-)	サイケンズミデス	...
...	...	...	...	...	...	...	...	...	...
2	19920611	1	2-5ASカツセイ		69	PMOL/DL			...
2	19941003	1	HCV5'NCR RT-PCR		(3+)				...
2	19950911	1	HCVテイリョウ(プローブ)		6.5	MEQ/ML			...
...	...	...	...	...	...	...	...	...	...

cleansing → conversion to table
→ averaging → discretization

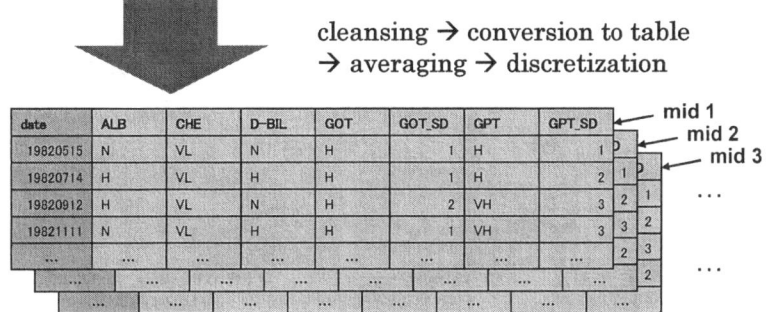

mid 1
mid 2
mid 3

date	ALB	CHE	D-BIL	GOT	GOT_SD	GPT	GPT_SD
19820515	N	VL	N	H	1	H	1
19820714	H	VL	H	H	1	H	2
19820912	H	VL	N	H	2	VH	3
19821111	N	VL	H	H	1	VH	3
...	...	...	...	...	...	...	...

Fig. 9. Averaging and discretization of inspection data

two categories. The first category includes administrative information such as patient's information (age and date of birth), pathological classification of the disease, date of biopsy and its result, and the effectiveness of interferon therapy. The second category includes temporal record of blood test and urinalysis. It contains the result of 983 types of both in- and out-hospital examinations.

4.1   Cleansing and Conversion to Table

In numeric attributes, letters and symbols such as H, L, or + are deleted. Values in nominal attributes are left as they are.

When converting the given data into an attribute-value table, both a masked patient ID (MID) and a date of inspection are used as search keys and an inspection item is defined as an attribute. Since it is not necessary that all patients must take all inspections, there are many missing values after this data conversion. No attempt is made to estimate these values and those missing values are not represented in graph-structured data in the following experiments. In future, it is necessary to consider the estimation of missing values.

Averaging and Discretization. This step is necessary due to the following two reasons: 1) obvious change in inspection across successive visits may not be found because the progress of hepatitis is slow, and 2) the date of visit is not synchronized across different patients. In this step, the numeric attributes are averaged and the most frequent value is used for nominal attributes over some interval. Further, for some inspections (GOT, GPT, TTT, and ZTT), standard deviations are calculated over six-month and added as new attributes.

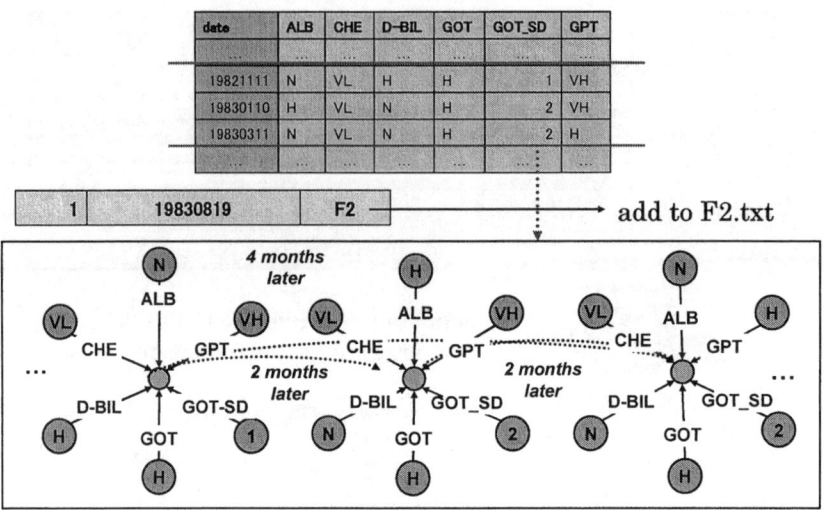

Fig. 10. An example of converted graph structured data

When we represent an inspection result as a node label, the number of node labels become too large and this lowers the efficiency of DT-GBI because frequent and discriminative patterns cannot be extracted properly. Therefore, we reduced the number of node labels by discretizing attribute values. For general numerical values, the normal ranges are specified and values are discretized into three ("L" for low, "N" for normal, and "H" for high). Based on the range, the standard deviations of GOT and GPT are discretized into five ("1" for the smallest deviation, "2", "3", "4", "5" for the largest deviation), while the standard deviations of TTT and ZTT are discretized into three ("1" for the smallest deviation, "2", "3" for the largest deviation). Figure 9 illustrates the mentioned four steps of data conversion.

Limiting Data Range. In our analysis it is assumed that each patient has one class label, which is determined at some inspection date. The longer the interval between the date when the class label is determined and the date of blood inspection is, the less reliable the correlation between them is. We consider that the pathological conditions remain the same for some duration and conduct the analysis for the data which lies in the range. Furthermore, although the original dataset contains hundreds of examinations, feature selection was conducted with the expert to reduce the number of attributes. The duration and attributes used depend on the objective of the analysis and are described in the following results.

Conversion to Graph Structured Data. When analyzing data by DT-GBI, it is necessary to convert the data to graph structure. One patient record is mapped into one directed graph. Assumption is made that there is no direct correlation between two sets of pathological tests that are more than a predefined interval (here, two years) apart. Hence, direct time correlation is considered only within this interval. Figure 10 shows an example of converted graph-structured data. In this figure, a star-shaped subgraph represents values of a set of pathological examination in a two-month interval. The center node of the subgraph is a hypothetical node for the interval. An edge pointing to a hypothetical node represents an examination. The node connected to the edge represents the value (preprocessed result) of the examination. The edge linking two hypothetical nodes represents time difference.

Class Label Setting. In the first and second experiments, we set the result (progress of fibrosis) of the first biopsy as class. In the third experiment, we set the subtype (B or C) as class. In the fourth experiment, the effectiveness of interferon therapy was used as class label.

5   Preliminary Results

5.1   Initial Settings

To apply DT-GBI, we use two criteria for selecting pairs as described before. One is frequency for selecting pairs to chunk, and the other is information gain [6] for finding discriminative patterns after chunking.

A decision tree was constructed in either of the following two ways: 1) apply chunking n_r=20 times at the root node and only once at the other nodes of a decision tree, 2) apply chunking n_e=20 times at every node of a decision tree. Decision tree pruning is conducted by postpruning: conduct pessimistic pruning by setting the confidence level to 25%.

We evaluated the prediction accuracy of decision trees constructed by DT-GBI by the average of 10 runs of 10-fold cross-validation. Thus, 100 decision trees were constructed in total. In each experiment, to determine an optimal beam width b, we first conducted 9-fold cross-validation for one randomly chosen 9 folds data (90% of all data) of the first run of the 10 runs of 10-fold cross-validation varying b from 1 to 15, and then adopted the narrowest beam width that brings to the lowest error rate.

In the following subsections, both the average error rate and examples of decision trees are shown in each experiment together with examples of extracted patterns. Two decision trees were selected out of the 100 decision trees in each experiment: one from the 10 trees constructed in the best run with the lowest error rate of the 10 runs of 10-fold cross validation, and the other from the 10 trees in the worst run with the highest error rate. In addition, the contingency tables of the selected decision trees for test data in cross validation are shown as well as the overall contingency table, which is calculated by summing up the contingency tables for the 100 decision trees in each experiment.

5.2   Classifying Patients with Fibrosis Stages

For the analysis in subsection 5.2 and subsection 5.3, the average was taken for two-month interval. As for the duration of data considered, data in the range

Table 1. Size of graphs (fibrosis stage)

stage of fibrosis	F0	F1	F2	F3	F4	Total
No. of graphs	4	125	53	37	43	262
Avg. No. of nodes	303	304	308	293	300	303
Max. No. of nodes	349	441	420	414	429	441
Min. No. of nodes	254	152	184	182	162	152

from 500 days before to 500 days after the first biopsy were extracted for the analysis of the biopsy result. When biopsy was operated for several times on the same patient, the treatment (*e.g.*, interferon therapy) after a biopsy may influence the result of blood inspection and lower the reliability of data. Thus, the date of first biopsy and the result of each patient are searched from the biopsy data file. In case that the result of the second biopsy or after differs from the result of the first one, the result from the first biopsy is defined as the class of that patient for the entire 1,000-day time-series.

Fibrosis stages are categorized into five stages: F0 (normal), F1, F2, F3, and F4 (severe = cirrhosis). We constructed decision trees which distinguish the patients at F4 stage from the patients at the other stages. In the following two experiments, we used 32 attributes. They are: ALB, CHE, D-BIL, GOT, GOT_SD, GPT, GPT_SD, HBC-AB, HBE-AB, HBE-AG, HBS-AB, HBS-AG, HCT, HCV-AB, HCV-RNA, HGB, I-BIL, ICG-15, MCH, MCHC, MCV, PLT, PT, RBC, T-BIL, T-CHO, TP, TTT, TTT_SD, WBC, ZTT, and ZTT_SD. Table 1 shows the size of graphs after the data conversion.

As shown in Table 1, the number of instances (graphs) in cirrhosis (F4) stage is 43 while the number of instances (graphs) in non-cirrhosis stages (F0 + F1 + F2 + F3) is 219. Unbalance in the number of instances may cause a biased decision tree. In order to relax this problem, we limited the number of instances to the 2:3 (cirrhosis:non-cirrhosis) ratio which is the same as in [12]. Thus, we used all instances from F4 stage for cirrhosis class (represented as LC) and select 65 instances from the other stages for non-cirrhosis class(represented as non-LC), 108 instances in all. How we selected these 108 instances is described below.

Experiment 1: F4 Stage vs {F0+F1} Stages

All 4 instances in F0 and 61 instances in F1 stage were used for non-cirrhosis class in this experiment. The beam width b was set to 15. The overall result is summarized in the left half of Table 2. The average error rate was 15.00% for n_r=20 and 12.50% for n_e=20. Figures 11 and 12 show one of the decision trees each from the best run with the lowest error rate (run 7) and from the worst run with the highest error rate (run 8) for n_e=20, respectively. Comparing these two decision trees, we notice that three patterns that appeared at the upper levels of each tree are identical. The contingency tables for these decision trees and the overall one are shown in Table 3. It is important not to diagnose non-LC patients as LC patients to prevent unnecessary treatment, but it is more important to classify LC patient correctly because F4 (cirrhosis) stage might lead to hepatoma. Table 3 reveals that although the number of misclassified instances for LC (F4)

Table 2. Average error rate (%) (fibrosis stage)

run of 10 CV	F4 vs.{F0,F1} $n_r=20$	F4 vs.{F0,F1} $n_e=20$	F4 vs.{F2,F3} $n_r=20$	F4 vs.{F2,F3} $n_e=20$
1	14.81	11.11	27.78	25.00
2	13.89	11.11	26.85	25.93
3	15.74	12.03	25.00	19.44
4	16.67	15.74	27.78	26.68
5	16.67	12.96	25.00	22.22
6	15.74	14.81	23.15	21.30
7	12.96	9.26	29.63	25.93
8	17.59	15.74	25.93	22.22
9	12.96	11.11	27.78	21.30
10	12.96	11.1	27.78	25.00
average	15.00	12.50	26.67	23.52
Standard Deviation	1.65	2.12	1.80	2.39

Table 3. Contingency table with the number of instances (F4 vs. {F0+F1})

Actual Class	Predicted Class					
	decision tree in Figure 11		decision tree in Figure 12		Overall	
	LC	non-LC	LC	non-LC	LC	non-LC
LC	3	1	4	1	364	66
non-LC	1	5	4	3	69	581

LC = F4, non-LC = {F0+F1}

and non-LC ({F0+F1}) are almost the same, the error rate for LC is larger than that for non-LC because the class distribution of LC and non-LC is unbalanced (note that the number of instances is 43 for LC and 65 for non-LC). The results are not favorable in this regards. Predicting minority class is more difficult than predicting majority class. This tendency holds for the remaining experiments. By regarding LC (F4) as positive and non-LC ({F0+F1}) as negative, decision trees constructed by DT-GBI tended to have more false negative than false positive.

Experiment 2: F4 Stage vs {F3+F2} Stages

In this experiment, we used all instances in F3 and 28 instances in F2 stage for non-cirrhosis class. The beam width b was set to 14. The overall result is summarized in the right-hand side of Table 2. The average error rate was 26.67% for $n_r=20$ and 23.52% for $n_e=20$. Figures 15 and 16 show examples of decision trees each from the best run with the lowest error rate (run 3) and the worst run with the highest error rate (run 4) for $n_e=20$, respectively. Comparing these two decision trees, we notice that two patterns that appeared at the upper levels of each tree are identical. The contingency tables for these decision trees and the overall one are shown in Table 4. Since the overall error rate in experiment 2 was larger than that of experiment 1, the number of misclassified instances

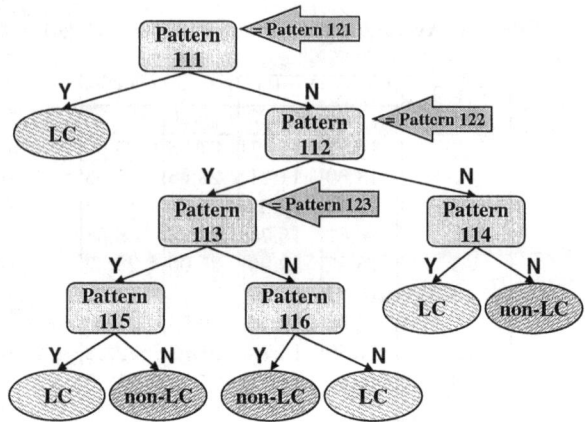

Fig. 11. One of the ten trees from the best run in exp.1 (n_e=20)

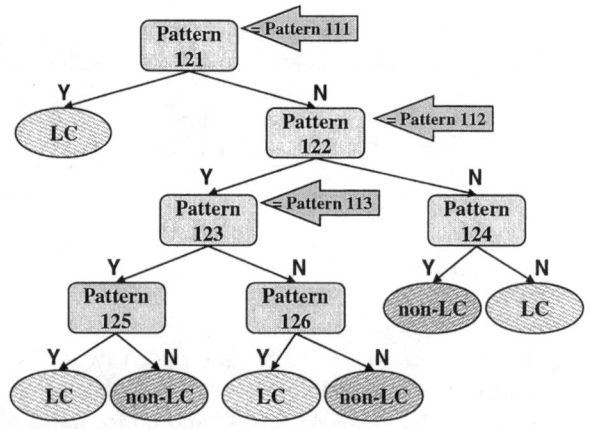

Fig. 12. One of the ten trees from the worst run in exp.1 (n_e=20)

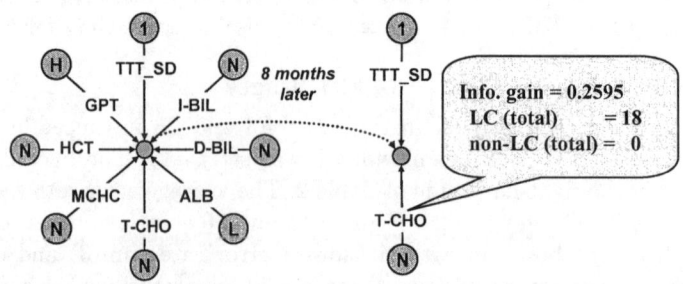

Fig. 13. Pattern 111 = Pattern 121 (if exist then LC)

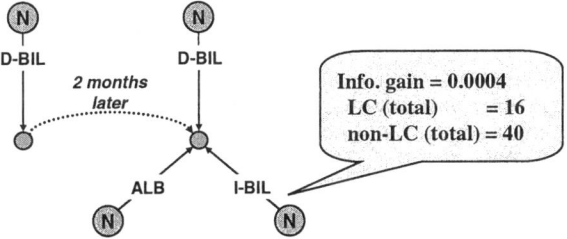

Fig. 14. Pattern 112 = Pattern 122

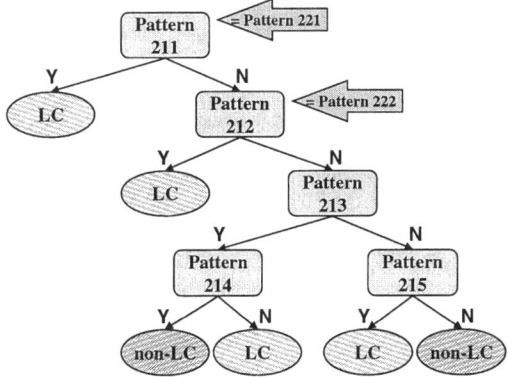

Fig. 15. One of the ten trees from the best run in exp.2 (n_e=20)

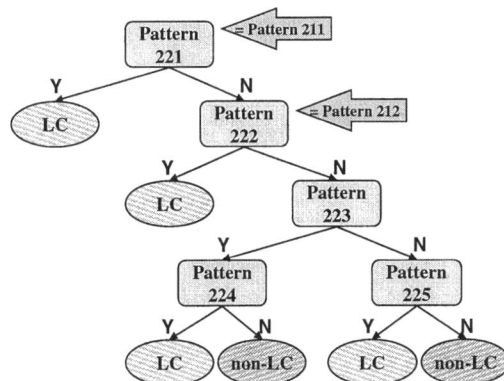

Fig. 16. One of the ten trees from the worst run in exp.2 (n_e=20)

increased. By regarding LC (F4) as positive and non-LC ({F3+F2}) as negative as described in experiment 1, decision trees constructed by DT-GBI tended to have more false negative than false positive for predicting the stage of fibrosis. This tendency was more prominent in experiment 2 than in experiment 1.

142   W. Geamsakul et al.

Table 4. Contingency table with the number of instances (F4 vs. {F3+F2})

Actual Class	Predicted Class					
	decision tree in Figure 15		decision tree in Figure 16		Overall	
	LC	non-LC	LC	non-LC	LC	non-LC
LC	3	1	2	2	282	148
non-LC	2	5	3	4	106	544

LC = F4, non-LC = {F3+F2}

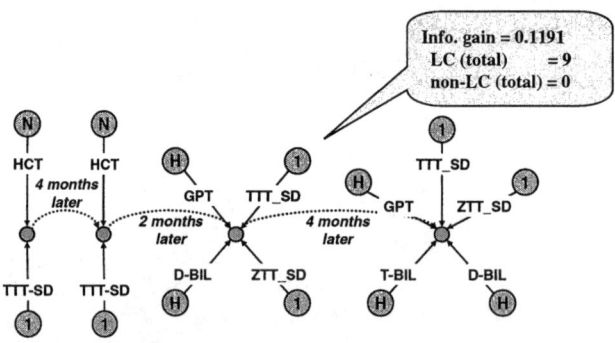

Fig. 17. Pattern 211 = Pattern 221 (if exist then LC)

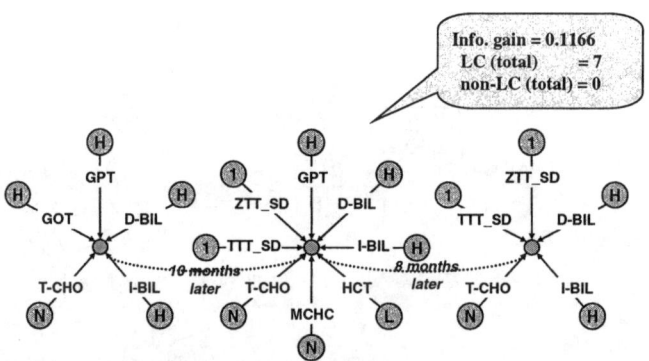

Fig. 18. Pattern 212 = Pattern 222

Discussion for the Analysis of Fibrosis Stages. The average prediction error rate in the first experiment is better than that in the second experiment, as the difference in characteristics between data in F4 stage and data in {F0+F1} stages is intuitively larger than that between data in F4 stage and data in {F3+F2}. The averaged error rate of 12.50% in experiment 1 is fairly comparable to that of 11.8% obtained by the decision tree reported in [12].

Patterns shown in Figures 13, 14, 17 and 18 are sufficiently discriminative since all of them are used at the nodes in the upper part of all decision trees.

date	ALB	D-BIL	GPT	HCT	I-BIL	MCHC	T-CHO	TTT_SD	...
19930517	L	N	H	N	N	N	N		1	...
19930716	L	L	H	N	N	N	N			...
19930914	L	L	H	N	N	N	N		1	...
19931113	L	N	H	N	N	N	N			...
19940112	L	L	H	N	N	N	N		1	...
19940313	L	N	N	N	N	N	N		1	...
19940512	L	N	H	N	N	N	N		1	...
19940711	L	N	H	N	N	N	N		1	...
19940909	L	L	H	N	N	N	N		1	...
19941108	L	N	N	N	N	N	N		1	...
19950107	L	N	N	L	N	N	N		1	...
19950308	L	N	N	N	N	N	N		1	...
19950507	L	N	H	N	N	N	N		1	...
19950706	L	N	N	L	N	N	N		1	...
19950904	L	L	N	L	N	L	N		1	...
19951103	L	L	N	N	N	N	N		1	...

Fig. 19. Data of No.203 patient

The certainty of these patterns is ensured as, for almost patients, they appear after the biopsy. These patterns include inspection items and their values that are typical of cirrhosis. These patterns may appear only once or several times in one patient. Figure 19 shows the data of a patient for whom pattern 111 exists. As we made no attempt to estimate missing values, the pattern was not counted even if the value of only one attribute is missing. At data in the Figure 19, pattern 111 would have been counted four if the value of TTT_SD in the fourth line had been "1" instead of missing.

5.3   Classifying Patients with Types (B or C)

There are two types of hepatitis recorded in the dataset; B and C. We constructed decision trees which distinguish between patients of type B and type C. As in subsection 5.2, the examination records from 500 days before to 500 days after the first biopsy were used and average was taken for two-month interval. Among the 32 attributes used in subsection 5.2, the attributes of antigen and antibody (HBC-AB, HBE-AB, HBE-AG, HBS-AB, HBS-AG, HCV-AB, HCV-RNA) were not included as they obviously indicate the type of hepatitis. Thus, we used the following 25 attributes: ALB, CHE, D-BIL, GOT, GOT_SD, GPT, GPT_SD, HCT, HGB, I-BIL, ICG-15, MCH, MCHC, MCV, PLT, PT, RBC, T-BIL, T-CHO, TP, TTT, TTT_SD, WBC, ZTT, and ZTT_SD. Table 5 shows the size of graphs after the data conversion. To keep the number of instances at 2:3 ratio [12], we used all of 77 instances in type B as "Type B" class and 116 instances in type C as "Type C" class. Hence, there are 193 instances in all. The beam width b was set to 5 in this experiment (Experiment 3).

Table 5. Size of graphs (hepatitis type)

hepatitis type	Type B	Type C	Total
No. of graphs	77	185	262
Avg. No. of nodes	238	286	272
Max. No. of nodes	375	377	377
Min. No. of nodes	150	167	150

Table 6. Average error rates (%) (hepatitis type)

run of	Type B vs. Type C	
10 CV	$n_r=20$	$n_e=20$
1	21.76	18.65
2	21.24	19.69
3	21.24	19.17
4	23.32	20.73
5	25.39	22.80
6	25.39	23.32
7	22.28	18.65
8	24.87	19.17
9	22.80	19.69
10	23.83	21.24
Average	23.21	20.31
Standard Deviation	1.53	1.57

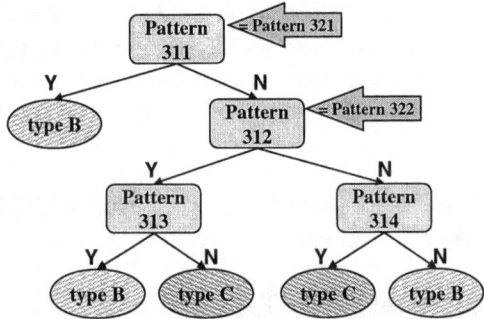

Fig. 20. One of the ten trees from the best run in exp.3 ($n_e=20$)

Table 7. Contingency table with the number of instances (hepatitis type)

		Predicted Class				
Actual	decision tree in Figure 20		decision tree in Figure 21		Overall	
Class	Type B	Type C	Type B	Type C	Type B	Type C
Type B	6	2	7	1	559	211
Type C	0	11	4	7	181	979

The overall result is summarized in Table 6. The average error rate was 23.21% for $n_r=20$ and 20.31% for $n_e=20$. Figure 20 and Figure 21 show samples of decision trees from the best run with the lowest error rate (run 1) and the worst run with the highest error rate (run 6) for $n_e = 20$, respectively. Comparing these two decision trees, two patterns (shown in Figures 22 and 23) were identical and used at the upper level nodes. There patterns also appeared at

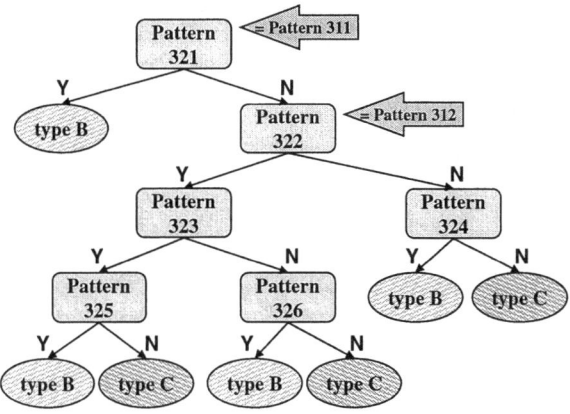

Fig. 21. One of the ten trees from the worst run in exp.3 (n_e=20)

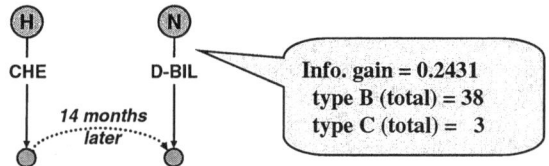

Fig. 22. Pattern 311 = Pattern 321 (if exist then Type B)

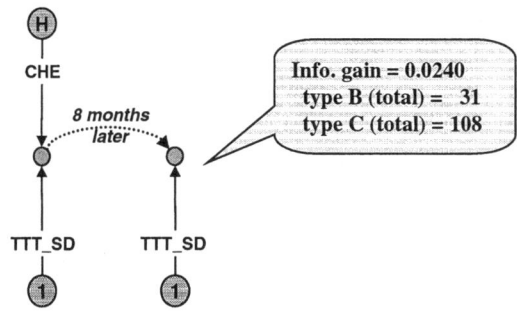

Fig. 23. Pattern 312 = Pattern 322

almost all the decision trees and thus are considered sufficiently discriminative. The contingency tables for these decision trees and the overall one are shown in Table 7. Since the hepatitis C tends to become chronic and can eventually lead to hepatoma, it is more valuable to classify the patient of type C correctly. The results are favorable in this regards because the minority class is type B in this experiment. Thus, by regarding type B as negative and type C as positive, decision trees constructed by DT-GBI tended to have more false positive than false negative for predicting the hepatitis type.

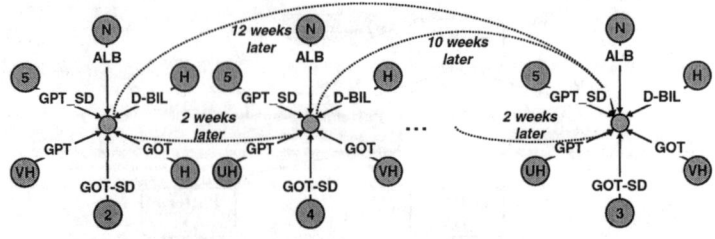

Fig. 24. An example of graph structured data for the analysis of interferon therapy

Table 8. Class label for interferon therapy

label	
R	virus disappeared (Response)
N	virus existed (Non-response)
?	no clue for virus activity
R?	R (not fully confirmed)
N?	N (not fully confirmed)
??	missing

Table 9. Size of graphs (interferon therapy)   **Table 10.** Average error rate (%) (interferon therapy)

effectiveness of interferon therapy	R	N	Total
No. of graphs	38	56	94
Avg. No. of nodes	77	74	75
Max. No. of nodes	123	121	123
Min. No. of nodes	41	33	33

run of 10 CV	$n_e=20$
1	18.75
2	23.96
3	20.83
4	20.83
5	21.88
6	22.92
7	26.04
8	23.96
9	23.96
10	22.92
Average	22.60
Standard Deviation	1.90

5.4   Classifying Interferon Therapy

An interferon is a medicine to get rid of the hepatitis virus and it is said that the smaller the amount of virus is, the more effective interferon therapy is. Unfortunately, the dataset provided by Chiba University Hospital does not contain the examination record for the amount of virus since it is expensive. However, it is believed that experts (medical doctors) decide when to administer an interferon by estimating the amount of virus from the results of other pathological exami-

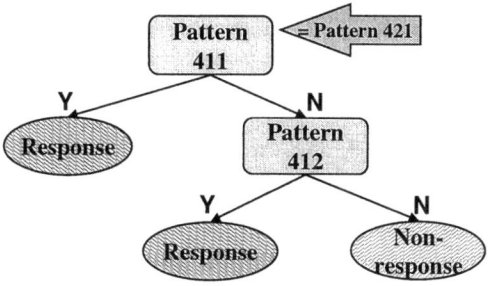

Fig. 25. One of the ten trees from the best run in exp.4

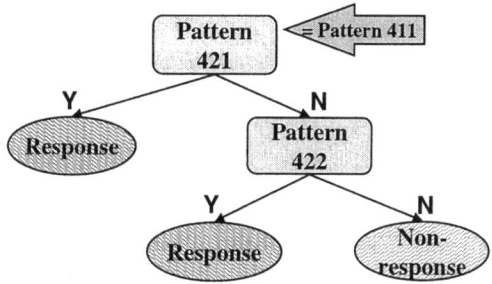

Fig. 26. One of the ten trees from the worst run in exp.4

Table 11. Contingency table with the number of instances (interferon therapy)

Actual Class	Predicted Class					
	decision tree in Figure25		decision tree in Figure26		Overall	
	R	N	R	N	R	N
R	3	1	2	2	250	130
N	0	6	4	2	83	477

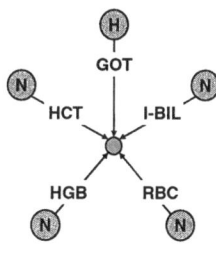

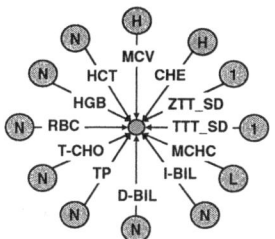

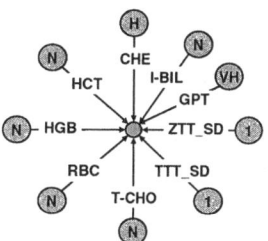

Fig. 27. Pattern 411 = Pattern 421 (if exist then R)

Fig. 28. Pattern 412 (if exist then R, if not exist then N)

Fig. 29. Pattern 422 (if exist then R, if not exist then N)

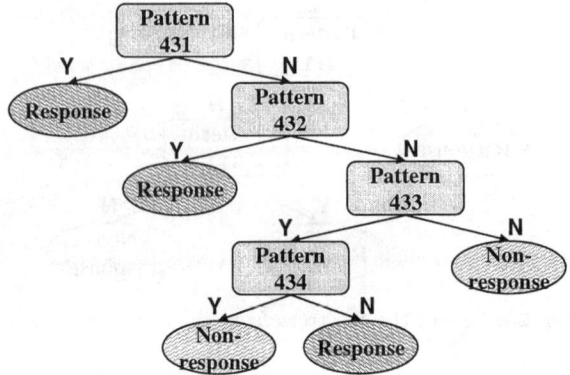

Fig. 30. Example of decision tree with time interval edge in exp.4

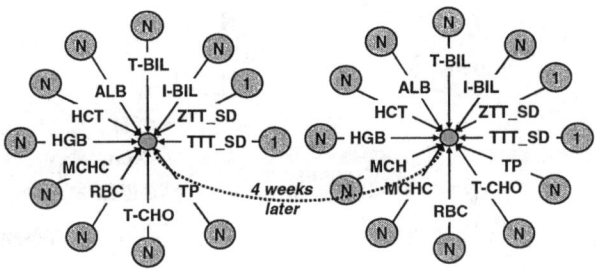

Fig. 31. Pattern 431 (if exist then R)

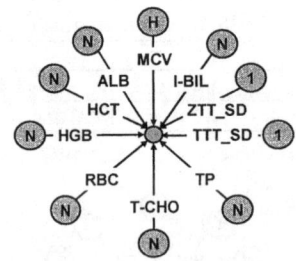

Fig. 32. Pattern 432 (if exist then R, if not exist then N)

nations. Response to interferon therapy was judged by a medical doctor for each patient, which was used as the class label for interferon therapy. The class labels specified by the doctor for interferon therapy are summarized in Table 8. Note that the following experiments (Experiment 4) were conducted for the patients with label R (38 patients) and N (56 patients). Medical records for other patients were not used.

To analyze the effectiveness of interferon therapy, we hypothesized that the amount of virus in a patient was almost stable for a certain duration just before the interferon injection in the dataset. Data in the range of 90 days to 1 day before the administration of interferon were extracted for each patient and average was taken for two-week interval. Furthermore, we hypothesized that each pathological condition in the extracted data could directly affect the pathological condition just before the administration. To represent this dependency, each subgraph was directly linked to the last subgraph in each patient. An example of converted graph-structured data is shown in Figure 24.

As in subsection 5.2 and subsection 5.3, feature selection was conducted to reduce the number of attributes. Since the objective of this analysis is to predict the effectiveness of interferon therapy without referring to the amount of virus, the attributes of antigen and antibody (HBC-AB, HBE-AB, HBE-AG, HBS-AB, HBS-AG, HCV-AB, HCV-RNA) were not included. Thus, as in subsection 5.3 we used the following 25 attributes: ALB, CHE, D-BIL, GOT, GOT_SD, GPT, GPT_SD, HCT, HGB, I-BIL, ICG-15, MCH, MCHC, MCV, PLT, PT, RBC, T-BIL, T-CHO, TP, TTT, TTT_SD, WBC, ZTT, and ZTT_SD. Table 9 shows the size of graphs after the data conversion. The beam width b was set to 3 in experiment 4.

The results are summarized in Table 10 and the overall average error rate was 22.60% (in this experiment we did not run the cases for n_r=20). Figures 25 and 26 show examples of decision trees each from the best run with the lowest error rate (run 1) and the worst run with the highest error rate (run 7) respectively. Patterns at the upper nodes in these trees are shown in Figures 27, 28 and 29. Although the structure of decision tree in Figure 25 is simple, its prediction accuracy was actually good (error rate=10%). Furthermore, since the pattern shown in Figure 27 was used at the root node of many decision trees, it is considered as sufficiently discriminative for classifying patients for whom interferon therapy was effective (with class label R).

The contingency tables for these decision trees and the overall one are shown in Table 11. By regarding the class label R (Response) as positive and the class label N (Non-response) as negative, the decision trees constructed by DT-GBI tended to have more false negative for predicting the effectiveness of interferon therapy. As in experiments 1 and 2, minority class is more difficult to predict. The patients with class label N are mostly classified correctly as "N", which will contribute to reducing the fruitless interferon therapy of patients, but some of the patients with class label R are also classified as "N", which may lead to miss the opportunity of curing patients with interferon therapy.

Unfortunately, only a few patterns contain time interval edges in the constructed decision trees, so we were unable to investigate how the change or stability of blood test will affect the effectiveness of interferon therapy. Figure 30 is an example of decision tree with time interval edges for the analysis of interferon therapy and some patterns in this tree are shown in Figures 31 and 32.

6   Conclusion

This paper has proposed a method called DT-GBI, which constructs a classifier (decision tree) for graph-structured data by GBI. Substructures useful for classification task are constructed on the fly by applying repeated chunking in GBI during the construction process of a decision tree. A beam search is very effective in increasing the predictive accuracy.

DT-GBI was applied to analyze a real-world hepatitis dataset which was provided by Chiba University Hospital as a part of evidence-based medicine. Four experiments were conducted on the hepatitis dataset and both constructed decision trees and their predictive accuracies were reported. DT-GBI was able to extract discriminative patterns that reflect both intra-correlation of individual inspection and inter-correlation among inspections at different time points and use them as attributes for classification. Some of the extracted patterns match medical experts' experience. The obtained prediction error rate results are thought satisfactory considering the various kinds of noises embedded in the data. We thus believe that DT-GBI is a useful tool for practicing evidence-based medicine.

General finding is that the decision trees constructed by DT-GBI tended to misclassify more instances with minority class than with the majority class. Incorporating cost-sensitive learning might be effective to take into account the imbalance in class distribution and different penalties for misclassification error.

Immediate future work includes to incorporate more sophisticated method for determining the number of cycles to call GBI at each node to improve prediction accuracy. Utilizing the rate of change of information gain by successive chunking is a possible way to automatically determine the number. Effectiveness of DT-GBI against the hepatitis data set with another way of preparing data should be examined, *e.g.*, estimating missing values, randomly selecting instances from non-cirrhosis class both for training and testing, etc. The validity of extracted patterns is now being evaluated and discussed by the domain experts (medical doctors).

Acknowledgment

This work was partially supported by the grant-in-aid for scientific research 1) on priority area "Realization of Active Mining in the Era of Information Flood" (No. 13131101, No. 13131206) and 2) No. 14780280 funded by the Japanese Ministry of Education, Culture, Sport, Science and Technology.

References

1. L. Breiman, J. H. Friedman, R. A. Olshen, and C. J. Stone. *Classification and Regression Trees.* Wadsworth & Brooks/Cole Advanced Books & Software, 1984.
2. S. Fortin. The graph isomorphism problem, 1996.
3. T. B. Ho, T. D. Nguyen, S. Kawasaki, S.Q. Le, D. D. Nguyen, H. Yokoi, and K. Takabayashi. Mining hepatitis data with temporal abstraction. In *Proc. of the 9th ACM SIGKDD International Conference on Knowledge Discovery and Data Mining*, pages 369–377, August 2003.

4. T. Matsuda, T. Yoshida, H. Motoda, and T. Washio. Knowledge discovery from structured data by beam-wise graph-based induction. In *Proc. of the 7th Pacific Rim International Confernce on Artificial Intelligence (Springer Verlag LNAI2417)*, pages 255–264, 2002.
5. M. Ohsaki, Y. Sato, H. Yokoi, and T. Yamaguchi. A rule discovery support system for sequential medical data - in the case study of a chronic hepatitis dataset -. In *Working note of International Workshop on Active Mining (AM2002)*, pages 97–102, 2002.
6. J. R. Quinlan. Induction of decision trees. *Machine Learning*, 1:81–106, 1986.
7. J. R. Quinlan. *C4.5:Programs For Machine Learning*. Morgan Kaufmann Publishers, 1993.
8. R. C. Read and D. G. Corneil. The graph isomorphism disease. *Journal of Graph Theory*, 1:339–363, 1977.
9. S. Tsumoto, K. Takabayashi, M. Nagira, and S. Hirano. Trend-evaluation multiscale analysis of the hepatitis dataset. In *Project "Realization of Active Mining in the Era of Information Flood" Report*, pages 191–197, March 2003.
10. G. Warodom, T. Matsuda, T. Yoshida, H. Motoda, and T. Washio. Classifier construction by graph-based induction for graph-structured data. In *Proc. of the 7th Pacific-Asia Conference on Knowledge Discovery and Data Mining (Springer Verlag LNAI2637)*, pages 52–62, 2003.
11. G. Warodom, T. Matsuda, T. Yoshida, H. Motoda, and T. Washio. Performance evaluation of decision tree graph-based induction. In *Proc. of the 6th Pacific-Asia Conference on Discovery Science (Springer Verlag LNAI2843)*, pages 128–140, 2003.
12. Y. Yamada, E. Suzuki, H. Yokoi, and K. Takabayashi. Decision-tree induction from time-series data based on a standard-example split test. In *Proc. of the 12th International Conference on Machine Learning*, pages 840–847, August 2003.
13. K. Yoshida and H. Motoda. Clip : Concept learning from inference pattern. *Journal of Artificial Intelligence*, 75(1):63–92, 1995.

Data Mining Oriented CRM Systems Based on MUSASHI: C-MUSASHI*

Katsutoshi Yada[1], Yukinobu Hamuro[2], Naoki Katoh[3], Takashi Washio[4],
Issey Fusamoto[1], Daisuke Fujishima[1], and Takaya Ikeda[1]

[1] Faculty of Commerce, Kansai University,
3-3-35, Yamate, Suita, Osaka 564-8680, Japan
{yada, da00587, da00591, da00039}@kansai-u.ac.jp
http://www2.ipcku.kansai-u.ac.jp/~yada/
[2] Department of Business administration, Osaka Sangyo University,
3-1-1 Nakagaito, Daito, Osaka, 567-8530 Japan
hamuro@adm.osaka-sandai.ac.jp
[3] Graduate School of Engineering, Kyoto University,
Kyoto University Katsura, Nishikyo-ku, Kyoto, 615-8540 Japan
naoki@archi.kyoto-u.ac.jp
[4] Institute for the Scientific and Industrial Research, Osaka University
8-1 Mihogaoka, Ibaraki, Osaka, 567-0047 Japan
washio@sanken.osaka-u.ac.jp

Abstract. MUSASHI is a set of commands which enables us to efficiently execute various types of data manipulations in a flexible manner, mainly aiming at data processing of huge amount of data required for data mining. Data format which MUSASHI can deal with is either an XML table written in XML or plain text file with table structure. In this paper we shall present a business application system of MUSASHI, called C-MUSASHI, dedicated to CRM oriented systems. Integrating a large amount of customer purchase histories in XML databases with the marketing tools and data mining technology based on MUSASHI, C-MUSASHI offers various basic tools for customer analysis and store management based on which data mining oriented CRM systems can be developed at extremely low cost. We apply C-MUSASHI to supermarkets and drugstores in Japan to discover useful knowledge for their marketing strategy and present possibility to construct useful CRM systems at extremely low cost by introducing MUSASHI.

1 Introduction

MUSASHI is an open-source software that provides a set of commands with which various types of data manipulations for a large amount of data mainly required for data mining in business field can be executed in an flexible manner

---

* Research of this paper is partly supported by the Grant-in-Aid for Scientific Research on Priority Areas (2) by the Ministry of Education, Science, Sports and Culture of Japan and the Kansai University Special Research fund, 2002.

S. Tsumoto et al. (Eds.): AM 2003, LNAI 3430, pp. 152–173, 2005.

[11][3][4][5]. We have developed a data mining oriented CRM system that runs on MUSASHI by integrating several marketing tools and data mining technology. Discussing the cases regarding simple customer management in Japanese supermarkets and drugstores, we shall describe general outlines, components, and analytical tools for CRM system which we have developed.

With the progress of deflation in recent Japanese economy, retailers in Japan are now under competitive environment and severe pressure. Many of these enterprises are now trying to encompass and maintain their loyal customers through the introduction of FSP (Frequent Shoppers Program) [6][14]. FSP is defined as one of the CRM systems to accomplish effective sales promotion by accumulating purchase history of the customers with membership cards in its own database and by recognizing the nature and the behavior of the loyal customers. However, it is very rare that CRM system such as FSP has actually contributed to successful business activities of the enterprises in recent years.

There are several reasons why the existing CRM system cannot contribute to the acquisition of customers and to the attainment of competitive advantage in the business. First of all, the cost to construct CRM system is very high. In fact, some of the enterprises have actually spent a large amount of money merely for the construction of data warehouse to accumulate purchase history data of the customers and, as a result, no budget is left for carrying out customer analysis. Secondly, it happens very often that although data are actually accumulated, techniques, software and human resources in their firms to analyze these data are in shortage, and thus the analysis of the customers is not in progress. Therefore, in many cases, enterprises are simply accumulat-ing the data but do not carry out the analysis of the customers.

In this paper, we shall introduce a CRM system, named C-MUSASHI, which can be constructed at very low cost by the use of the open-source software MUSASHI, and thus can be adopted freely even by a small enterprise. C-MUSASHI consists of three components, basic tools for customer analysis, store management systems and data mining oriented CRM systems. These components have been developed through joint research activities with various types of enterprises. With C-MUSASHI, it is possible to carry out the analysis of the customers without investing a large amount of budget for building up a new analytical system. In this paper we will explain the components of C-MUSASHI and cases where C-MUSASHI is applied to a large amount of customer history data of supermarkets and drugstores in Japan to discover useful knowledge for marketing strategy.

2   C-MUSASHI in Retailers

2.1   MUSASHI and Operation Systems

MUSASHI, the Mining Utilities and System Architecture for Scalable processing of Historical data, is a data mining platform [3][5] that efficiently and flexibly processes large-scale data that has been described in XML data. One of its remarkable advantages lies in the powerful and flexible ability to preprocess various amounts of raw data in the knowledge discovery process. The development of MUSASHI has been progressed as an open source software, and thus everybody can download it freely from [11].

MUSASHI has a set of small data processing commands designed for retrieving and processing large datasets efficiently for various purposes such as data extraction, cleaning, reporting and data mining. Such data processing can be executed simply by running MUSASHI commands as a shell script. These commands also includes various data mining commands such as sequential mining, association rule, decision tree, graph mining and clustering commands.

MUSASHI uses XML as a data structure to integrate multiple databases, by which various types of data can be represented. MUSASHI makes it feasible to carry out the flexible and low-cost integration of the structured and vast business data in companies.

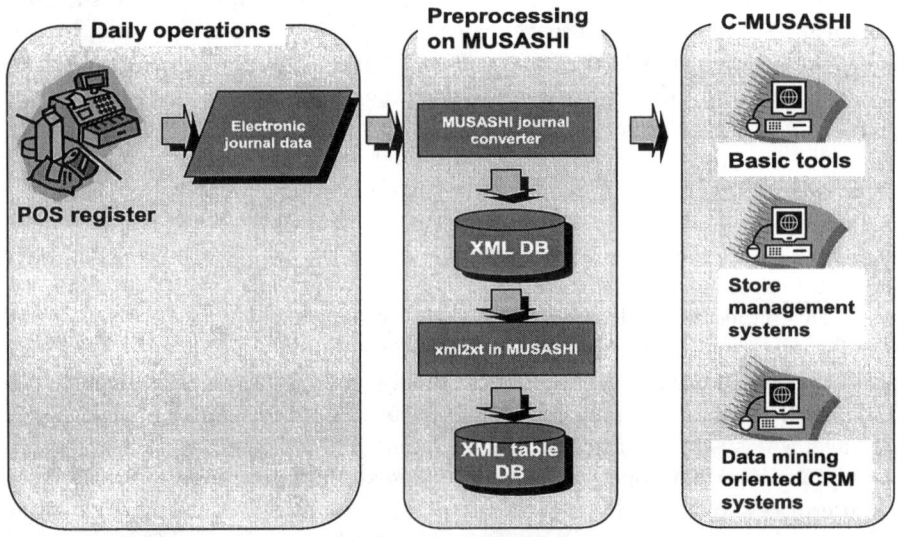

Fig. 1. C-MUSASHI system in the retailers

C-MUSASHI is a CRM system that runs on MUSASHI, by which it is possible to process the purchase history of a large number of customers and to analyze consumer behavior in detail for an efficient and effective customer control. Figure 1 shows the positioning of C-MUSASHI in a system for daily operation of the retailers. By using C-MUSASHI, everybody can build up a CRM system through the processes given below without introducing commercial data warehouse. POS (point of sales) registers used in recent years output the data called electronic journal, in which all operation logs are recorded. Store controller collects the electronic journals from the registers in the stores and accumulates them. The electronic journal data is then converted by "MUSASHI journal converter" to

XML data with minimal data loss. Figure 2 shows a sample of XML data that is converted from electronic journal data output. It is clear that operations in detail on POS cash registers are accumulated as XML data structure.

```
<?xml version="1.00" encoding="euc-jp"?>
<date="20011206" time=101545>
  <receipt="198765">
    <items>
      <JAN>4901984625422</JAN>
      <name>bread</name>
      <vol>1</vol>
      <unit>109 </unit>
    </items>
    <card>
      <customer>2101205787635 </customer>
      <name>Kandai Taro</name>
      <address>Osaka Susita 3-3-35</address>
    </customer>
    <items>
      <JAN>3053289502011</JAN>
      <name>milk</name>
      <vol>2</vol>
      <unit>149 </unit>
    </items>
    <accounts>
      <total>407</total>
      <deposit>1000</deposit>
      <balance>593</balance>
  </receipt>
```

Fig. 2. XML data that is converted from electronic journal data

However, if all operation logs at POS registers are accumulated on XML data, the amount of data may become enormous which in turn leads to the decrease of the processing speed. In this respect, we define a table-type data structure called XML table (see Figure 3). It is easy for users to transform XML data into XML table data by using "xml2xt" command in MUSASHI. The XML table is an XML document such that the root element named <xmltbl> has two elements, <header> and <body>. The table data is described in the body element using a very simple text format with one record on each line, and each field within that record separated by a comma. Names and positional information relating to each of the fields are described in the <field> element. Therefore it is possible to access data via field names. The data title and comments are displayed in their respective <title> and <comment> fields. A system is built up by combining XML data such as operation logs with XML data and XML table data. Thus, by properly using pure XML and XML table depending on the purposes, it is to construct an efficient system with high degree of freedom.

```
<?xml version="1.0" encoding="euc-jp"?>
<xmltbl version="1.1">
<header>
<title>Sales Transactions</title>
<field no="1" name="customer"/>
<field no="2" name="date"/>
<field no="3" name="JAN"/>
<field no="4" name="vol"/>
</header>
<body><![CDATA[
2101205787635 20011206 4901984625422 1
2101205787635 20011206 3053289502011 2
]]></body>
</xmltbl>
```

Fig. 3. Sales data which has been converted into an XML table

2.2   Components of C-MUSASHI

C-MUSASHI is a business application for customer relationship management and is composed of three components, basic tools for customer analysis, store management systems and data mining oriented CRM systems. The first provides basic information necessary for the implementation of store management and customer management.

The second is a store management system based on the methodology "Store Portfolio Management (SPM)" which is newly proposed in this paper aiming to support the   headquarter of chain store for controlling many stores. By using this system, it is possible to implement the appropriate strategy depending on the circumstance of each store. The third is a data mining oriented CRM system which discovers useful knowledge from customer purchase history data for the effective customer relationship management by using data mining techniques. It includes many data mining algorithms we developed to extract meaningful rules from a large amount of customer purchase history data. No other existing CRM system has the same functions and advanced data mining algorithms for customer relationship management. We will introduce these components in the subsequent sections.

3   Basic Tools for Customer Analysis

In this section, we shall introduce the tools for basic customer analysis in C-MUSASHI. Such tools are usually incorporated in existing CRM systems. Here we will explain some of such tools: decile analysis, RFM analysis, customer attrition analysis, and LTV (life time value) measurement. C-MUSASHI also has many other tools for customer analysis. We will present here only a part of them here.

3.1   Decile Analysis

In decile analysis, based on the ranking of the customers derived from the amount of purchase, customers are divided into ten groups of equal size, and then basic indices such as average amount of purchase, number of visits to the store, etc. are computed for each group [6][14]. From this report, it can be understood that all customers do not have an equal value for the store, but only a small fraction of the customers contribute to most of the profit in the store.

3.2   RFM Analysis

RFM analysis [14][8] is one of the tools most frequently used in the application purpose such as direct-mail marketing. The customers are classified according to three factors, i.e. recency of the last date of purchase, frequency of purchase, and monetary factor (purchase amount). Based on this classification, adequate sales promotion is executed for each customer group. For instance, in a supermarket, if a customer had the highest purchase frequency and the highest purchase amount, and did not visit to the store within one month, sufficient efforts must be made to bring back this customer from the stores of the competitors.

3.3   Customer Attrition Analysis

This analysis indicates which fraction of customers in a certain customer group would continuously visit the store in the next period (e.g. one month later) [8]. In other words, this is an analysis to predict how many customers will go away to the other stores. These output are also used for the calculation of LTV as described below.

3.4   LTV (Life Time Value)

LTV is a net present value of the profit which an average customer in a certain customer group brings to a store (an enterprise) within a given period [8][1]. It is calculated from the data such as sales amount of the customer group, customer maintaining rate, and discount rate such as the rate of interest on a national bond. Long-term customer strategy should be set up based on LTV, and it is an important factor relating to CRM system. However, the component for calculation of LTV prepared in C-MUSASHI is currently very simple and it must be customized depending on enterprises to use it.

These four tools are minimally required as well as very important for CRM in business field. It is possible to set up various types of marketing strategies based on the results of analysis. However, they are general and conventional, and then do not necessarily bring new knowledge to support differentiation strategy of the enterprise.

4   Store Management Systems Based on SPM

Store management systems in C-MUSASHI are to support for strategic planning of chain stores based on Store Portfolio Management (SPM) we proposed. SPM is the strategic store management methods based on Product Portfolio Management in strategic management theory in order to support for planning chain store strategy from the viewpoints of an overall firm to provide significant information of stores such as store ' s profitability and effectiveness of store sales promotion.

4.1   Product Portfolio Management in Strategic Management

Product Portfolio Management (PPM) is the strategic method for optimal allocation of management resources among multiple SBU (Strategic Business Units) in an enterprise to understand demand and supply of cash flow in each SBU [7]. It is not easy to completely understand demand and supply of cash flow in each SBU because of the multiplicity and the diversity of the circumstances of SBU. So "Growth-Share Matrix" has been employed in PPM in order to recognize clusters of SBU which exhibit the similar tendency of cash flow (See Figure 4). The growth-share matrix has two dimensions; the one is the growth dimension which is ratio of market growth in which each SBU belongs to, and the other is the share dimension which is relative market share of SBU to the rival company. These two dimensions come from the product lifecycle theory and the experience curve theory. Product lifecycle theory is to explain the dynamics of a product market by comparing a product to a living creature, and to propose that the growth process of product market is composed of four stages; introduction, growth, maturity and decline. In PPM the ratio of market growth in these four stages are associated with demand and supply of cash flow in each SBU. In the stage of introduction, the rate of market growth is high and the growth increases demand of cash flow to expand overall market and to penetrate their products into the market, while the market growth rate is low in stages of maturity and decline which decreases demand of cash flow. Based on the market growth dimension, it is possible to relatively evaluate which SBU demands cash flow in their enterprises.

Experience curve has been known as the linear relationship between the costs of production and the cumulative production quantity, which was first observed by a management consultant at the Boston Consulting Group in 1960s. It appears that the real value-added production cost decline by 20 to 30 percent for each doubling of cumulative production quantity. If a firm could acquire more experience of production by increasing its market share, it could achieve a cost advantage in its market (industry). Therefore high relative market share to a rival company which emerges a cost advantage is associated with capability of SBU to supply cash flow.

Four cells of the Growth-Share Matrix in Figure 4 are named such as "stars" "cash cows," "question marks" and "dogs". SBU in stars which has high market share and high growth rate, not only generates large amounts of cash, but also

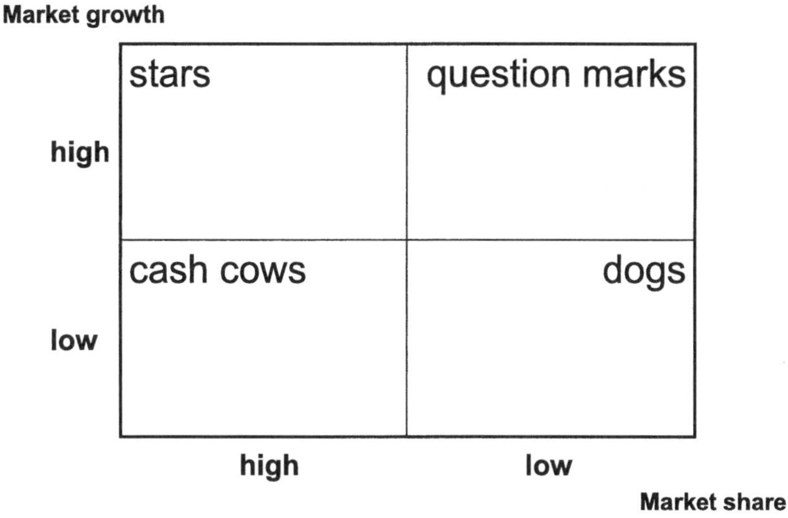

Market growth

stars	question marks
high	
cash cows	dogs
low	

high   **low**

Market share

Fig. 4. The Growth-Share Matrix in PPM

consume large amounts of cash because of high growth market. "Cash cows" with high market share and low growth of market, exhibit the excess cash. "Question marks" which have low market share and high market growth consume large amounts of cash in order to gain market share and to become stars. "Dogs" with low market share and slow growth neither generate nor consume a large amount of cash. In PPM the strategy of each SBU is determined by whether its market share is high or low, and its ratio of market growth is high or not.

4.2 Store Portfolio Management for Chain Store Management

Based on the idea of the above PPM, we propose Store Portfolio Management (SPM) which is a methodology to support for strategic planning of chain stores management. The SPM provides useful information of each store such as store's profitability and effectiveness of store sales promotion from the viewpoints of the headquarter of an overall chain store. It is impossible to completely understand each situation of many stores and, even if it is possible, it is impossible to implement different marketing strategy corresponding to each store. The purpose of SPM is to plan different marketing strategy of each store cluster which has faced with the similar situation and markets. Here we the situations and markets of stores are measured by using various di-mensions.

Various kinds of evaluation dimensions can be employed in SPM such as profitability, sales amount, the number of visiting customers and an average of sales amount per customer (See Table 1). Users can select appropriate dimensions corresponding to their situations and industry. In SPM each evaluation criterion has been associated with each marketing strategy. For example, if a store is

Table 1. List of store's evaluation dimensions which can be used in SPM

Name of dimension	Function
Profitability	The ratio of profit to sales amount of a store
Sales amount	Sales amount per store and month
# of customers	The number of visiting customer in a month
Sales / a customer	An average of sales amount per customer in a month
Effectiveness of sales promotion	The ratio of waste sales promotion to all sales promotion of the store in a month

recognized as low profitability store, an appropriate pricing strategy has to be implemented to improve the profitability.

4.3   Store Evaluation

It is difficult for the marketing stuff of a chain store to categorize their stores into a number of clusters by using all the above dimensions because of low interpretability of the resulting clusters. According to our experience, it seems to be appropriate way to use two or three dimensions to clustering stores into some meaningful groups.

Store Evaluation by Using Two-dimensional Matrix. Figure 5 shows a typical case of store clusters by using two dimensions; profitability and sales amount. All stores have been classified into one of four clusters in comparison with an average of overall chain stores in Figure 5. Cluster A is "star store" cluster with high profitability and high sales amount. Stores in cluster B classified as "cash cows" exhibit high profitability and low sales amount. Stores in B have to increase market share in the local area by using more sales promotion strategies. Stores in cluster C classified as "Question marks" have low profitability and high sales amount and thus have to improve profitability. Cluster D is "dog store" with low profitability and sales amount. Marketing stuff of chain store has to consider whether these stores of D are to be scrapped or rebuilt under new store concept depending on the environment.

Figure 6 shows an example of store cluster of a drugstore chain in Japan by using above Profitability-Sales amount matrix. In this drugstore chain the number of stores classified into cluster A is small and the number of stores in cluster C or D is relatively large because this chain decreases competitiveness in each local area.

Store management system based on SPM which we developed has modules for analyzing the classified clusters in more details. Users can get useful information for the effective marketing strategy by using these modules. In fact, for this

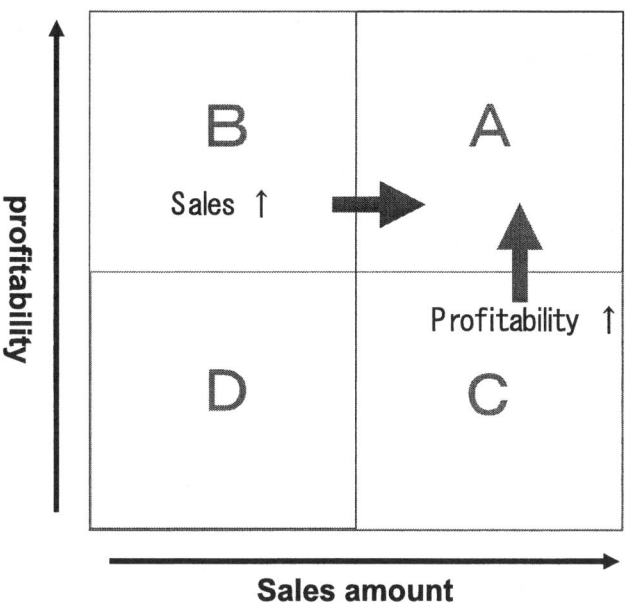

Fig. 5. A sample of store clusters by using Profitability-Sales amount matrix

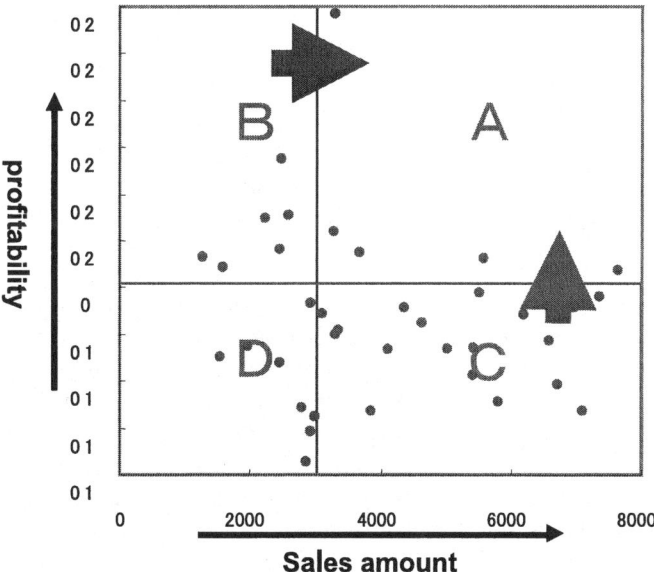

Fig. 6. An example of store clusters in a drugstore chain in Japan

drugstore chain, we found that the reason of the low profitability in these drug-stores is ineffectiveness of sales promotion in each store. We then determined which product categories have to be improved for the effectiveness of sales pro-motion.One of the modules caluculates the number of days for each product category that the sales amount when sold at a discounted price is less than the average sales amount at regular price. Such promotion sales is called "waste sales promotion". Figure 7 shows the results obtained for three stores S_1, S_2, S_3. It is observed from the figure that the number of waste sales promotions in store A's soap category (See figure 7) is larger than that of other shops and the number of waste sales promotions in mouth care category of store B is large. The marketing stuff in the headquarters of drugstore can plan different sales strategy for each store to focus on the specific categories depending on these data.

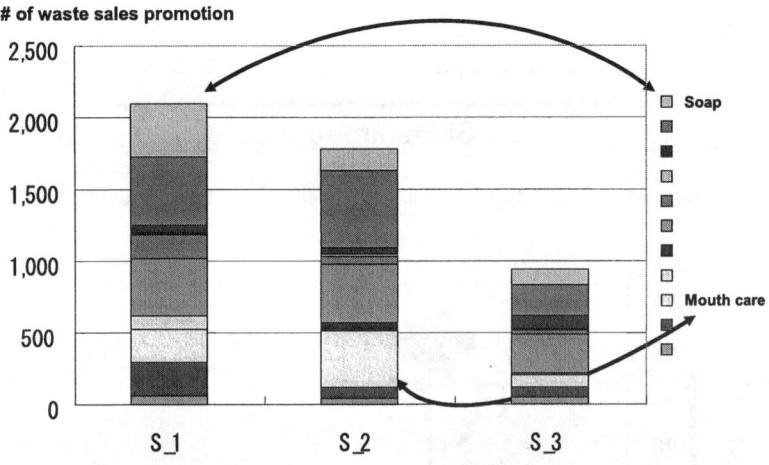

Fig. 7. The number of products with waste sales promotions of each store

Store Evaluation by Using Three-Dimensional Diagrams. Users can use more evaluation dimensions for analyzing situations of each store in detail. Figure 8 shows store evaluation by using threedimensions; profitability, an average of sales amount per customer and the number of visiting customers. It is observed in store S_1 that the number of visiting customers is large, but sales amount per customer and profitability is lower than other stores. We can guess that ratio of bargain hunters who purchase only discounted goods is high. In store S_2 the number of customers is small, but an average of sales amount per customer is very high compared to other stores. Store S_2 maybe has small number of loyal customer who contributes to almost profit of a store and acquire no sufficient newcomers from rival stores.

We can plan effective and appropriate store management strategy for each store clusters to understand each situation of stores by using the store manage-

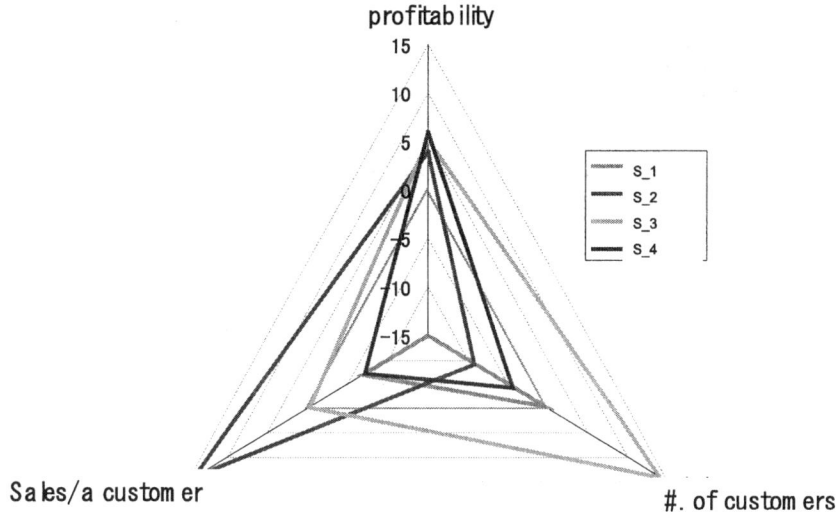

Fig. 8. Store evaluation by using three dimension diagrams

ment systems. Currently these store management systems can deal with the data of less than 100 stores and be applied to supermarket and drugstore chain.

5 Data Mining Oriented CRM Systems

In this section data mining oriented CRM system will be presented, which discovers new knowledge useful for implementing effective CRM strategy from the purchase data of the customers. General CRM systems commercially available simply comprise the functions of retrieval and aggregation as basic tools of C-MUSASHI, and there are very few CRM systems in which an analytical system that can deal with large-scale data equipped with data mining engine is available. In this section, we explain our system that can discover useful customer knowledge by integrating the data mining technique with CRM system.

5.1 Systems Structure and Four Modules of Data Mining Oriented CRM Systems

Figure 9 shows a structure of data mining oriented CRM system in C-MUSASHI. Customer purchase history data accumulated as XML table is preprocesses by a core system of MUSASHI. The preprocessed data is then provided as retail support information in two different ways.

In the first approach, the data preprocessed at the core of MUSASHI is received through WEB server. Then, the data is analyzed and provided to the

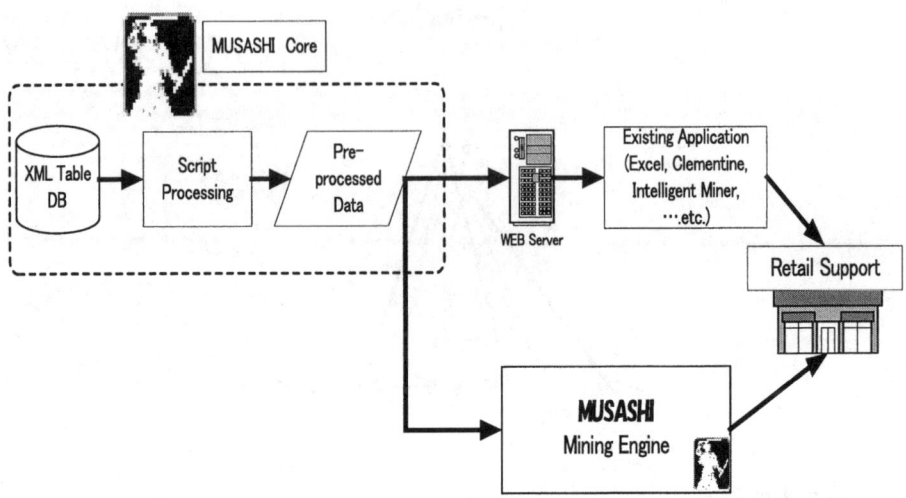

Fig. 9. Configuration of data mining oriented CRM systems

retail stores by using existing application software such as spread-sheet or data mining tools. In this case, C-MUSASHI is only in charge of preprocessing of a large amount of data.

In the second approach, the data is directly received from the core system of MUSASHI. Rules are extracted by the use of data mining engine in MUSASHI, and useful knowledge is obtained from them. In this case, C-MUSASHI carries out a series of processing to derive prediction model and useful knowledge. Whether one of these approaches or both should be adopted by the enterprise should be determined according to the existing analytical environment and daily business activities.

CRM system in C-MUSASHI which integrates the data mining technique consists of four modules corresponding to the life cycle of the customers [1][12][13]. Just as each product has its own life cycle, each customer has life cycle as a growth model. Figure 10 shows the time series change of the amount of money used by a typical customer. Just like the life cycle of the product, it appears that the customer life cycle has the stages of introduction, growth, maturation, and decline.

It is not that all customers should be treated on equal basis. Among the customers, there are bargain hunters who purchase only the commodities at the discounted price and also the loyal customers who make great contribution to the profit of the store. In the first stage, it is important to find the customers who will become loyal from among the new customers for effective sales promotion. So we developed an early discovery module to detect such customers in order to attract the customers who may bring higher profitability.

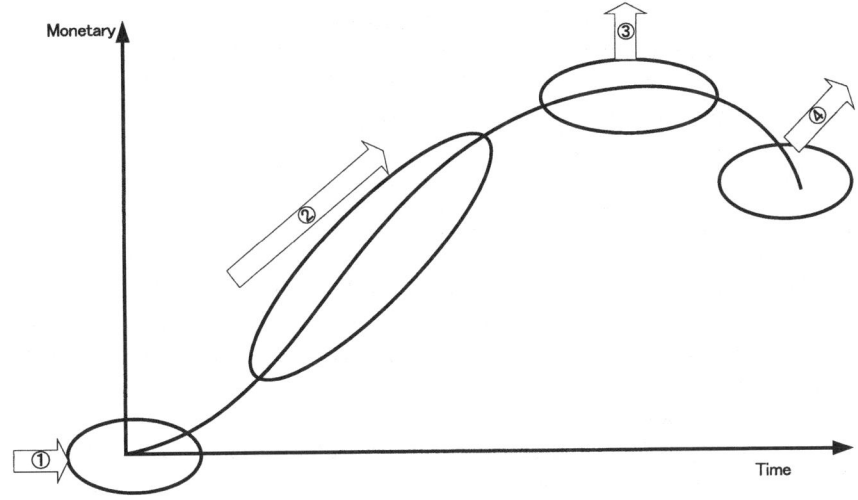

Fig. 10. Customer life cycle and four CRM modules

In the second stage, an analysis is required to promote new customers and to turn quasi-loyal customers to the loyal customers. For this purpose, we developed a decile switch analysis module. In the third stage, merchandise assortment is set up to meet the requirements of the loyal customers. A basket analysis module is prepared for the loyal customers in order to attain higher satisfaction and to raise the sales for them. In the final stage, for the purpose of preventing the loyal customers from going away to the other competitive stores, the analysis using the customer attrition analysis module is performed. Detailed description will be given below on these modules.

5.2 Early Discovery Module to Detect Loyal Customers from Newcomers

This module is a system for constructing a predictive model to discover from new customers within short time after the first visit to the store those who will become loyal customers in future and to acquire knowledge to capture these customers [9][10]. The user can select the preferred range of the customer groups classified by basic tools explained in Sections 3.1 and 3.2 and the period to be analyzed.

The explanatory attributes are prepared from the purchase data during the specified period such as one month or during the first five visits from the first one to the store. Sales ratio of the product category for each customer (the ratio of sales amount of the product category to total sales amount) is computed in the module. A model for predicting loyal customers will then be constructed from the above data joined together by using MUSASHI's command "xtclassify".

As a result, the model tells us which category of purchasing features these new prospective loyal customers have. Such information provides valuable implication as to how loyal customers are obtained from the competitive stores or to determine on which product category the emphasis should be put when a new store will be opened.

5.3   Decile Switch Analysis Module

Decile switch analysis module is a system to find out what kind of changes of purchase behavior of each of ten customer groups computed by decile analysis gives strong influence on the sales of the store. Given two periods, the following processing will be automatically started: First the customers who visited the store in the first period are classified into ten groups by decile analysis. The customers in each group are then classified into 10 groups again according to the decile analysis in the second period. When a customer did not visit the store in the second period, he/she does not belong to any decile group and thus classified as another group. Thus, the customers are classified into 11 groups. Since the customers are classified into 10 groups in the first stage, they are classified into 110 groups in total.

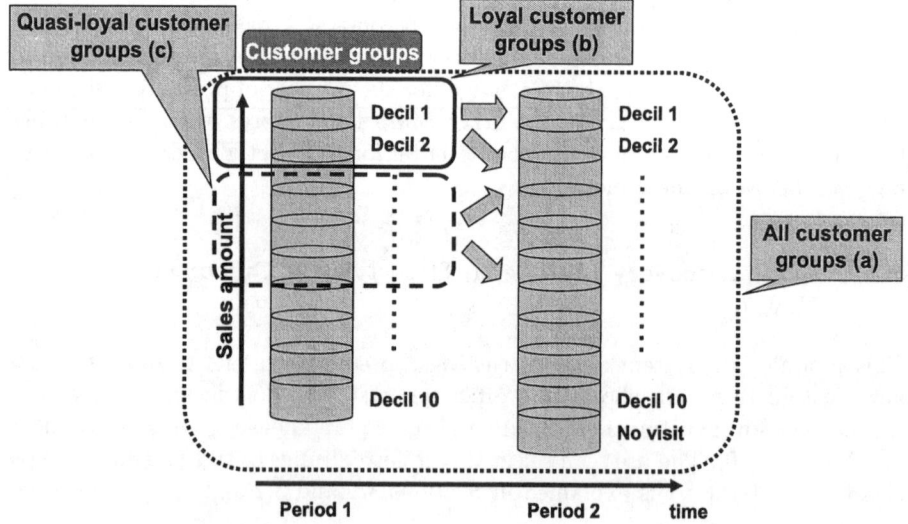

Fig. 11. The framework of decile switch analysis

For each of these customer groups, the difference between the purchase amount in the preceding period and that in the subsequent period is calculated. We then compute the changes of sales amount of which customer groups give strong influence on total sales amount of the store.

Next, judging from the above numerical values (influence on total sales amount of the store), the user decides which of the following data he/she wants to see, e.g., decile switch of (a) all customers, (b) loyal customers of the store, or (c) quasi-loyal customers (See Figure 11). If the user wants to see the decile switch of quasi-loyal customers, sales ratio of each product category for the relevant customer group in the preceding period is calculated, and a decision tree is generated, which shows the difference in the purchased categories between the quasi-loyal customers whose decile increased in the subsequent period (decile-up) and those whose decile value decreased (decile-down). Based on the rules obtained from the decision tree, the user can judge which product category should be recommended to quasi-loyal customers in order to increase the total sales of the store in future.

5.4   Basket Analysis Module of the Loyal Customer

For the purpose of increasing the sales amount of a store, it is the most important and also minimally required to keep loyal customers exclusively for a store. In general, the loyal customers have the tendency to continue to visit a particular store. As far as the merchandises and services to satisfy these customers are provided, it is easy to continuously keep these customers to the store than to make efforts to acquire the new customers from the rival stores. This module is to find out the merchandises preferred by loyal customers according to the result of the basket analysis on their purchase data [2].

From the results obtained by this module, it is possible not only to find out which product category the loyal customer prefers, but also to extract the most frequently purchased merchandise and to indicate the product belonging to C rank in ABC analysis. In the store control practiced in the past, if sales amount of the products preferred by the loyal customers is not very large, then the product often tends to disappear from the sales counter. Based on such information extracted from this module, the store manager can display the particular merchandise on the sales counter which loyal customer prefers and can pay special attention so that the merchandise will not be out of stock.

5.5   Module for Customer Attrition Analysis

Customer attrition analysis module is a system for extracting the purchase behavior of the loyal customers who left the store and to provide information for effective sales promotion in order to keep such loyal customers. When the user defines the loyal customers, the group of the customers is extracted, who had been loyal customers continuously for the past few months and had gone thereafter to the other stores. Using the sales ratio of product category preceding the attrition of the customers as explanatory variable, a classification model of the customer group is generated. By elucidating which group of customers is more easily diverted to the other store and which category of products these customers had been purchasing, the store manager can obtain useful information on the improvement of merchandise lineup at the store to keep loyal customers.

Four modules explained above are briefly summarized in Table 2.

Table 2. The summary of four modules in data mining oriented CRM systems

Name of module	The purpose of module
Early discovery of loyal customer	To construct a prediction model to discover potential loyal customers from newcomers.
Decile switch analysis	To find out what kind of changes of purchase behavior of customer groups derived from decile analysis give strong effects on the sales of the store.
Basket analysis for loyal customer	To discover the merchandises preferred by loyal customers according to the result of the basket analysis to keep them to the store.
Customer attrition analysis	To extract the purchase behavior of loyal customers who left the store and to provide information for effective sales promotion in order to keep loyal customers.

6   Case Studies of C-MUSASHI in Japanese Supermarket

In this section we will discuss the cases of C-MUSASHI in real business world. Since we cannot deal with all of the cases of the four modules in this paper, we will introduce the cases of decile switch analysis and customer attrition analysis modules in a large-scale supermarket.

6.1   The Case of Customer Growth by Using Decile Switch Analysis Module in a Supermarket

There is a chain store of supermarket in Japan, selling a wide range of goods including fresh foods, groceries and medicine. Recently, the sales amount in almost all stores of them has been decreased because of the price reduction under local competitive market and deflation in Japan. However, one store gradually increased the sales amount more than those of the other stores during the period we are concerned with in this case. The purpose of this analysis is to find out which customer groups had positive effects on sales amount of the store and then to discover the feature of the product categories they purchased, in order to implement the effective sales promotions in other stores for increasing total sales of a chain store.

First, two periods, i.e. April and May of 2003, were set up for analysis by the marketing stuff in this supermarket. Figure 12 shows the number of customers categorized in each decile switch group. There are many customers staying in decile 1 in both April and May, who are the most important loyal customers to the store. However they do not have so strong effects on sales of this store though the number of them is larger than that of the other decile switch groups.

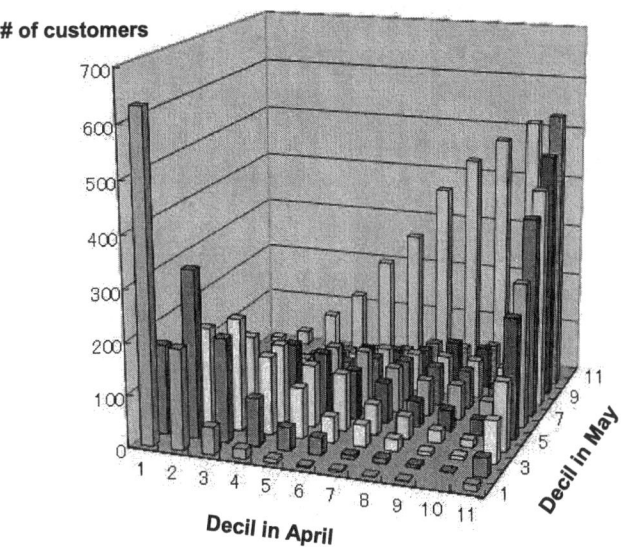

Fig. 12. The number of customers in each decile group

Figure 13 shows the changes of the purchase amounts in April and May of the customer groups classified according to the decile values of both periods. In the figure, the portion indicated by a circle shows that the sales for the quasi-loyal customer groups (the customers with decile 2-4) in April increases in May. From the figure, it is easy to observe that the sales increase of quasi-loyal customers makes great contribution to the increase of the total sales amount of the store.

Next, focusing on the quasi-loyal customers based on the above information, we carried out decile switch analysis by using decision tree to classify them into decile-up or decile-down customer groups. In the rules obtained from the decision tree, we found some interesting facts (See Figure 14). For instance, it was found that the customer who had exhibited higher purchase percentage of the product category such as milk, eggs, yoghurt, etc., which are easily perishable, shows high purchase amount in the subsequent period. Also, it was discovered that the customers who had been purchasing drugs such as medicine for colds or headache exhibited the increase in decile value in the subsequent period.

The store manager interpreted these rules as follows: If a customer is inclined to purchase daily foodstuffs at a store, total purchase amount of the customer

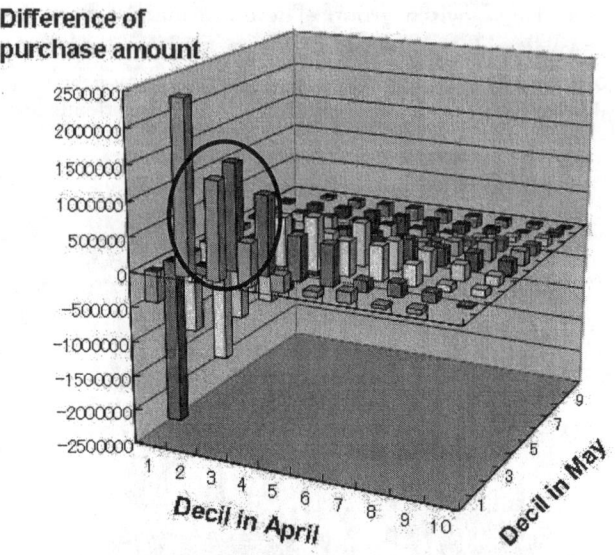

Fig. 13. Changes of sales amount for each decile group

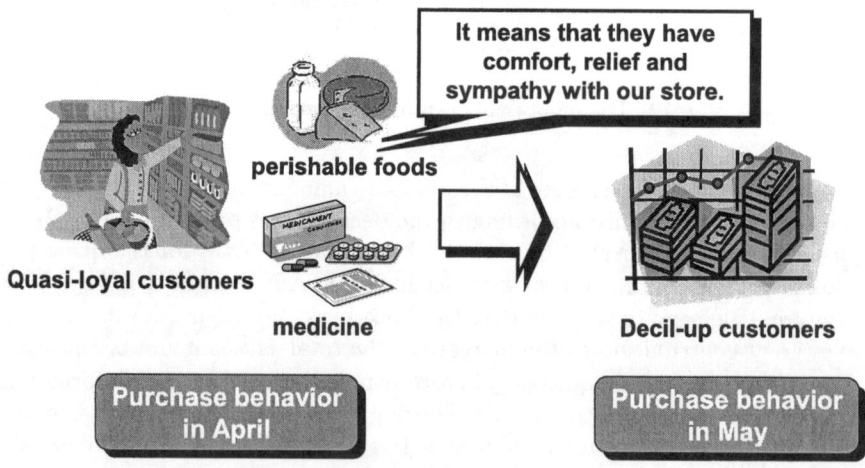

Fig. 14. The rules obtained from the decision tree by using decile switch analysis module

including other categories can be maintained at high level. As a result, the customer may have a sense of comfort, relief and sympathy with the store and would be more likely to buy other goods relating to health such as drugs. Based on such information, the store manager is carrying out sales promotion to keep the store in such atmosphere as to give the customers a sense of comfort, relief and sympathy to the store.

6.2   The Case of Customer Attrition Analysis

Due to the recent rapid change of economic circumstances, it has become important to manage loyal customers who contribute to profits of the store. The most important required term is to keep loyal customers of a store to increase the sales amount under these environments. However there exists a part of them who leave the store and switch to the rival store. The purpose of this analysis is to present analysis process to manage attrition customer by using customer attrition analysis module and to extract the purchase behavior of the loyal customers who left the store to provide useful information for effective sales promotion to keep such loyal customers. If we discover the distinctive purchase behavior of them before leaving the store, it is possible to implement sales promotion strategies to keep them to the store.

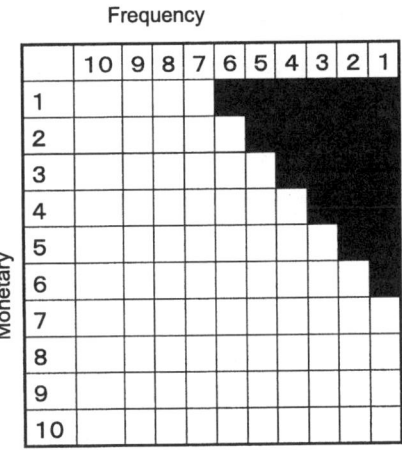

Fig. 15. The definition of loyal customer by using frequency and monetary dimensions

A user can define the loyal customer segments by using frequency and monetary dimensions (balck sells in Figure 15 illustrates an example of the loyal customer segments). After defining them, two customer groups are extracted; the first group called "fixed loyal customers" is defined as those who had been loyal customers continuously for the past four months in the target periods and the second called "attrition customers" is defined as those who had been loyal customers continuously for first three months and had gone to the other stores at the final month. We used four months of purchase data from Sep. 2002 through Dec. 2002 of a supermarket in Japan. The number of the fixed loyal customers is 1918, and that of attrition customers is 191. Using the sales ratios of rough product categories as explanatory variables, a classification model is generated which characterizes the distinction between the attrition customers and the fixed customers.

Figure 16 shows a part of results extracted from the derived decision tree. In this figure it was observed that the customer whose ratio of fruit category in his/her purchases had not been exceeding 5 percents and that of meat category had not been exceeding 15 percents, became an attrition customer after one month at the ratio of about 66 percents (44/67). Executing additional analysis, the marketing stuff in the store interpreted these rules as follows: The customers who have children have a tendency to leave the store. Depending on these findings, the new sales promotion strategy for a family with children has been planned in the store.

```
if($fruit<=0.05)
  then if($meat<=0.15)
    then $class="attrition customer" (hit/sup)=(44/67)
    else $class="fixed customer"     (hit/sup)=(147/273)
        ⋮
```

Fig. 16. A part of results extracted from purchase data of target customer groups

7   Conclusion

In this paper, we have introduced a CRM system called C-MUSASHI which can be constructed at very low cost by the use of the open-source software MUSASHI. We have explained components and software tools of C-MUSASHI. In particular, C-MUSASHI contains several data mining tools which can be used to analyze purchase behavior of customers in order to increase the sales amount of a retail store. However, we could not explain the details of all of the modules in this paper. In some of the modules, sufficient analysis cannot be carried out in actual business. We will try to offer these modules to the public as soon as possible so that those who are concerned in business field would have an advantage to use the modules. In future, we will continue to make improvement for the construction of effective CRM systems by incorporating the comments and advices from the experts in this field.

In C-MUSASHI, a typical decision tree tool and basket analysis tool were used as data mining technique. A number of useful data mining algorithms are now provided by the researchers. We will continuously try to utilize and incorporate these techniques into C-MUSASHI, and we will act as a bridge between the research field and actual business activities.

References

1. Blattberg, R. C., Getz, G., Thomas, J. S.: Customer Equity: Building and Managing Relationships as Valuable Assets. Harvard Business School Press. (2001)
2. Fujisawa, K., Hamuro, Y., Katoh, N., Tokuyama, T. and Yada, K.: Approximation of Optimal Two-Dimensional Association Rules for Categorical Attributes Using Semidefinite Programming. Lecture Notes in Artificial Intelligence **1721**. Proceedings of First International Conference DS'99. (1999) 148–159
3. Hamuro, Y., Katoh, N. and Yada, K.: Data Mining oriented System for Business Applications. Lecture Notes in Artificial Intelligence 1532. Proceedings of First International Conference DS'98. (1998) 441–442
4. Hamuro, Y., Katoh, N., Matsuda, Y. and Yada, K.: Mining Pharmacy Data Helps to Make Profits. Data Mining and Knowledge Discovery. **2** (1998) 391–398
5. Hamuro, Y., Katoh, N. and Yada, K.: MUSASHI: Flexible and Efficient Data Preprocessing Tool for KDD based on XML. DCAP2002 Workshop held in conjunction with ICDM2002. (2002) 38–49
6. Hawkins, G. E.: Building the Customer Specific Retail Enterprise. Breezy Heights Publishing. (1999)
7. Hedley, B.: Strategy and the business portfolio. Long Range Planning. **10** 1 (1977) 9–15
8. Hughes, A. M.: Strategic Database Marketing. The McGraw-Hill. (1994)
9. Ip, E., Johnson, J., Yada, K., Hamuro, Y., Katoh, N. and Cheung, S.: A Neural Network Application to Identify High-Value Customer for a Large Retail Store in Japan. Neural Networks in Business: Techniques and Applications. Idea Group Publishing. (2002) 55–69
10. Ip, E., Yada, K., Hamuro, Y. and Katoh, N.: A Data Mining System for Managing Customer Relationship. Proceedings of the 2000 Americas Conference on Information Systems. (2000) 101–105
11. MUSASHI: Mining Utilities and System Architecture for Scalable processing of Historical data. URL: http://musashi.sourceforge.jp/.
12. Reed, T.: Measure Your Customer Lifecycle. DM News 21. **33** (1999) 23
13. Rongstad, N.: Find Out How to Stop Customers from Leaving. Target Marketing 22. **7** (1999) 28–29
14. Woolf, B. P.: Customer Specific Marketing. Teal Books. (1993)

Investigation of Rule Interestingness
in Medical Data Mining

Miho Ohsaki[1], Shinya Kitaguchi[2], Hideto Yokoi[3], and Takahira Yamaguchi[4]

[1] Doshisha University, Faculty of Engineering,
1-3 Tataramiyakodani, Kyotanabe-shi, Kyoto 610-0321, Japan
mohsaki@mail.doshisha.ac.jp
[2] Shizuoka University, Faculty of Information,
3-5-1 Johoku, Hamamatsu-shi, Shizuoka 432-8011, Japan
kitaguchi@ks.cs.inf.shizuoka.ac.jp
[3] Chiba University Hospital, Medical Informatics,
1-8-1 Inohana, Chuo-ku, Chiba-shi, Chiba 260-0856, Japan
yokoih@telemed.ho.chiba-u.ac.jp
[4] Keio University, Faculty of Science and Technology,
3-14-1 Hiyoshi, Kohoku-ku, Yokohama-shi, Kanagawa 223-8522, Japan
yamaguti@ae.keio.ac.jp

Abstract. This research experimentally investigates the performance of conventional rule interestingness measures and discusses their usefulness for supporting KDD through human-system interaction in medical domain. We compared the evaluation results by a medical expert and those by selected sixteen kinds of interestingness measures for the rules discovered in a dataset on hepatitis. χ^2 measure, recall, and accuracy demonstrated the highest performance, and specificity and prevalence did the lowest. The interestingness measures showed a complementary relationship for each other. These results indicated that some interestingness measures have the possibility to predict really interesting rules at a certain level and that the combinational use of interestingness measures will be useful. We then discussed how to combinationally utilize interestingness measures and proposed a post-processing user interface utilizing them, which supports KDD through human-system interaction.

1   Introduction

Medical data mining is one of active research fields in Knowledge Discovery in Databases (KDD) due to its scientific and social contribution. We have been conducted case studies to discovery new knowledge on the symptom of hepatitis which is a progressive liver disease, since grasping the symptom of hepatitis is essential for its medical treatment. We have repeated obtaining rules to predict prognosis from a clinical dataset and their evaluation by a medical expert, improving the mining system and conditions. In this iterative process, we recognized the significance of system-human interaction to enhance rule quality by reflecting the domain knowledge and the requirement of a medical expert. We

S. Tsumoto et al. (Eds.): AM 2003, LNAI 3430, pp. 174–189, 2005.

then began to focus on the issue to semi-automatically support system-human interaction [1].

Rule interestingness is also an important field in KDD, and there have been many studies that formulated interestingness measures and evaluated rules with them instead of humans. Some latest studies made a survey on individually proposed interestingness measures and tried to analyze them [5, 6, 7]. However, they were mainly based on mathematical analysis, and little attention has been given to how much interestingness measures can reflect real human interest.

These two backgrounds led us to have the following purposes in this research: (1) investigating the conventional interestingness measures and comparing them with the evaluation results of rules by a medical expert, and (2) discussing whether they are useful to support system-human interaction in medical KDD. In this paper, Section 2 introduces our previous research on medical data mining dealing with hepatitis as a subject matter and reports our survey of conventional interestingness measures. It also selects interestingness measures suitable to our purpose. Section 3 shows the experiment that evaluated rules on hepatitis with the selected interestingness measures and compared the evaluation results by them with those by a medical expert. Section 4 discusses how conventional interestingness measures can be applied to supporting KDD through system-human interaction. Finally, Section 5 concludes the paper and comments on the future work.

2 Related Work

2.1 Our Previous Research on Medical Data Mining

We have conducted case studies [1] to discover the rules predicting prognosis based on diagnosis in a dataset of the medical test results on viral chronic hepatitis. The dataset was open as the common one of data mining contests [8, 9]. We repeated the set of rule generation by our mining system and rule evaluation by a medical expert two times, and the repetition made us discover the rules highly valued by the medical expert. We finely pre-processed the dataset based on medical expert's advice, since such a real medical dataset is ill-defined and has many noises and missing values. We then performed a popular time-series mining technique, which extracts representative temporal patterns from a dataset by clustering and learns rules consisting of extracted patterns by a decision tree [11]. we did not treat the subsequence extraction with a sliding window used in the literature [11] to avoid STS clustering problem pointed out in the literature [12]. We simply extracted subsequences at the starting point of medical tests from the dataset of medical test results. In the first mining, we used EM algorithm [2] for clustering and C4.5 [3] for learning. In the second mining, we used K-means algorithm [4] for clustering to remove the problem that EM algorithm is not easily understandable and adjustable for medical experts.

The upper graph in Fig. 1 shows one of the rules, which the medical expert focused on, in the first mining. It estimates the future trend of GPT, one of major medical tests to grasp hepatitis symptom, in the future one year by using the

176 M. Ohsaki et al.

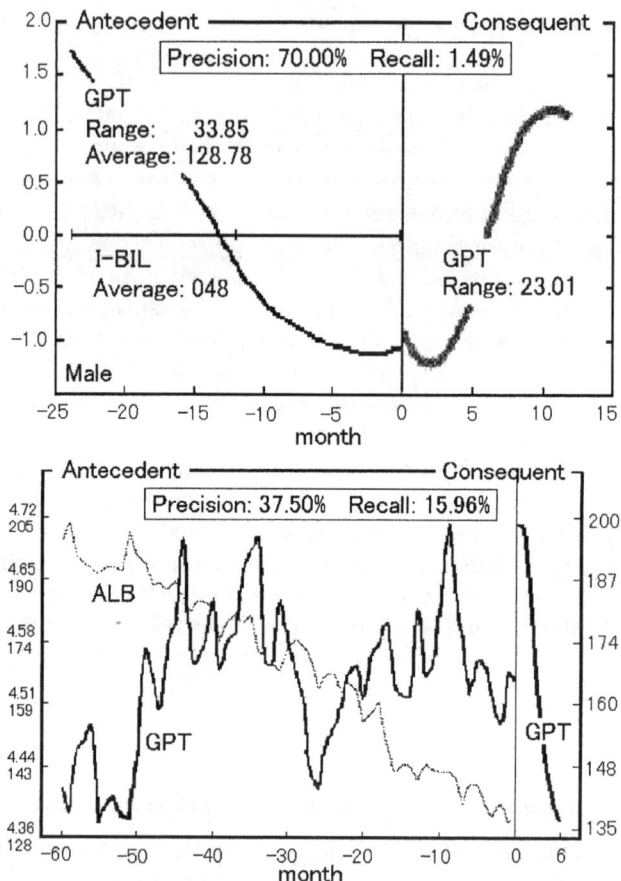

Fig. 1. Highly valued rules in the first (upper) and the second mining (lower)

change of several medical test results in the past two years. The medical expert commented on it as follows: the rule offers a hypothesis that GPT value changes with an about three-years cyclic, and the hypothesis is interesting since it differs from the conventional common sense of medical experts that GPT value basically decreases in a monotone. We then improved our mining system, extended the observation term, and obtained new rules. The lower graph in Fig. 1 shows one of the rules, which the medical expert highly valued, in our second mining. The medical expert commented on it that it implies GPT value globally changes two times in the past five years and more strongly supports the hypothesis of GPT's cyclic change.

In addition to that, we obtained the evaluation results of rules by the medical expert. We removed obviously meaningless rules in which the medical test results stay in their normal ranges and presented remaining rules to the medical expert. He conducted the following evaluation tasks: For each mining, he checked all presented rules and gave each of them the comment on its medical interpretation

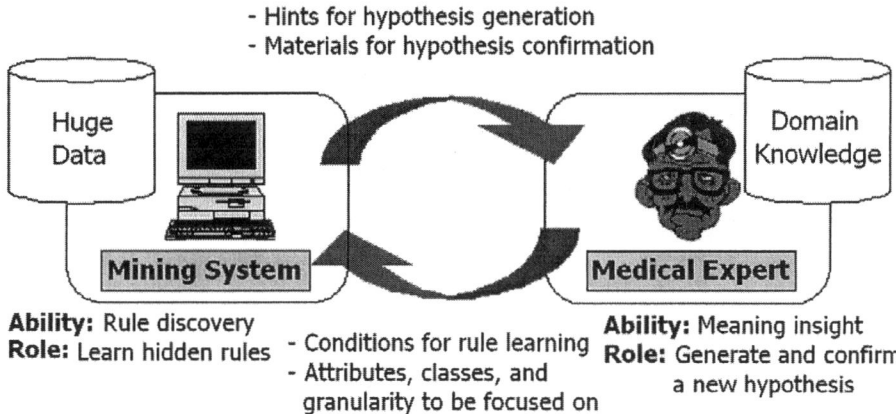

Fig. 2. Conceptual model of interaction between a mining system and a medical expert

and one of rule quality labels. The rule quality labels were Especially-Interesting (**EI**), Interesting (**I**), Not-Understandable (**NU**), and Not-Interesting (**NI**). **EI** means that the rule was a key to generate or confirm a hypothesis. As a consequence, we obtained a set of rules and their evaluation results by the medical expert in the first mining and that in the second mining. Three and nine rules received **EI** and **I** in the first mining, respectively. Similarly, two and six rules did in the second mining.

After we achieved some positive results, we tried to systematize the know-how and methodology obtained through the repetition of mining and evaluating process on the system-human interaction to polish up rules in medical domain. We made a conceptual model of interaction that describes the relation and media between a mining system and a medical expert (See Fig. 2). It also describes the ability and rule of a mining system and those of a medical expert.

A mining system learns hidden rules faithfully to the data structure and offers them to a medical expert as the hints and materials for hypothesis generation and confirmation (Note that the word 'confirmation' in this paper does not mean the highly reliable proof of a hypothesis by additional medical experiments under strictly controlled conditions. It means the additional information extraction from the same data to enhance the reliability of an initial hypothesis). While, a medical expert generates and confirms a hypothesis, namely a seed of new knowledge, by evaluating the rules based on his/her domain knowledge. A framework to support KDD through such human-system interaction should well-balancedly reflect the both of objective criteria (the mathematical features of data) and subjective criteria (domain knowledge, interest, and focus point of a medical expert) to each process of KDD, namely pre-processing, mining, and post-processing. It is important not to mix up the objective and subjective criteria to avoid too much biased unreliable results; The framework should explicit notify a mining system and a medical expert which criterion or which combination of criteria is used now. Following these backgrounds, this research focuses

Table 1. Factors to categorize conventional interestingness measures

Factors	Meaning	Sub-factors
Subject	Who evaluates?	Computer / Human user
Object	What is evaluated?	Association rule / Classification rule
Unit	By how many objects?	A rule / A set of rules
Criterion	Based on what criterion?	Absolute criterion / Relative criterion
Theory	Based on what theory?	Number of instances / Probability / Statistics / Information / Distance of rules or attributes / Complexity of a rule

on interestingness measures that represent the mathematical features of data as the objective criteria for human-system interaction.

2.2   Conventional Rule Interestingness Measures

We categorized conventional interestingness measures with the several factors in Table 1 based on the results of our and other researchers' surveys [5, 6, 7]. The subject to evaluate rules, a computer or human user, is the most important categorization factor. Interestingness measures by a computer and human user are called objective and subjective ones, respectively. There are more than forty objective measures at least. They estimate how a rule is mathematically meaningful based on the distribution structure of the instances related to the rule. They are mainly used to remove meaningless rules rather than to discover really interesting ones for a human user, since they do not include domain knowledge [13, 14, 15, 16, 17, 18, 19, 20, 21, 22, 23, 24]. In contrast, there are only a dozen of subjective measures [25, 26, 27, 28, 29, 30, 31, 32].

They estimate how a rule fits to a belief, a bias, and/or a rule template formulated beforehand by a human user. Although the initial conditions such as a belief are given by a human user, the estimation of how a rule fits to them is based on a mathematically defined distance. They are useful to discover really interesting rules to some extent due to their built-in domain knowledge. However, they depend on the precondition that a human user can clearly formulate his/her own interest and do not discover absolutely unexpected knowledge. Few subjective measures adaptively learn real human interest through human-system interaction.

The conventional interestingness measures, not only objective but also subjective, do not directly reflect the interest that a human user really has. To avoid the confusion of real human interest, objective measure, and subjective measure, we clearly differentiate them. **Objective Measure**: The feature such as the correctness, uniqueness, and strength of a rule, calculated by the mathematical analysis. It does not include human evaluation criteria. **Subjective Measure**: The similarity or difference between the information on interestingness given beforehand by a human user and those obtained from a rule. Although it includes human evaluation criteria in its initial state, the calculation of similarity or difference is mainly based on the mathematical analysis. **Real Human Interest**:

Table 2. The objective measures of rule interestingness used in this research. **N:** Number of instances included in the antecedent and/or consequent of a rule. **P:** Probability of the antecedent and/or consequent of a rule. **S:** Statistical variable based on P. **I:** Information of the antecedent and/or consequent of a rule

Measure Name / Theory	Evaluation Criterion / Formula
Coverage / P	Generality of the antecedent of a rule. / $P(A)$, $P(A)$: Probability of antecedent.
Prevalence / P	Generality of the consequent of a rule. / $P(C)$, $P(C)$: Probability of consequent.
Precision / P	Performance of a rule to predict its consequent. / $P(C\|A)$, $P(C\|A)$: Conditional probability of consequent for antecedent.
Recall / P	Performance of a rule not to leak its consequent. / $P(A\|C)$, $P(A\|C)$: Conditional probability of antecedent for consequent.
Support / P	Generality of a rule. / $P(A\cap C)$, $P(A\cap C)$: Probability of antecedent and consequent.
Specificity / P	Performance of a rule to leak the negation of its consequent. / $P(\overline{A}\|\overline{C})$
Accuracy / P	Summation of the support of a rule and that of its reverse. / $P(A\cap C)+P(\overline{A}\cap\overline{C})$, $P(\overline{A}\cap\overline{C})$: Probability of the negation of antecedent and the negation of consequent.
Lift / P	Dependency between the antecedent and consequent of a rule. / $P(C\|A)/P(C)$
Leverage / P	Dependency between the antecedent and consequent of a rule. / $P(C\|A)-P(A)*P(C)$
GOI (GOI-D, GOI-G) [19] / P	Multiplication of the antecedent-consequent dependency and generality of a rule. / $((\frac{P(C\|A)}{P(A)*P(C)})^k-1)*((P(A)*P(C))^m$ / k,m: Coefficients of dependency and generality, respectively. $k=2m$ for GOI-D. $m=2k$ for GOI-G.
χ^2-M [20] / S	Dependency between the antecedent and consequent of a rule. / $\sum_{event}\frac{(T_{event}-O_{event})^2}{T_{event}}$, event: $A\to C, A\to\overline{C}, \overline{A}\to C, \overline{A}\to\overline{C}$ / T_{event}: Theoretical number of instances in $event$. O_{event}: Observed number of instances in $event$.
J-M [14] / I	Dependency between the antecedent and consequent of a rule. / $P(A)*(I_{diff}(C\|A;C)+I_{diff}(\overline{C}\|A;\overline{C}))$ / $I_{diff}(X;Y)=P(X)*\log_2\frac{P(X)}{P(Y)}$
K-M / I	Dependency between the antecedent and consequent of a rule. / $I_{diff}(C\|A;C)+I_{diff}(\overline{C}\|A;\overline{C}))-I_{diff}(C\|A;\overline{C}))-I_{diff}(\overline{C}\|A;C))$
PSI [13] / N	Dependency between the antecedent and consequent of a rule. / $N(A\cap C)-\frac{N(A)*N(C)}{N(U)}$, $N(A),N(C),N(A\cap C),N(U)$: The number of instances in the antecedent, consequent, antecedent and consequent, and universe, respectively.
Credibility [16] / P, N	Multiplication of the generality of a rule and the uniqueness of its consequent. / $\beta_i*P(C)*\|P(R_i\|C)-P(R_i)\|*T(R_i)$, $\beta_i=\frac{1}{2*P(R_i)*(1-P(R_i))}$ / β_i: Coefficient of normalization. $P(R_i)$: Probability of the rule $R_i=P(A\cap C)$. $T(R_i)$: Threshold number of instances in the rule R_i.

The interest which a human user really feels for a rule in his/her mind. It is formed by the synthesis of cognition, domain knowledge, individual experiences, and the influences of the rules that he/she evaluated before.

This research specifically focuses on objective measures and investigates the relation between them and real human interest. We then explain the details of objective measures here. They can be categorized into some groups with the criterion and theory for evaluation. Although the criterion is absolute or relative as shown in Table 1, the majority of present objective measures are based on an absolute criterion. There are several kinds of criterion based on the following factors: Correctness – How many instances the antecedent and/or consequent of a rule support, or how strong their dependence is [13, 14, 20, 23], Generality – How similar the trend of a rule is to that of all data [18] or the other rules, Uniqueness – How different the trend of a rule is from that of all data [17, 21, 24] or the other rules [18, 20], and Information Richness – How much information a rule possesses [15]. These factors naturally prescribe the theory for evaluation and the interestingness calculation method based on the theory. The theory includes the number of instances [13], probability [19, 21], statistics [20, 23], information [14, 23], the distance of rules or attributes [17, 18, 24], and the complexity of a rule [15] (See Table 1).

We selected the basic objective measures shown in Table 2 for the experiment in Section 3. Some objective measures in Table 2 are expediently written in abbreviations: GOI means "Gray and Orlowska's Interestingness" [19], and we call GOI with the dependency coefficient value at the double of the generality one GOI-D, and vice versa for GOI-G. χ^2-M means "χ^2 Measure using all four quadrants, $A \rightarrow C$, $A \rightarrow \overline{C}$, $\overline{A} \rightarrow C$, and $\overline{A} \rightarrow \overline{C}$" [20]. J-M and K-M mean "J Measure" [14] and "our original measure based on J-M" (we used 'K' for the name of this measure, since 'K' is the next alphabet to 'J'). PSI means "Piatetsky-Shapiro's Interestingness" [13]. Although we actually used other objective measures on reliable exceptions [33, 34, 35], they gave all rules the same lowest evaluation values due to the mismatch of their and our evaluation objects. This paper then does not mention their experimental results.

Now we explain the motivation of this research in detail. Objective measures are useful to automatically remove obviously meaningless rules. However, some factors of evaluation criterion have contradiction to each other such as generality and uniqueness and may not match with or contradict to real human interest. In a sense, it may be proper not to investigate the relation between objective measures and real human interest, since their evaluation criterion does not include the knowledge on rule semantics and are obviously not the same of real human interest. However, our idea is that they may be useful to support KDD through human-system interaction if they possess a certain level of performance to detect really interesting rules. In addition to that, they may offer a human user unexpected new viewpoints. Although the validity of objective measures has been theoretically proven and/or experimentally discussed using some benchmark data [5, 6, 7], very few attempts have been made to investigate their comparative performance and the relation between them and real human interest for a real application. Our investigation will be novel in this light.

3   Experiment to Compare Objective Interestingness Measures with Real Human Interest

3.1   Experimental Conditions

The experiment examined the performance of objective measures to estimate real human interest by comparing the evaluation by them and a human user. Concretely speaking, the selected objective measures and a medical expert evaluated the same rules, and their evaluation values were qualitatively and quantitatively compared. We used the objective measures in Table 2 and the rules and their evaluation results in our previous research (Refer Section 2.1).

The evaluation procedure of objective measures was designed as follows: For each objective measure, the same rules as in our previous research were evaluated by the objective measure, sorted in the descending order of evaluation values, and assigned the rule quality labels. The rules from the top to the m-th were assigned **EI**, where m was the number of **EI** rules in the evaluation by the medical expert. Next, the rules from the $(m + 1)$-th to the $(m + n)$-th were assigned **I**, where n was the number of **I** rules in the evaluation by the medical expert. The assignment of **NU** and **NI** followed the same procedure. We dared not to do evaluation value thresholding for the labeling. The first reason was that it is quite difficult to find the optimal thresholds for the all combinations of labels and objective measures. The second reason was that although our labeling procedure may not be precise, it can set the conditions of objective measures at least equal through simple processing. The last reason was that our number-based labeling is more realistic than threshold-based labeling. The number of rules labeled with **EI** or **I** by a human user inevitably stabilizes at around a dozen in a practical situation, since the number of evaluation by him/her has a severe limitation caused by his/her fatigue.

Table 3. The total rank of objective measures through first and second mining

Total Rank	Averaged Meta Criterion	Measure Name	Averaged Rank	Measure Name
1	0.63	χ^2-M	3.0	χ^2-M, Recall
2	0.62	Recall	3.5	Accuracy
3	0.59	Accuracy	4.5	Lift
4	0.58	Lift	5.0	K-M
5	0.55	Credibility, K-M	6.5	Credibility
12	0.35	Leverage	9.5	GOI-G, Precision
13	0.29	GOI-D	10.0	Leverage
14	0.25	Precision	10.5	Coverage, GOI-D
15	0.23	Specificity	11.0	Specificity
16	0.11	Prevalence	14.0	Prevalence

3.2   Results and Discussion

Fig. 3 and 4 show the experimental results in the first and second mining, respectively. We analyzed the relation between the evaluation results by the medical expert and the objective measures qualitatively and quantitatively. As the qual-

Rule ID	2 3 11 4 5 8 12 13 22 23 24 27 6 17 21 1 7 9 10 14 15 16 18 19 20 25 26 28 29 30	#1	#2	#3	#4	Meta
Expert	EI EI EI I I I I I I I I I NU NU NU NU NI NI NI NI NI NI NI NI NI NI NI NI NI NI					
Recall		8/12+	2/3+	22/30+	+0.48+	0.67
χ2-M		8/12+	1/3	22/30+	+0.38+	0.63
J-M		7/12+	2/3+	20/30+	+0.36+	0.60
K-M		7/12+	1/3	20/30+	+0.14+	0.55
Accuracy		6/12+	1/3	18/30+	+0.25+	0.50
Lift		6/12+	1/3	18/30+	+0.15+	0.49
Precision		6/12+	0/3	18/30+	+0.23+	0.46
Support		5/12+	1/3	16/30+	+0.13+	0.43
PSI		5/12+	1/3	16/30+	+0.13+	0.43
Specificity		6/12+	0/3	17/30+	-0.04	0.42
GOI-D		5/12+	1/3	15/30	0.00	0.40
Leverage		5/12+	0/3	16/30+	+0.13+	0.39
GOI-G		5/12+	0/3	16/30+	-0.02	0.38
Credibility		5/12+	0/3	16/30+	+0.01+	0.38
Coverage		4/12	1/3	14/30	+0.08+	0.36
Prevalence		2/12	1/3	10/30	-0.20	0.21

Fig. 3. The evaluation results by a medical expert and objective measures for the rules in first mining. Each column represents a rule, and each row represents the set of evaluation results by an objective measure. The rules are sorted in the descending order of the evaluation values given by the medical expert. The objective measures are sorted in the descending order of the meta criterion values. A square in the left-hand side surrounds the rules labeled with **EI** or **I** by the medical expert. White and black cells mean that the evaluation by an objective measure was and was not the same by the medical expert, respectively. The five columns in the right side show the performance on the four comprehensive criteria and the meta one. '+' means the value is greater than that of random selection

Rule ID	13 21 14 15 16 17 18 19 20 1 2 3 4 5 6 7 8 9 10 11 12	#1	#2	#3	#4	Meta
Expert	EI EI I I I I I I I NU NI NI NI NI NI NI NI NI NI NI NI					
Credibility		6.00/8+	1/2+	17.00/21+	+0.46+	0.72
Accuracy		6.00/8+	0/2	17.00/21+	+0.48+	0.67
Lift		6.00/8+	0/2	17.00/21+	+0.36+	0.66
χ2-M		6.00/8+	0/2	15.00/21+	+0.36+	0.62
Recall		4.00/8+	2/2+	13.00/21+	+0.27+	0.57
K-M		5.00/8+	0/2	15.00/21+	+0.11+	0.55
GOI-G		5.00/8+	0/2	13.00/21+	+0.19+	0.52
Coverage		3.00/8	2/2+	11.00/21	-0.13	0.45
Support		2.00/8	1/2+	9.00/21	-0.24	0.30
Leverage		2.00/8	1/2+	9.00/21	-0.17	0.30
PSI		2.00/8	1/2+	9.00/21	-0.17	0.30
J-M		2.00/8	0/2	9.00/21	-0.20	0.25
GOI-D		1.00/8	1/2+	7.00/21	-0.50	0.18
Precision		0.00/8	0/2	5.00/21	-0.51	0.04
Specificity		0.00/8	0/2	4.00/21	-0.47	0.03
Prevalence		0.00/8	0/2	4.00/21	-0.65	0.01

Fig. 4. The evaluation results by a medical expert and objective measures for the rules in second mining. See the caption of Fig. 3 for the details

itative analysis, we visualized their degree of agreement to easily grasp its trend. We colored the rules with agreement white and those with disagreement black. The pattern of white and black cells for an objective measure describes how its evaluation matched with those by the medical expert. The more the number of white cells in the left-hand side, the better its performance to estimate real human interest. For the quantitative analysis, we defined four comprehensive criteria to evaluate the performance of an objective measure. #1: Performance on **I** (the number of rules labeled with **I** by the objective measure over that by the medical expert. Note that **I** includes **EI**). #2: Performance on **EI** (the number of rules labeled with **EI** by the objective measure over that by the medical expert). #3: Number-based performance on all evaluation (the number of rules with the same evaluation results by the objective measure and the medical expert over that of all rules). #4: Correlation-based performance on all evaluation (the correlation coefficient between the evaluation results by the objective measure and those by the medical expert). The values of these criteria are shown in the right side of Fig. 3 and 4. The symbol '+' besides a value means that the value is greater than that in case rules are randomly selected as **EI** or **I**. Therefore, an objective measure with '+' has higher performance than random selection does at least. To know the total performance, we defined the weighted average of the four criteria as a meta criterion; we assigned 0.4, 0.1, 0.4, and 0.1 to #1, #2, #3, and #4, respectively, according to their importance. The objective measures were sorted in the descending order of the values of meta criterion.

The results in the first mining in Fig. 3 show that Recall demonstrated the highest performance, χ^2-M did the second highest, and J-M did the third highest. Prevalence demonstrated the lowest performance, Coverage did the second lowest, and Credibility and GOI-G did the third lowest. The results in the second mining in Fig. 4 show that Credibility demonstrated the highest performance, Accuracy did the second highest, and Lift did the third highest. Prevalence demonstrated the lowest performance, Specificity did the second lowest, and Precision did the third lowest. To understand the whole trend, we calculated the total rank of objective measures through first and second mining and summarized it in Table 3. We averaged the value of meta criterion in first mining and that in second mining for each objective measure and sorted the objective measures with the averages. Although we carefully defined the meta criterion, it is hard to say that the meta criterion perfectly expresses the performance of objective measures. We then also did the same calculation on the ranks in first and second mining for multidirectional discussions. As shown in Table 3, in either case of averaged meta criterion or averaged rank, χ^2-M, Recall, and Accuracy maintained their high performance through the first and second mining. On the other hand, Prevalence and Specificity maintained their low performance. The other objective measures slightly changed their middle performance.

Some objective measures – χ^2-M, Recall, and Accuracy – showed constantly high performance; They had comparatively many white cells and '+' for all comprehensive criteria. The results and the medical expert's comments on them imply that his interest consisted of not only the medical semantics but also the statistical characteristics of rules. The patterns of white and black cells are mosaic-like in Fig. 3 and 4. They imply that the objective measures had almost complementary relationship for each other and that the combinational use of objective measures may achieve a higher performance. For example, the logical addition of Recall and χ^2-M in Fig. 3 increases the value of correct answer rate #3 from $22/30 = 73.3\%$ to $29/30 = 96.7\%$. Now we summarize the experimental results as follows: some objective measures will work at a certain level in spite of no consideration of domain semantics, and the combinational use of objective measures will work better. Although the experimental results are specific to the experimental conditions, they gave us the possibility to utilize objective measures that have not been given by the conventional theoretical studies on objective measures.

4   Further Discussion and Proposal

Inspired by the experimental results, we propose a post-processing user interface that utilizes objective measures for supporting KDD through human-system interaction. We designed it as shown in Fig. 5. The solid and dotted lines express the output from a mining system to a human user and the input from a human user to a mining system through the user interface, respectively. In the user interface, a human user can select one among the objective measures stored in a repository by clicking a button corresponding to the one. The user interface presents the mined rules sorted with the evaluation results by the selected objective measure. This function recommends possibly interesting rules and helps the human user see and think them explicitly changing his/her viewpoint. Consequently, this multi-view discussion will contribute to the hypothesis generation by the human user (Refer Fig. 2); The human user can organize a new knowledge with the pieces of knowledge given by the rules. The human user also can input his/her own evaluation results for the rules as numerical values into the user interface. An evaluation learning algorithm behind the user interface gradually models the interest of the human user using the repository of objective measures through human-system interaction (We explain the evaluation learning algorithm in the next paragraph). Once the model is obtained, the human user can select the model as a newly learned objective measure and sort the rules with it. This function helps the human user explicitly grasp his/her own implicit evaluation criteria by looking at the sorted rules. Consequently, this awareness will contribute to the hypothesis confirmation by the human user. We have already developed the prototype of user interface and got some favorable comments on it from a medical expert: A user interface that helps a human user see and think rules meets the needs of medical experts, because the burden of rule evaluation on medical experts is quite heavy at present. The functions to let a human user actively select and sort rules will be useful to give the human user unexpected viewpoints and ideas.

We here explain the evaluation learning algorithm embedded in the post-processing user interface. Our idea is that the interest of a human user can be

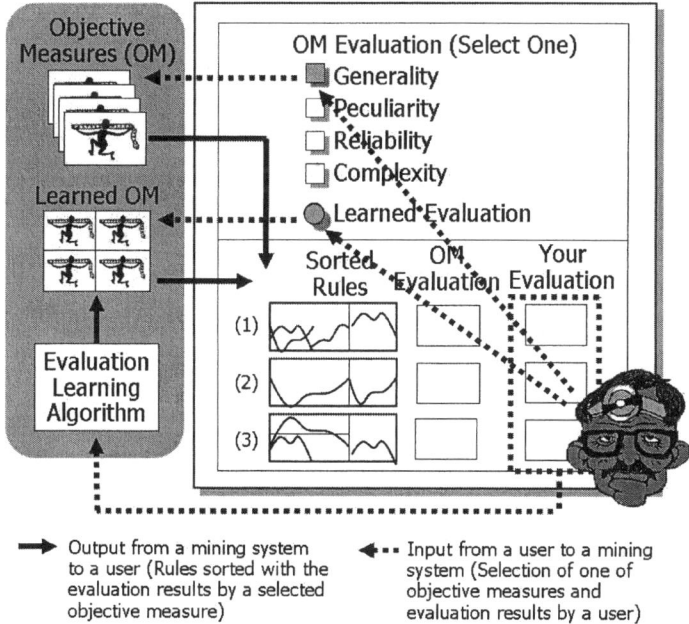

Output from a mining system
to a user (Rules sorted with the
evaluation results by a selected
objective measure)

Input from a user to a mining
system (Selection of one of
objective measures and
evaluation results by a user)

Fig. 5. Post-processing user interface utilizing objective measures

Table 4. The performance of evaluation learning algorithms in our latest research

Evaluation Learning Algorithm	First Mining				Second Mining			
	Training Data			Leave-	Training Data			Leave-
	#1	#2	#3	one-out	#1	#2	#3	one-out
C4.5	83.33	66.67	93.33	50.00	100.00	100.00	90.48	76.19
neural network	100.00	100.00	100.0	36.67	100.00	100.00	100.00	66.67
linear regression	100.00	100.00	100.00	23.33	100.00	100.00	100.00	76.19
objective measure with the highest performance	66.67	66.67	73.33	–	75.00	50.00	80.95	–

learned with a conventional learning algorithm using the evaluation results by all
objective measures in the repository as inputs and those by the human user as
outputs. The most simple method is to formulate a function, $y = f(x_1, x_2, ..., x_n)$,
where y is a evaluation result by a human user, x_i is that by i-th objective measure, and n is the number of objective measures. We can realize it with linear
regression [37] by regarding the function as a summation of weighted values of
objective measures. We also can do that with neural network by regarding the
function as a mapping among the evaluation results – Three-layered backpropagation neural network [36], which is the most popular one, will work well –.
Other method is to organize a tree structure expressing a relation among the
evaluation results with C4.5 [3].

The conceivable bottleneck is that the modeling by an evaluation learning
algorithm does not succeed due to the inadequate quality and quantity of eval-

uation results by a human user. Especially, the problem of their quantity may be serious; The number of evaluation results by a human user may be too small for machine learning. This kind of problems frequently appears in the intelligent systems including human factors such as interactive evolutionary computation [38, 32]. However, our purpose to use an evaluation learning algorithm is not highly precise modeling but roughly approximative modeling to support the thinking process of a human user through human-system interaction. Therefore, we judged that the modeling by an evaluation learning algorithm is worth trying.

In our latest research, we actually made the models with C4.5, neural network, and linear regression. We briefly report their performance estimated in the latest research using the rules and their evaluation results obtained in our past research [1] that was introduced in Section 2.1. As shown in Table 4, their performance in the first mining, which was the phase of hypothesis generation, was considerably low due to the fluctuation of evaluation by a human user. On the other, C4.5 and linear regression outperformed an objective measure with the highest performance for #1 and #2 in the second mining, which was the phase of hypothesis confirmation. These results indicates that although the modeling will not work well in the phase of hypothesis generation, that by C4.5 and linear regression as evaluation learning algorithms will work to a certain level in the phase of hypothesis confirmation.

5   Conclusions and Future Work

We investigated how objective measures can estimate real human interest in medical domain in an experiment comparing the evaluation results of rules by selected objective measures and those by a medical expert. As the experimental results, the best objective measures, χ^2 measure, recall, and accuracy had a considerably high performance. In addition to that, the objective measures used here showed a complementary relationship for each other. Therefore, it was indicated that the objective measures with the highest performance and the

Table 5. Outlines of issues in our future work

Issue (i) Investigation/analysis of objective measures and real human interest.
Sub-issue (i)-1 Experiments with different objective measures, datasets, and medical experts.
Sub-issue (i)-2 Mathematical analysis of objective measures.
Sub-issue (i)-3 Reductive analysis of real human interest using the combination of objective measures.

Issue (ii) Utilization of objective measures for KDD support based on human-system interaction.
Sub-issue (ii)-1 Development of a post-processing user interface.
Sub-issue (ii)-2 Development of a comprehensive KDD environment.

combinational use of objective measures will be useful to support medical KDD through human-system interaction. We then finally proposed a post-processing user interface utilizing objective measures and discussed how to realize it.

Our future work will be directed to two issues including some sub-issues as shown in Table 5. We describe their outlines. On Issue (i) the investigation/analysis of objective measures and real human interest, Sub-issue (i)-1 and (i)-2 are needed to generalize the current experimental results and to grasp the theoretical possibility and limitation of objective measures, respectively. Sub-issue (i)-3 is needed to establish the method to predict real human interest. We have already finished an experiment on Sub-issue (i)-1, and will show the results soon. Sub-issue (i)-2 and (i)-3 are now under discussion. The outcome of those empirical and theoretical researches will contribute to solving Issue (ii).

Issue (ii) the utilization of objective measures for KDD support based on human-system interaction, assumes that the smooth interaction between a human user and a mining system is a key to obtain really interesting rules for the human user. Our previous research in Section 2.1 [1] and others' researches using the same dataset of ours [10] led us to this assumption. We think that smooth human-system interaction stimulates the hypothesis generation and confirmation of a human user, and actually it did in our previous research. Sub-issue (ii)-1 is needed to support such a thinking process in the post-processing phase of data mining. As mentioned in Section 4, we have already developed the prototype of post-processing user interface utilizing objective measures. We will improve and evaluate it. Sub-issue (ii)-2 is the extension of Sub-issue (ii)-1; It focuses on the spiral KDD process of pre-processing, mining, and post-processing. As the one of Sub-issue (ii)-2 solutions, we are developing a comprehensive KDD environment based on constructive meta learning scheme [39, 40].

References

1. Ohsaki, M., Sato, Y., Yokoi, H., Yamaguchi, T.: A Rule Discovery Support System for Sequential Medical Data, – In the Case Study of a Chronic Hepatitis Dataset –. Proceedings of International Workshop on Active Mining AM-2002 in IEEE International Conference on Data Mining ICDM-2002 (2002) 97–102

2. Dempster, A. P., Laird,N. M., and Rubin, D. B.: Maximum Likelihood from Incomplete Data via the EM Algorithm. Journal of the Royal Statistical Society, vol.39, (1977) 1–38.

3. Quinlan, J. R.: C4.5 – Program for Machine Learning –, Morgan Kaufmann (1993).

4. MacQueen, J. B.: Some Methods for Classification and Analysis of Multivariate Observations. Proceedings of Berkeley Symposium on Mathematical Statistics and Probability, vol.1 (1967) 281–297.

5. Yao, Y. Y. Zhong, N.: An Analysis of Quantitative Measures Associated with Rules. Proceedings of Pacific-Asia Conference on Knowledge Discovery and Data Mining PAKDD-1999 (1999) 479–488

6. Hilderman, R. J., Hamilton, H. J.: Knowledge Discovery and Measure of Interest. Kluwer Academic Publishers (2001)

188   M. Ohsaki et al.

7. Tan, P. N., Kumar V., Srivastava, J.: Selecting the Right Interestingness Measure for Association Patterns. Proceedings of International Conference on Knowledge Discovery and Data Mining KDD-2002 (2002) 32–41
8. Hepatitis Dataset for Discovery Challenge. in Web Page of European Conference on Principles and Practice of Knowledge Discovery in Databases PKDD-2002 (2002) http://lisp.vse.cz/challenge/ecmlpkdd2002/
9. Hepatitis Dataset for Discovery Challenge. European Conf. on Principles and Practice of Knowledge Discovery in Databases (PKDD'03), Cavtat-Dubrovnik, Croatia (2003) http://lisp.vse.cz/challenge/ecmlpkdd2003/
10. Motoda, H. (eds.): Active Mining, IOS Press, Amsterdam, Holland (2002).
11. Das, G., King-Ip, L., Heikki, M., Renganathan, G., Smyth, P.: Rule Discovery from Time Series. Proceedings of International Conference on Knowledge Discovery and Data Mining KDD-1998 (1998) 16–22
12. Lin, J., Keogh, E., Truppel, W.: (Not) Finding Rules in Time Series: A Surprising Result with Implications for Previous and Future Research. Proceedings of International Conference on Artificial Intelligence IC-AI-2003 (2003) 55–61
13. Piatetsky-Shapiro, G.: Discovery, Analysis and Presentation of Strong Rules. in Piatetsky-Shapiro, G., Frawley, W. J. (eds.): Knowledge Discovery in Databases. AAAI/MIT Press (1991) 229–248
14. Smyth, P., Goodman, R. M.: Rule Induction using Information Theory. in Piatetsky-Shapiro, G., Frawley, W. J. (eds.): Knowledge Discovery in Databases. AAAI/MIT Press (1991) 159–176
15. Hamilton, H. J., Fudger, D. F.: Estimating DBLearn's Potential for Knowledge Discovery in Databases. Computational Intelligence, 11, 2 (1995) 280–296
16. Hamilton, H. J., Shan, N., Ziarko, W.: Machine Learning of Credible Classifications. Proceedings of Australian Conference on Artificial Intelligence AI-1997 (1997) 330–339
17. Dong, G., Li, J.: Interestingness of Discovered Association Rules in Terms of Neighborhood-Based Unexpectedness. Proceedings of Pacific-Asia Conference on Knowledge Discovery and Data Mining PAKDD-1998 (1998) 72–86
18. Gago, P., Bento, C.: A Metric for Selection of the Most Promising Rules. Proceedings of European Conference on the Principles of Data Mining and Knowledge Discovery PKDD-1998 (1998) 19–27
19. Gray, B., Orlowska, M. E.: CCAIIA: Clustering Categorical Attributes into Interesting Association Rules. Proceedings of Pacific-Asia Conference on Knowledge Discovery and Data Mining PAKDD-1998 (1998) 132–143
20. Morimoto, Y., Fukuda, T., Matsuzawa, H., Tokuyama, T., Yoda, K.: Algorithms for Mining Association Rules for Binary Segmentations of Huge Categorical Databases. Proceedings of International Conference on Very Large Databases VLDB-1998 (1998) 380–391
21. Freitas, A. A.: On Rule Interestingness Measures. Knowledge-Based Systems, vol.12, no.5 and 6 (1999) 309–315
22. Liu, H., Lu, H., Feng, L., Hussain, F.: Efficient Search of Reliable Exceptions. Proceedings of Pacific-Asia Conference on Knowledge Discovery and Data Mining PAKDD-1999 (1999) 194–203
23. Jaroszewicz, S., Simovici, D. A.: A General Measure of Rule Interestingness. Proceedings of European Conference on Principles of Data Mining and Knowledge Discovery PKDD-2001 (2001) 253–265
24. Zhong, N., Yao, Y. Y., Ohshima, M.: Peculiarity Oriented Multi-Database Mining. IEEE Transaction on Knowledge and Data Engineering, 15, 4 (2003) 952–960

25. Klementtinen, M., Mannila, H., Ronkainen, P., Toivone, H., Verkamo, A. I.: Finding Interesting Rules from Large Sets of Discovered Association Rules. Proceedings of International Conference on Information and Knowledge Management CIKM-1994 (1994) 401–407
26. Kamber, M., Shinghal, R.: Evaluating the Interestingness of Characteristic Rules. Proceedings of International Conference on Knowledge Discovery and Data Mining KDD-1996 (1996) 263–266
27. Liu, B., Hsu, W., Chen, S., Mia, Y.: Analyzing the Subjective Interestingness of Association Rules. Intelligent Systems, 15, 5 (2000) 47–55
28. Liu, B., Hsu, W., Mia, Y.: Identifying Non-Actionable Association Rules. Proceedings of International Conference on Knowledge Discovery and Data Mining KDD-2001 (2001) 329–334
29. Padmanabhan, B., Tuzhilin, A.: A Belief-Driven Method for Discovering Unexpected Patterns. Proceedings of International Conference on Knowledge Discovery and Data Mining KDD-1998 (1998) 94–100
30. Sahara, S.: On Incorporating Subjective Interestingness into the Mining Process. Proceedings of IEEE International Conference on Data Mining ICDM-2002 (2002) 681–684
31. Silberschatz, A., Tuzhilin, A.: On Subjective Measures of Interestingness in Knowledge Discovery. Proceedings of International Conference on Knowledge Discovery and Data Mining KDD-1995 (1995) 275–281
32. Terano, T., Inada, M.: Data Mining from Clinical Data using Interactive Evolutionary Computation. in Ghosh, A., Tsutsui, S. (eds.): Advances in Evolutionary Computing. Springer (2003) 847–862
33. Suzuki, E. and Shimura M.: Exceptional Knowledge Discovery in Databases Based on an Information-Theoretic Approach. Journal of Japanese Society for Artificial Intelligence, vol.12, no.2 (1997) pp.305–312 (in Japanese).
34. Hussain, F., Liu, H., and Lu, H.: Relative Measure for Mining Interesting Rules. Proceedings of Workshop (Knowledge Management: Theory and Applications) in European Conference on Principles and Practice of Knowledge Discovery in Databases PKDD-2000 (2000).
35. Suzuki, E.: Mining Financial Data with Scheduled Discovery of Exception Rules. Proceedings of Discovery Challenge in 4th European Conference on Principles and Practice of Knowledge Discovery in Databases PKDD-2000 (2000).
36. Werbos, P. J.: The Roots of Backpropagation. Wiley-Interscience (1974/1994).
37. Fox, J.: Applied Regression Analysis, Linear Models, and Related Methods. Sage Publications (1997).
38. Takagi, H.: Interactive Evolutionary Computation: Fusion of the Capacities of EC Optimization and Human Evaluation. Proceedings of the IEEE, vol.89, no.9 (2001) 1275–1296.
39. H. Abe and T. Yamaguchi: Constructing Inductive Applications by Meta-Learning with Method Repositories, Progress in Discovery Science, LNAI2281 (2002) 576–585.
40. H. Abe and T. Yamaguchi: CAMLET, http://panda.cs.inf.shizuoka.ac.jp/japanese/study/KDD/camlet/

Experimental Evaluation of
Time-Series Decision Tree

Yuu Yamada[1], Einoshin Suzuki[1], Hideto Yokoi[2], and Katsuhiko Takabayashi[2]

[1] Electrical and Computer Engineering, Yokohama National University,
79-5 Tokiwadai, Hodogaya, Yokohama 240-8501, Japan
yuu@slab.dnj.ynu.ac.jp
suzuki@ynu.ac.jp
[2] Division for Medical Informatics, Chiba-University Hospital,
1-8-1 Inohana, Chuo, Chiba, 260-8677, Japan
yokoih@telemed.ho.chiba-u.ac.jp
takaba@ho.chiba-u.ac.jp

Abstract. In this paper, we give experimental evaluation of our time-series decision tree induction method under various conditions. Our time-series tree has a value (i.e. a time sequence) of a time-series attribute in its internal node, and splits examples based on dissimilarity between a pair of time sequences. Our method selects, for a split test, a time sequence which exists in data by exhaustive search based on class and shape information. It has been empirically observed that the method induces accurate and comprehensive decision trees in time-series classification, which has gaining increasing attention due to its importance in various real-world applications. The evaluation has revealed several important findings including interaction between a split test and its measure of goodness.

1   Introduction

Time-series data are employed in various domains including politics, economics, science, industry, agriculture, and medicine. Classification of time-series data is related to many promising application problems. For instance, an accurate classifier for liver cirrhosis from time-series data of medical tests might replace a biopsy which picks liver tissue by inserting an instrument directly into liver. Such a classifier is highly important since it would substantially reduce costs of both patients and hospitals.

Conventional classification methods for time-series data can be classified into a transformation approach and a direct approach. The former maps a time sequence to another representation. The latter, on the other hand, typically relies on a dissimilarity measure between a pair of time sequences. They are further divided into those which handle time sequences that exist in data [6] and those which rely on abstracted patterns [3, 4, 7].

Comprehensiveness of a classifier is highly important in various domains including medicine. The direct approach, which explicitly handles real time se-

S. Tsumoto et al. (Eds.): AM 2003, LNAI 3430, pp. 190–209, 2005.
© Springer-Verlag Berlin Heidelberg 2005

quences, has an advantage over other approaches. In our chronic hepatitis domain, we have found that physicians tend to prefer real time sequences instead of abstracted time sequences which can be meaningless. However, conventional methods such as [6] rely on sampling and problems related with extensive computation in such methods still remained unknown.

In [15], we have proposed, for decision-tree induction, a split test which finds the "best" time sequence that exists in data with exhaustive search. Our time-series decision tree represents a novel classifier for time-series classification. Our learning method for the time-series decision tree has enabled us to discover a classifier which is highly appraised by domain experts [15]. In this paper, we perform extensive experiments based on advice from domain experts, and investigate various characteristics of our time-series decision tree.

2   Time-Series Decision Tree

2.1   Time-Series Classification

A time sequence A represents a list of values $\alpha_1, \alpha_2, \cdots, \alpha_I$ sorted in chronological order. For simplicity, this paper assumes that the values are obtained or sampled with an equivalent interval $(= 1)$.

A data set D consists of n examples e_1, e_2, $\cdots$, e_n, and each example e_i is described by m attributes a_1, a_2, $\cdots$, a_m and a class attribute c. An attribute a_j can represent a time-series attribute which takes a time sequence as its value. The class attribute c represents a nominal attribute and its value is called a class. We show an example of a data set which consists of time-series attributes in Figure 1. In time-series classification, the objective represents induction of a classifier, which predicts the class of an example e, given a training data set D.

2.2   Dissimilarity Measure Based on Dynamic Time Warping

In this section, we overview two dissimilarity measures for a pair of time sequences. The first measure represents a Manhattan distance, which is calculated by taking all the vertical differences between a pair of data points of the time sequences, and then summing their absolute values together[1]. It should be noted that Manhattan distance as well as Euclidean distance cannot be applied to a pair of time sequences with different numbers of values, and the results can be counter-intuitive [10]. The main reason lies in the fact that these measures assume a fixed vertical correspondence of values, while a human being can flexibly recognize the shape of a time sequence.

The second measure is based on Dynamic Time Warping (DTW) [8, 13]. DTW can afford non-linear distortion along the time axis since it can assign multiple values of a time sequence to a single value of the other time sequence. This measure, therefore, can not only be applied to a pair of time sequences

---

[1] We can show Euclidean distance instead of Manhattan distance. Experiments, however, showed that there is no clear winner in accuracy.

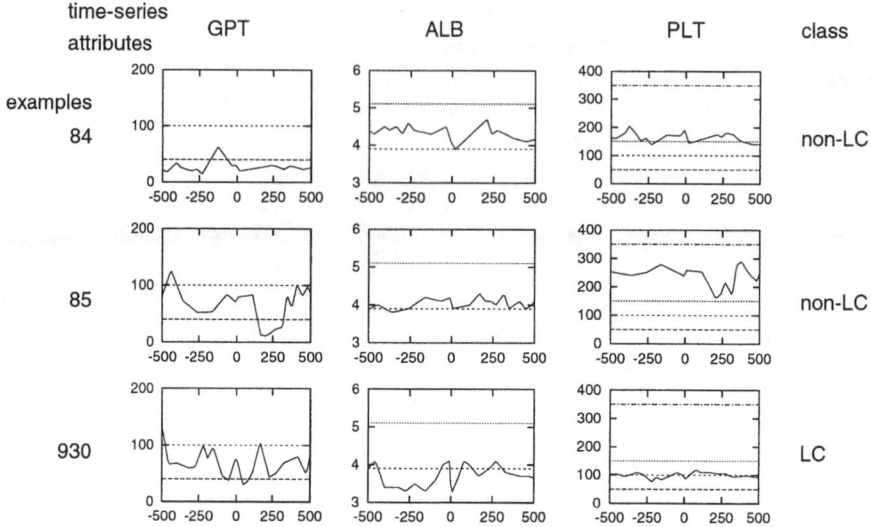

Fig. 1. Data set which consists of time-series attributes

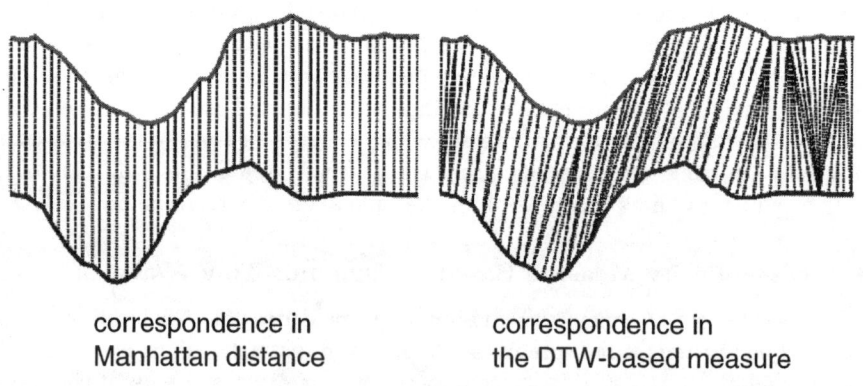

correspondence in
Manhattan distance

correspondence in
the DTW-based measure

Fig. 2. Correspondence of a pair of time sequences in the Manhattan distance and the DTW-based measure

with different numbers of values, but also fits human intuition. Figure 2 shows examples of correspondence in which the Euclidean distance and the dissimilarity measure based on DTW are employed. From the Figure, we see that the right-hand side seems more natural than the other.

Now we define the DTW-based measure $G(A, B)$ between a pair of time sequences $A = \alpha_1, \alpha_2, \cdots, \alpha_I$ and $B = \beta_1, \beta_2, \cdots, \beta_J$. The correspondence between A and B is called a warping path, and can be represented as a sequence of grids $F = f_1, f_2, \ldots, f_K$ on an $I \times J$ plane as shown in Figure 3.

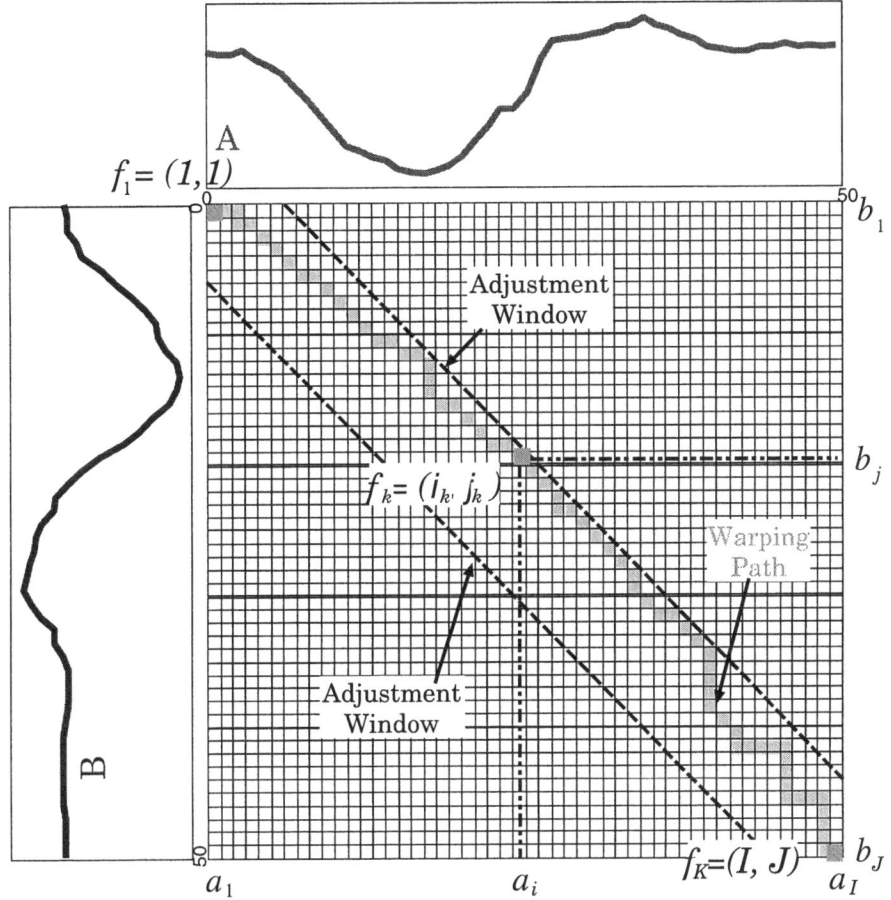

Fig. 3. Example of a warping path

Let the distance between two values α_{i_k} and β_{j_k} be $d(f_k) = |\alpha_{i_k} - \beta_{j_k}|$, then an evaluation function $\Delta(\boldsymbol{F})$ is given by $\Delta(\boldsymbol{F}) = 1/(I + J) \sum_{k=1}^{K} d(f_k)w_k$. The smaller the value of $\Delta(\boldsymbol{F})$ is, the more similar $\boldsymbol{A}$ and $\boldsymbol{B}$ are. In order to prevent excessive distortion, we assume an adjustment window $(|i_k - j_k| \leq r)$, and consider minimizing $\Delta(\boldsymbol{F})$ in terms of $\boldsymbol{F}$, where w_k is a positive weight for f_k, $w_k = (i_k - i_{k-1}) + (j_k - j_{k-1})$, $i_0 = j_0 = 0$. The minimization can be resolved without checking all possible $\boldsymbol{F}$ since dynamic programming, of which complexity is $O(IJ)$, can be employed. The minimum value of $\Delta(\boldsymbol{F})$ gives the value of $G(\boldsymbol{A}, \boldsymbol{B})$.

2.3   Learning Time-Series Decision Tree

Our time-series tree [15] has a time sequence which exists in data and an attribute in its internal node, and splits a set of examples according to the dissimilarity of their corresponding time sequences to the time sequence. The use of a time sequence which exists in data in its split node is expected to contribute to comprehensibility of the classifier, and each time sequence is obtained by exhaustive search. The dissimilarity measure is based on DTW described in section 2.2.

We call this split test a standard-example split test. A standard-example split test $\sigma(e, a, \theta)$ consists of a standard example e, an attribute a, and a threshold θ. Let a value of an example e in terms of a time-series attribute a be $e(a)$, then a standard-example split test divides a set of examples $e_1, e_2, \cdots, e_n$ to a set $S_1(e, a, \theta)$ of examples each of which $e_i(a)$ satisfies $G(e(a), e_i(a)) < \theta$ and the rest $S_2(e, a, \theta)$. We also call this split test a θ-guillotine cut.

As the goodness of a split test, we have selected gain ratio [12] since it is frequently used in decision-tree induction. Since at most $n - 1$ split points are inspected for an attribute in a θ-guillotine cut and we consider each example as a candidate of a standard example, it frequently happens that several split points exhibit the largest value of gain ratio. We assume that consideration on shapes of time sequences is essential in comprehensibility of a classifier, thus, in such a case, we define that the best split test exhibits the largest gap between the sets of time sequences in the child nodes. The gap $gap(e, a, \theta)$ of $\sigma(e, a, \theta)$ is equivalent to $G(e''(a), e(a)) - G(e'(a), e(a))$ where e' and e'' represent the example $e_i(a)$ in $S_1(e, a, \theta)$ with the largest $G(e(a), e_i(a))$ and the example $e_j(a)$ in $S_2(e, a, \theta)$ with the smallest $G(e(a), e_j(a))$ respectively. When several split tests exhibit the largest value of gain ratio, the split test with the largest $gap(e, a, \theta)$ among them is selected.

Below we show the procedure *standardExSplit* which obtains the best standard-example split test, where ω.gr and ω.gap represent the gain ratio and the gap of a split test ω respectively.

Procedure: *standardExSplit*
Input: Set of examples $e_1, e_2, \cdots, e_n$
Return value: Best split test ω
1   ω.gr $= 0$
2   **Foreach**(example e)
3   **Foreach**(time-series attribute a)
4   Sort examples $e_1, e_2, \cdots, e_n$ in the current node using $G(e(a), e_i(a))$ as a key to $\epsilon_1, \epsilon_2, \cdots, \epsilon_n$
5   **Foreach**(θ-guillotine cut ω' of $\epsilon_1, \epsilon_2, \cdots, \epsilon_n$)
6   **If** ω'.gr $> \omega$.gr
7                $\omega = \omega'$
8   **Else If** ω'.gr $== \omega$.gr **And** ω'.gap $> \omega$.gap
9                $\omega = \omega'$
10 **Return** ω

We have also proposed a cluster-example split test $\sigma'(e', e'', a)$ for comparison. A cluster-example split test divides a set of examples $e_1, e_2, \cdots, e_n$ into a set $U_1(e', e'', a)$ of examples each of which $e_i(a)$ satisfies $d(e'(a), e_i(a)) < d(e''(a), e_i(a))$ and the rest $U_2(e', e'', a)$. The goodness of a split test is equivalent to that of the standard-example split test without θ.

2.4   Conditions of the First Series of Experiments

In order to investigate the effectiveness of the proposed method, we performed experiments with real-world data sets. Chronic hepatitis data have been donated from Chiba University Hospital in Japan, and have been employed in [1]. The Australian sign language data[2] and the EEG data belong to the benchmark data sets in the UCI KDD archive [5].

For the chronic hepatitis data, we have settled a classification problem of predicting whether a patient is liver cirrhosis (the degree of fibrosis is F4 or the result of the corresponding biopsy is LC in the data). Since the patients underwent different numbers of medical tests, we have employed time sequences each of which has more than 9 test values during a period of before 500 days and after 500 days of a biopsy. As consequence, our data set consists of 30 LC-patients and 34 non-LC patients. Since the intervals of medical tests differ, we have employed liner interpolation between two adjacent values and transformed each time sequence to a time sequence of 101 values with a 10-day interval[3]. One of us, who is a physician, suggested to use in classification 14 attributes (GOT[4], GPT[5], ZTT, TTT, T-BIL, I-BIL, D-BIL, T-CHO, TP, ALB, CHE, WBC, PLT, HGB) which are important in hepatitis. We considered that the change of medical test values might be as important as the values, and have generated 14 novel attributes as follows. Each value $e(a, t)$ of an attribute a at time t is transformed to $e'(a, t)$ by $e'(a, t) = e(a, t) - \{l(e, a) + s(e, a)\}/2$, where $l(e, a)$ and $s(e, a)$ represent the maximum and the minimum value of a for e respectively. As consequence, another data set with 28 attributes was used in the experiments.

The Australian sign language data represent a record of hand position and movement of 95 words which were uttered several times by five people. In the experiments, we have chosen randomly five words "Norway", "spend", "lose", "forget", and "boy" as classes, and employed 70 examples for each class. Among the 15 attributes, 9 (x, y, z, roll, thumb, fore, index, ring, little) are employed and the number of values in a time sequence is 50[6]. The EEG data set is a record of brain waves represented in a set of 255-value time sequences obtained from 64 electrodes placed on scalps. We have agglomerated three situations for each patient and omitted examples with missing values, and obtained a data set of 192 attributes for 77 alcoholic people and 43 non-alcoholic people.

In the experiments, we tested two decision-tree learners with the standard-example split test (SE-split) and the cluster-example split test (CE-spit) presented in section 2.3. Throughout the experiments, we employed the pessimistic

---

[2] The original source is http://www.cse.unsw.edu.au/~ waleed/tml/data/.

[3] We admit that we can employ a different preprocessing method such as considering regularity of the tests.

[4] i.e. AST.

[5] i.e. ALT.

[6] For each time sequence, 50 points with an equivalent interval were generated by linear interpolation between two adjacent points.

pruning method [11] and the adjustment window r of DTW was settled to 10 % of the total length[7].

For comparative purpose, we have chosen methods presented in section 1. In order to investigate the effect of our exhaustive search and use of gaps, we tested modified versions of SE-split which select each standard example from randomly chosen 1 or 10 examples without using gaps as Random 1 and Random 10 respectively. Intuitively, the former corresponds to a decision-tree version of [6]. In our implementation of [4], the maximum number of segments was set to 3 since it outperformed the cases of 5, 7, 11. In our implementation of [7], we used average, maximum, minimum, median, and mode as global features, and Increase, Decrease, and Flat with 3 clusters and 10-equal-length discretization as its "parametrised event primitives". Av-split, and 1-NN represent the split test for the average values of time sequences, and the nearest neighbor method with the DTW-based measure respectively.

It is widely known that the performance of a nearest neighbor method largely depends on its dissimilarity measure. As the result of trial and error, the following dissimilarity measure $H(e_i, e_j)$ has been chosen since it often exhibits the highest accuracy.

$$H(e_i, e_j) = \sum_{k=1}^{m} \frac{G(e_i(a_k), e_j(a_k))}{q(a_k)},$$

where $q(a_k)$ is the maximum value of the dissimilarity measure for a time-series attribute a_k, i.e. $q(a_k) \geq \forall i \forall j \ G(e(a_i), e(a_j))$.

In the standard-example split test, the value of a gap $gap(e, a, \theta)$ largely depends on its attribute a. In the experiments, we have also tested to substitute $gap(e, a, \theta)/q(a)$ for $gap(e, a, \theta)$. We omit the results in the following sections since this normalization does not necessarily improve accuracy.

2.5   Results of the First Series of Experiments

We show the results of the experiments in Tables 1 and 2 where the evaluation methods are leave-one-out and 20×5-fold cross validation respectively. In the Tables, the size represents the average number of nodes in a decision tree, and the time is equal to {(the time for obtaining the DTW values of time sequences for all attributes and all pairs of examples) + (the time needed for leave-one-out or 20 times 5-fold cross validation)}/(the number of learned classifiers) in order to compare eager learners and a lazy learner. A PC with a 3-GHz Pentium IV CPU with 1.5G-byte memory was used in each trial. H1 and H2 represent the data sets with 14 and 28 attributes respectively both obtained from the chronic hepatitis data.

First, we briefly summarize comparison of our SE-split with other non-naive methods. From the Tables, our exhaustive search and use of gaps are justified since SE-split draws with Random 1 and 10 in accuracy but outperforms them in terms of tree sizes. Our SE-split draws with [4] in terms of these criteria but is

---

[7] A value less than 1 is round down.

Table 1. Results of experiments with leave-one-out

	accuracy (%)				time (s)				size			
method	H1	H2	Sign	EEG	H1	H2	Sign	EEG	H1	H2	Sign	EEG
SE-split	79.7	85.9	86.3	70.0	0.8	1.4	63.3	96.8	9.0	7.1	38.7	16.6
Random 1	71.9	68.8	85.7	54.2	0.2	0.5	1.2	50.9	15.6	12.9	69.5	33.7
Random 10	79.7	82.8	86.3	67.5	0.4	0.8	3.4	59.9	10.2	9.8	50.8	20.6
Geurts	75.0	78.1	-	-	26.2	41.1	-	-	10.2	9.5	-	-
Kadous	68.8	68.8	36.9	10.8	2.0	4.9	10.6	1167.0	9.2	10.8	39.5	40.0
CE-spit	65.6	73.4	85.4	63.3	1.3	1.3	1876.4	1300.5	9.4	7.2	42.8	23.4
Av-split	73.4	70.3	35.7	52.5	0.0	0.1	0.2	2.9	10.9	11.4	47.4	61.9
1-NN	82.8	84.4	97.4	60.8	0.2	0.4	0.1	47.5	N/A	N/A	N/A	N/A

Table 2. Results of experiments with 20×5-fold cross validation

	accuracy (%)				time (s)				size			
method	H1	H2	Sign	EEG	H1	H2	Sign	EEG	H1	H2	Sign	EEG
SE-split	71.1	75.6	85.9	63.8	0.5	0.8	28.3	51.1	8.3	7.5	32.5	13.4
Random 1	67.3	69.3	81.0	55.5	0.1	0.3	0.8	48.1	12.1	10.7	59.0	24.6
Random 10	73.8	72.2	84.2	60.5	0.2	0.5	2.6	64.5	9.0	8.4	41.1	16.5
Geurts	68.7	72.1	-	-	7.7	14.5	-	-	7.9	8.1	-	-
Kadous	68.1	67.7	36.2	41.1	2.1	4.7	10.4	642.9	7.9	8.7	33.5	26.8
CE-spit	69.1	69.0	86.2	58.5	0.6	1.5	966.9	530.0	7.9	7.4	36.0	19.9
Av-split	73.0	70.7	34.9	51.3	0.0	0.0	0.2	2.5	10.1	10.0	43.0	40.1
1-NN	80.9	81.5	96.6	61.8	2.2	4.4	9.3	1021.9	N/A	N/A	N/A	N/A

much faster[8]. We have noticed that [4] might be vulnerable to outliers but this should be confirmed by investigation. We attribute the poor performance of our [7] to our choice of parameter values, and consider that we need to tune them to obtain satisfactory results.

In terms of accuracy, Random 1, [7], and Av-split suffer in the EEG data set and the latter two in the Sign data set. This would suggest effectiveness of exhaustive search, small number of parameters, and explicit handling of time sequences. 1-NN exhibits high accuracy in the Sign data set and relatively low accuracy in the EEG data set. These results might come from the fact that all attributes are relevant in the sign data set while many attributes are irrelevant in the EEG data set.

CE-spit, although it handles the structure of a time sequence explicitly, almost always exhibits lower accuracy than SE-split. We consider that this is due to the fact that CE-split rarely produces pure child nodes[9] since it mainly di-

---

[8] We could not include the results of the latter for two data sets since we estimate them several months with our current implementation. Reuse of intermediate results, however, would significantly shorten time.

[9] A pure child node represents a node with examples belonging to the same class.

vides a set of examples based on their shapes. We have observed that SE-split
often produces nearly pure child nodes due to its use of the θ-guillotine cut.

Experimental results show that DTW is sometimes time-inefficient. It should
be noted that time is less important than accuracy in our problem. Recent
advances such as [9], however, can significantly speed up DTW.

In terms of the size a decision tree, SE-split, CE-split, and [4] constantly
exhibit good performance. It should be noted that SE-split and CE-split show
similar tendencies though the latter method often produces slightly larger trees
possibly due to the pure node problem. A nearest neighbor method, being a
lazy learner, has deficiency in comprehensiveness of its learned results. This
deficiency can be considered as crucial in application domains such as medicine
where interpretation of learned results is highly important.

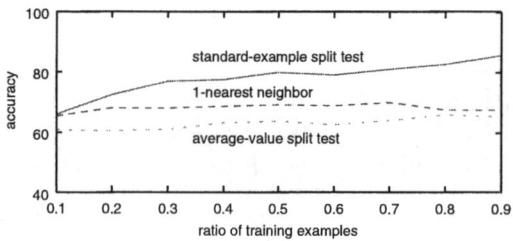

Fig. 4. Learning curve of each method for the EEG data

The difference between Tables 1 and 2 in time mainly comes from the number
of examples in the training set and the test set. The execution time of 1-NN,
being a lazy learner, is equivalent to the time of the test phase and is roughly
proportional to the number of test examples. As the result, it runs faster with
leave-one-out than 20 × 5-fold cross validation, which is the opposite tendency
of a decision-tree learner.

The accuracy of SE-split often degrades substantially with 20 × 5-fold cross
validation compared with leave-one-out. We attribute this to the fact that a
"good" example, which is selected as a standard example if it is in a training
set, belongs to the test set in 20 × 5-fold cross validation more frequently than in
leave-one-out. In order to justify this assumption, we show the learning curve[10]
of each method for EEG data, which consists of the largest number of examples
in the four data sets, in Figure 4. In order to increase the number of examples, we
counted a situation of a patient as an example. Hence an example is described by
64 attributes, and we have picked up 250 examples from each class randomly. We
omitted several methods due to their performance in Tables 1 and 2. From the
Figure, the accuracy of the decision-tree learner with the standard-example split
test degrades heavily when the number of examples is small. These experiments
show that our standard-example split test is appropriate for a data set with a
relatively large number of examples.

---

[10] Each accuracy represents an average of 20 trials.

2.6   Knowledge Discovery from the Chronic Hepatitis Data

Chronic hepatitis represents a disease in which liver cells become inflamed and harmed by virus infection. In case the inflammation lasts a long period, the disease comes to an end which is called a liver cirrhosis. During the process to a liver cirrhosis, the degree of fibrosis represents an index of the progress, and the degree of fibrosis consists of five stages ranging from F0 (no fiber) to F4 (liver cirrhosis). The degree of fibrosis can be inspected by biopsy which picks liver tissue by inserting an instrument directly into liver. A biopsy, however, cannot be frequently performed since it requires a short-term admission to a hospital and involves danger such as hemorrhage. Therefore, if a conventional medical test such as a blood test can predict the degree of fibrosis, it would be highly beneficial in medicine since it can replace a biopsy.

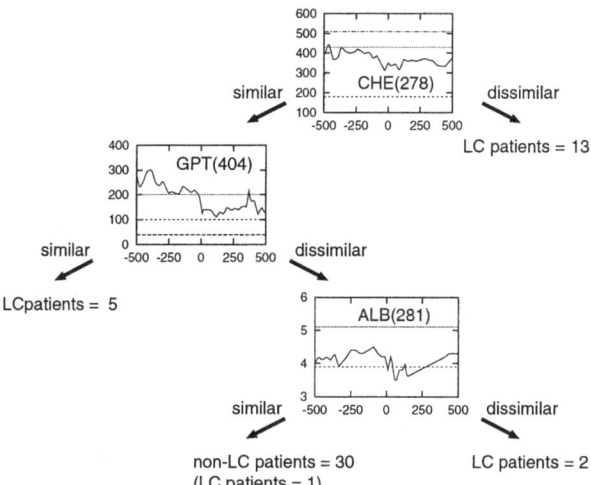

Fig. 5. Time-series tree learned from H0 (chronic hepatitis data of the first biopsies)

The classifier obtained below might realize such a story. We have prepared another data set, which we call H0, from the chronic hepatitis data by dealing with the first biopsies only. H0 consists of 51 examples (21 LC patients, and 30 non-LC patients) each of which is described with 14 attributes. Since a patient who underwent a biopsy is typically subject to various treatments such as interferon, the use of the first biopsies only enables us to analyze a more natural stage of the disease than in H1 and H2. We show the decision tree with the standard-example split test learned from H0 in Figure 5. In the Figure, a number described subsequent to an attribute in parentheses represents a patient ID, and a leaf node predicts its majority class. A horizontal dashed line in a graph represents a border value of two categories (e.g. normal and high) of the corresponding medical test.

Table 3. Experimental results with H0 using leave-one-out

method	accuracy (%)	time (s)	size
SE-split	88.2	0.5	6.9
Random 1	74.5	0.1	8.4
Random 10	78.4	0.3	7.4
Geurts	84.3	12.5	7.4
Kadous	78.4	1.6	5.1
CE-spit	62.7	0.5	8.5
Av-split	82.4	0.0	10.1
1-NN	74.5	0.1	N/A

The decision tree and the time sequences employed in the Figure have attracted interests of physicians, and were recognized as an important discovery. The time-series tree investigates potential capacity of a liver by CHE and predicts patients with low capacity as liver cirrhosis. Then the tree investigates the degree of inflammation for other patients by GPT, and predicts patients with heavy inflammation as liver cirrhosis. For other patients, the tree investigates another sort of potential capacity of a liver by ALB and predicts liver cirrhosis based on the capacity. This procedure highly agrees with routine interpretation of blood tests by physicians. Our proposed method was highly appraised by them since it discovered results which are highly consistent to knowledge of physicians by only using medical knowledge on relevant attributes. They consider that we need to verify plausibility of this classifier in terms of as much information as possible from various sources then eventually move to biological tests.

During the quest, there was an interesting debate among the authors. Yamada and Suzuki, as machine learning researchers, proposed abstracting the time sequences in Figure 5. Yokoi and Takabayashi, who are physicians, however, insisted to use time sequences that exist in the data set[11]. The physicians are afraid that such abstracted time sequences are meaningless, and claim that the use of real time sequences is appropriate from the medical point of view.

We show the results of the learning methods with H0 in Table 3. Our time-series tree outperforms other methods in accuracy[12], and in tree size except for [7]. Test of significance based on two-tailed t-distribution shows that the differences of tree sizes are statistically significant. We can safely conclude that our method outperforms other methods when both accuracy and tree sizes are considered. Moreover, inspection of mis-predicted patients in leave-one-out revealed that most of them can be considered as exceptions. This shows that our method is also effective in detecting exceptional patients.

---

[11] Other physicians supported Yokoi and Takabayashi. Anyway they are not reluctant to see the results of abstracted patterns too.

[12] By a binary test with correspondence, however, we cannot reject, for example, the hypothesis that SE-split and Av-split differ in accuracy. We need more examples to show superiority of our approach in terms of accuracy.

We obtained the following comments from medical experts who are not authors of our articles.

- The proposed learning method exhibits novelty and is highly interesting. The splits in the upper parts of the time-decision trees are valid, and the learning results are surprisingly well as a method which employs domain knowledge on attributes only.
- Medical test values which are measured after a biopsy are typically influenced by treatment such as interferon (IFN). It would be better to use only medical test values which were measured before a biopsy.
- 1000 days are long as a period of measurement since the number n of patients is small. It would be better to use shorter periods such as 365 days.
- The number of medical tests might be possibly reduced to 4 per year. Prediction from a smaller number of medical tests has a higher impact on clinical treatment[13].
- A medical expert is familiar with sensitivity, specificity, and an ROC curve as evaluation indices of a classifier. It causes more problems to overlook an LC patient than mistake a non-LC patient.

3   Experiments for Misclassification Costs

3.1   Conditions of Experiments

Based on one of the comments in the previous section, we evaluated our time-series decision tree without using medical test data after a biopsy. For a continuous attribute, C4.5 [12] employs a split test which verifies whether a value is greater than a threshold. This split test will be called an average-split test in this paper. We call our approach which employs both the standard-example split test and the average-split test a combined-split test. For the sake of comparison, we also employed the average-split test alone and a line-split test, which replaces a standard example by a line segment. A line segment in the latter method is obtained by discretizing test values by an equal-frequency method with $\alpha - 1$ bins, and connecting two points (l_1, p_1) and (l_2, p_2) where l_1 and l_2 represent the beginning and the end of a measurement respectively. Each of p_1 and p_2 represents one of the end values of discretized bins. For instance, it considers 25 line segments if $\alpha = 5$. The cluster-example split test was not employed since it exhibited poor performance in section 2.

We show a confusion matrix in Table 4. As the domain experts stated, it is important to decrease the number FN of overlooked LC patients than the number FP of mistaken non-LC patients. Therefore, we employ sensitivity, specificity, and (misclassification) cost in addition to predictive accuracy as evaluation indices. The added indices are considered to be important in the following order.

$$Cost = \frac{C\ FN + FP}{C(TP + FN) + (TN + FP)} \qquad (1)$$

---

[13] We admit that this remains for future work.

Table 4. Confusion matrix

	LC	non-LC
LC (Prediction)	TP	FP
non-LC (Prediction)	FN	TN

Table 5. Data sets employed in the experiments

experiments for	data (# of non-LC patients : # of LC patients)
the number of medical tests	180BCp6i5 (68:23), 180BCp3i5 (133:40), 180BCp2i5 (149:42)
the selected period	90BCp3i5 (120:38), 180BCp6i5 (68:23), 270BCp9i5 (39:15), 360BCp12i5 (18:13)
the interpolation interval	180BCp6i2, 180BCp6i4, 180BCp6i6, 180BCp6i8, 180BCp6i10 (all 68:23)

$$Sensitivity \text{ (True Positive Rate)} = \frac{TP}{TP + FN} \tag{2}$$

$$Specificity \text{ (True Negative Rate)} = \frac{TN}{TN + FP} \tag{3}$$

where C represents a user-specified weight. We settled $C = 5$ throughout the experiments, and employed a leave-one-out method. Note that $Cost$ is normalized in order to facilitate comparison of experimental results from different data sets.

It is reported that Laplace correction is effective in decision tree induction for cost-sensitive classification [2]. We obtained the probability $\Pr(a)$ of a class a when there are $\nu(a)$ examples of a among ν examples as follows.

$$\Pr(a) = \frac{\nu(a) + l}{\nu + 2l} \tag{4}$$

where l represents a parameter of the Laplace correction. We settled $l = 1$ unless stated.

We modified data selection criteria in each series of experiments and prepared various data sets as shown in Table 5. In a name of a data set, the first figure represents the number of days of the selected period of measurement before a biopsy, the figure subsequent to a "p" represents the number of required medical tests, and the figure subsequent to an "i" represents the number of days of an interval in interpolation. Since we employed both B-type patients and C-type patients in all experiments, each name of a data set contains a string "BC". Since we had obtained novel data of biopsies after [15], we employed an integrated version in the experiments.

3.2   Experimental Results

Firstly, we modified the required number of medical tests to 6, 3, 2 under a 180-day period and a 5-day interpolation interval. We show the results in

Table 6. Results of experiments for test numbers, where data sets p6, p3, and p2 represent 180BCp6i5, 180BCp3i5, and 180BCp2i5 respectively

method	accuracy (%)			size			cost			sensitivity			specificity		
	p6	p3	p2	p6	p3	p2	p6	p3	p2	p6	p3	p2	p6	p3	p2
Combined	78.0	75.7	80.6	10.9	20.5	18.9	0.35	0.35	0.33	0.52	0.53	0.52	0.87	0.83	0.89
Average	83.5	82.1	87.4	3.2	24.7	7.4	0.39	0.27	0.27	0.39	0.63	0.57	0.99	0.88	0.96
Line	84.6	82.7	85.9	9.0	22.7	3.6	0.30	0.27	0.34	0.57	0.63	0.43	0.94	0.89	0.98

Table 7. Results for accuracy, size, and cost of experiments for periods, where data sets 90, 180, 270, and 360 represent 90BCp3i5, 180BCp6i5, 270BCp9i5, and 360BCp12i5 respectively

method	accuracy (%)				size				cost			
	90	180	270	360	90	180	270	360	90	180	270	360
Combined	77.8	78.0	64.8	45.2	19.5	10.9	8.5	5.5	0.36	0.35	0.52	0.69
Average	79.7	83.5	79.6	71.0	23.7	3.2	8.7	6.4	0.30	0.39	0.41	0.40
Line	77.2	84.6	74.1	48.4	18.7	9.0	8.7	6.5	0.41	0.30	0.40	0.58

Table 8. Results for sensitivity and specificity of experiments for periods

method	sensitivity				specificity			
	90	180	270	360	90	180	270	360
Combined	0.50	0.52	0.33	0.23	0.87	0.87	0.77	0.61
Average	0.61	0.39	0.40	0.54	0.86	0.99	0.95	0.83
Line	0.39	0.57	0.47	0.38	0.89	0.94	0.85	0.56

Table 9. Results for accuracy, size, and cost of experiments for intervals, where data sets i2, i4, i6, i8, and i10 represent 180BCp6i2, 180BCp6i4, 180BCp6i6, 180BCp6i8, and 180BCp6i10 respectively

method	accuracy (%)					size					cost				
	i2	i4	i6	i8	i10	i2	i4	i6	i8	i10	i2	i4	i6	i8	i10
Combined	85.7	85.7	82.4	81.3	82.4	10.9	10.9	12.4	12.3	12.4	0.29	0.31	0.33	0.33	0.33
Average	84.6	84.6	83.5	84.6	82.4	3.0	3.0	3.2	3.9	5.1	0.36	0.36	0.39	0.36	0.39
Line	85.7	83.5	83.5	84.6	79.1	9.0	9.0	8.9	9.1	11.2	0.29	0.32	0.32	0.30	0.32

Table 6. From the Table, we see that the average-split test and the line-split test outperform other methods in cost for p2 and p6 respectively. For p3, the methods exhibit the same cost and outperform our standard-example split test. We believe that the poor performance of our method is due to lack of information on shapes of time sequences and the number of examples. We interpret the results that lack of the former information in p2 favors the average-split test, while lack of the latter information in p6 favors the line-split test. If simplicity

Table 10. Results for sensitivity and specificity of experiments for intervals

method	sensitivity					specificity				
	i2	i4	i6	i8	i10	i2	i4	i6	i8	i10
Combined	0.57	0.52	0.52	0.52	0.52	0.96	0.97	0.93	0.91	0.93
Average	0.43	0.43	0.39	0.43	0.39	0.99	0.99	0.99	0.99	0.97
Line	0.57	0.52	0.52	0.57	0.57	0.96	0.94	0.94	0.94	0.87

Table 11. Results of experiments for Laplace correction values with 180BCp6i6, where methods C, A, and L represent Combined, Average, and Line respectively

value	accuracy (%)			size			cost			sensitivity			specificity		
	C	A	L	C	A	L	C	A	L	C	A	L	C	A	L
0	86.8	85.7	82.4	10.9	10.8	7.4	0.28	0.29	0.33	0.57	0.57	0.52	0.97	0.96	0.93
1	82.4	83.5	83.5	12.4	3.2	8.9	0.33	0.39	0.32	0.52	0.39	0.52	0.93	0.99	0.94
2	81.3	83.5	80.2	9.1	3.0	9.0	0.36	0.39	0.38	0.48	0.39	0.43	0.93	0.99	0.93
3	83.5	73.6	83.5	9.1	2.5	9.0	0.30	0.63	0.34	0.57	0.00	0.48	0.93	0.99	0.96
4	81.3	83.5	79.1	9.2	2.6	8.9	0.36	0.39	0.39	0.48	0.39	0.43	0.93	0.99	0.91
5	82.4	83.5	82.4	9.1	2.7	8.9	0.35	0.39	0.37	0.48	0.39	0.43	0.94	0.99	0.96

of a classifier is also considered, the decision tree learned with the average-split test from p2 would be judged as the best.

Secondly, we modified the selected period to 90, 180, 270, 360 days under an interpolation interval 5 days and the number of required medical tests per 30 days 1. We show the results in Tables 7 and 8. From Table 7, we see that the average-split test and the line-split test almost always outperform our standard-example split test in cost though there is no clear winner between them. We again attribute these to lack of information on shapes of time sequences and the number of examples. Our standard-example split test performs relatively well for 90 and 180 and this would be due to their relatively large numbers of examples. If simplicity of a classifier is also considered, the decision tree learned with the line-split test from 180 would be judged as the best.

Thirdly, we modified the interpolation intervals to 2, 4, $\cdots$, 10 days under a 180-day period and the required number of medical tests 6. We show the results in Tables 9 and 10. From Table 9, we see that our standard-example split test and the line-split test outperform the average-split test in cost though there is no clear winner between them. Since a 180 in Tables 7 and 8 represents 180BCp6i5, it would be displayed as i5 in this Table. Our poor performance of cost 0.35 for i5 shows that our method exhibits good performance for small and large intervals, and this fact requires further investigation. If simplicity of a classifier is also considered, the line-split test is judged as the best and we again attribute this to lack of information for our method.

Lastly, we modified the Laplace correction parameter l to 0, 1, $\cdots$, 5 under a 180-day period, the required number of medical tests 6, and a 6-day interpolation interval. We show the results in Table 11. From the Table, we see that the Laplace correction increases cost for our standard-example split test and the line-split test contrary to our expectation. Even for the average-split test, the case without the Laplace correction ($l = 0$) rivals the best case with the Laplace correction ($l = 1$). The Table shows that these come from the fact that the Laplace correction lowers sensitivity but this requires further investigation.

3.3   Analysis of Experiments

First of all, our time-series tree uses time sequences which exist in data thus is free from the problem of using a time sequence which can be meaningless. However, its predictive power is not as high as we have expected[14].

In the experiments of section 2, we employed longer time sequences and a larger number of training examples than in this paper. It should be also noted that the class ratio in section 2 was nearly equivalent. We believe that our time-series decision tree is adequate for this kind of classification problems. The classification problems in this section, since they neglect medical tests data after a biopsy, exhibit opposite characteristics, favoring a robust method such as the average-split test. Though it is appropriate to neglect medical tests data after a biopsy from medical viewpoint, the effect is negative for our time-series decision tree.

The decision trees which were constructed using the split tests contain many LC-leaves, especially those with the combined-split test. Most of the leaves contain a small number of training examples, thus they rarely correspond to a test example. This observation led us to consider modifying tree-structures in order to decrease cost.

4   Experiments for Goodness of a Split Test

4.1   Motivations

From the discussions in the previous section, we considered to use the medical tests data after a biopsy and to replace gain ratio by gain. The former was realized by using the data sets employed in section 2. For the latter, consider their characteristics as goodness of a split test with tests 1 and 2 in Table 12. Tests 1 and 2 are selected with gain ratio and gain respectively. As stated in [12], gain ratio tends to select an unbalanced split test where a child node has an extremely small number of examples. We believe that example 1 corresponds to this case and decided to perform a systematic comparison of the two criteria.

4.2   Experiments

We have compared our standard-example split test, the cluster-example split test, the average-split test, a method by Geurts [4], and a method by Kadous [7]. We settled $N_{max} = 5$ in the method of Geurts, and the number of discretized

---

[14] It should be noted that the obtained accuracy can be counter-intuitive in this kind of experiments.

Table 12. Two examples of a split test

Split test	Left	Right	gain	gain ratio
test 1	6 (0, 6)	113 (76, 37)	0.078	0.269
test 2	47 (42, 5)	72 (34, 38)	0.147	0.152

Table 13. Experimental results with gain and gain ratio

method	goodness	accuracy (%) H1	H2	size H1	H2	cost H1	H2	sensitivity H1	H2	specificity H1	H2
SE-split	gain	64.1	78.1	10.6	7.2	0.34	0.25	0.67	0.73	0.62	0.82
	gain ratio	79.7	85.9	9.0	7.1	0.24	0.18	0.73	0.80	0.85	0.91
CE-split	gain	81.2	76.6	9.0	8.7	0.20	0.23	0.80	0.77	0.82	0.76
	gain ratio	65.6	73.4	9.4	7.2	0.36	0.31	0.63	0.67	0.68	0.79
AV-split	gain	79.7	79.7	7.8	10.8	0.22	0.24	0.77	0.73	0.82	0.85
	gain ratio	73.4	70.3	10.9	11.4	0.31	0.39	0.67	0.57	0.79	0.82
Geurts	gain	68.8	70.3	10.1	9.7	0.28	0.32	0.73	0.67	0.65	0.74
	gain ratio	71.9	67.2	10.0	9.2	0.29	0.29	0.70	0.73	0.74	0.62
Kadous	gain	65.6	62.5	12.6	12.0	0.38	0.41	0.60	0.57	0.71	0.68
	gain ratio	71.9	65.6	8.8	13.2	0.29	0.27	0.70	0.77	0.74	0.56
1-NN		82.8	84.4	N/A	N/A	0.19	0.18	0.80	0.80	0.85	0.88

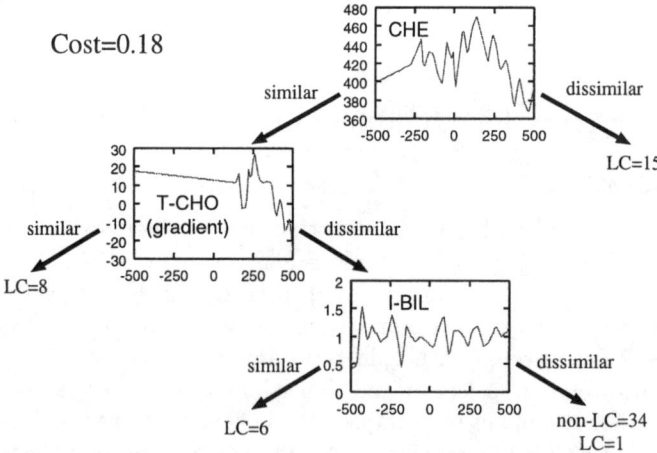

Fig. 6. SE-split decision tree (H2, GainRatio)

bins 5 and the number of clusters 5 in the method of Kadous. Experiments were performed with a leave-one-out method, and without the Laplace correction.

We show the results in Table 13, and the decision trees learned from all data with the standard-example split test, the cluster-example split test, and the average-split test in Figures 6, 7, and 8 respectively. The conditions are chosen so that each of them exhibits the lowest cost for the corresponding method.

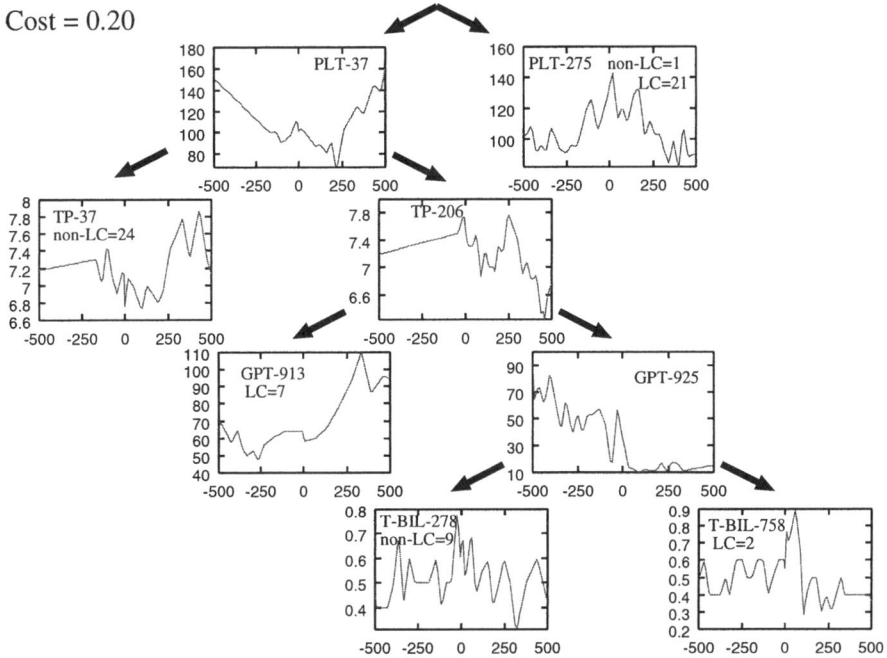

Fig. 7. CE-split decision tree (H1, Gain)

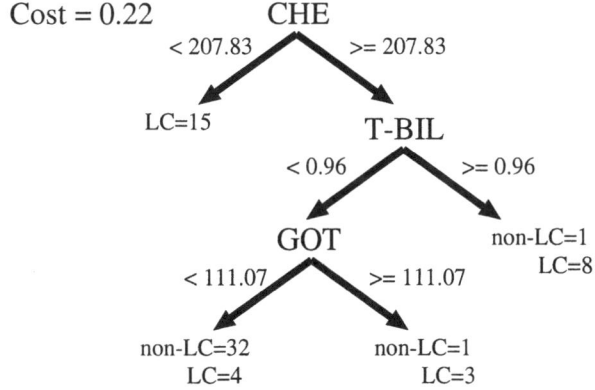

Fig. 8. AV-split decision tree (H1, Gain)

From the Table, we see that our standard-example split test performs better with gain ratio, and the cluster-example split test and the average-split test perform better with gain. We think that the former is due to affinity of gain ratio, which tends to select an unbalanced split, to our standard-example split test, which splits examples based on their similarities or dissimilarities to its standard example. Similarly, we think that the latter is due to affinity of gain, which is known to exhibit no such tendency, to the cluster-example split test and the average-split test, both of which consider characteristics of two children nodes in split. Actually, we have confirmed that a split test tends to produce a small-sized leaf with gain ratio while a split test tends to construct a relatively balanced split with gain.

5   Conclusions

For our time-series decision tree, we have investigated the case in which medical tests before a biopsy are neglected and the case in which goodness of a split test is altered. In the former case, our time-series decision tree is outperformed by simpler decision trees in misclassification cost due to lack of information on sequences and examples. In the latter case, our standard-example split test performs better with gain ratio, and the cluster-example split test and the average-split test perform better with gain probably due to affinities in each combination. We plan to extend our approach as both a cost-sensitive learner and a discovery method.

In applying a machine learning algorithm to real data, one often encounters the problems of quantity, quality, and form. Data are massive (quantity), noisy (quality), and in various shapes (form). Recently, the third problem has motivated several researchers to propose classification from structured data including time-series, and we believe that this tendency will continue in the near future.

Information technology in medicine has spread its target to multimedia data such as time-series data and image data from string data and numerical data in the last decade, and aims to support the whole process of medicine which handles various types of data [14]. Our decision-tree induction method which handles the shape of a time sequence explicitly, has succeeded in discovering results which were highly appraised by physicians. We anticipate that there is a long way toward an effective classification method which handles various structures of multimedia data explicitly, but our method can be regarded as an important step toward this objective.

Acknowledgement

This work was partially supported by the grant-in-aid for scientific research on priority area "Active Mining" from the Japanese Ministry of Education, Culture, Sports, Science and Technology.

References

1. P. Berka. ECML/PKDD 2002 discovery challenge, download data about hepatitis. http://lisp.vse.cz/challenge/ ecmlpkdd2002/, 2002. (current September 28th, 2002).

2. J. P. Bradford, C. Kunz, R. Kohavi, C. Brunk, and C. E. Brodley. Pruning decision trees with misclassification costs. In *Proc. Tenth European Conference on Machine Learning (ECML)*, pages 131–136. 1998.

3. C. Drücker et al. "as time goes by" - using time series based decision tree induction to analyze the behaviour of opponent players. In *RoboCup 2001: Robot Soccer World Cup V, LNAI 2377*, pages 325–330. 2002.

4. P. Geurts. Pattern extraction for time series classification. In *Principles of Data Mining and Knowledge Discovery (PKDD), LNAI 2168*, pages 115–127. 2001.

5. S. Hettich and S. D. Bay. The UCI KDD archive. http://kdd.ics.uci.edu, 1999. Irvine, CA: University of California, Department of Information and Computer Science.

6. J. J. Rodríguez, C. J. Alonso, and H. Bostrvm. Learning first order logic time series classifiers. In *Proc. Work-in-Progress Track at the Tenth International Conference on Inductive Logic Programming*, pages 260–275. 2000.

7. M. W. Kadous. Learning comprehensible descriptions of multivariate time series. In *Proc. Sixteenth International Conference on Machine Learning (ICML)*, pages 454–463. 1999.

8. E. J. Keogh. Mining and indexing time series data. http://www.cs.ucr.edu/%7Eeamonn/tutorial_on_time_series.ppt, 2001. Tutorial at the 2001 IEEE International Conference on Data Mining (ICDM).

9. E. J. Keogh. Exact indexing of dynamic time warping. In *Proc. 28th International Conference on Very Large Data Bases*, pages 406–417. 2002.

10. E. J. Keogh and M. J. Pazzani. Scaling up dynamic time warping for datamining application. In *Proc. Sixth ACM SIGKDD International Conference on Knowledge Discovery and Data Mining (KDD)*, pages 285–289. 2000.

11. J. Mingers. An empirical comparison of pruning methods for decision tree induction. *Machine Learning*, 4, 1989.

12. J. R. Quinlan. *C4.5: Programs for Machine Learning*. Morgan Kaufmann, San Mateo, Calif., 1993.

13. H. Sakoe and S. Chiba. Dynamic programming algorithm optimization for spoken word recognition. *IEEE Transaction on Acoustics, Speech, and Signal Processing*, ASSP-26, 1978.

14. H. Tanaka. *Electronic Patient Record and IT Medical Treatment*. MED, Tokyo, 2001. (in Japanese).

15. Y. Yamada, E. Suzuki, H. Yokoi, and K. Takabayashi. Decision-tree induction from time-series data based on a standard-example split test. In *Proc. Twentieth International Conference on Machine Learning (ICML)*, pages 840–847. 2003.

Spiral Multi-aspect Hepatitis Data Mining

Muneaki Ohshima[1], Tomohiro Okuno[1], Yasuo Fujita[1],
Ning Zhong[1], Juzhen Dong[1], and Hideto Yokoi[2]

[1] Dept. of Information Engineering, Maebashi Institute of Technology,
460-1 Kamisadori-cho, Maebashi 371-0816, Japan
[2] School of Medicine, Chiba University,
1-8-1 Inohana, Chuo-ku, Chiba 260-8677, Japan

Abstract. When therapy using IFN (interferon) medication for chronic hepatitis patients, various conceptual knowledge/rules will benefit for giving a treatment. The paper describes our work on cooperatively using various data mining agents including the GDT-RS inductive learning system for discovering decision rules, the LOI (learning with ordered information) for discovering ordering rules and important features, as well as the POM (peculiarity oriented mining) for finding peculiarity data/rules, in a spiral discovery process with multi-phase such as pre-processing, rule mining, and post-processing, for multi-aspect analysis of the hepatitis data and meta learning. Our methodology and experimental results show that the perspective of medical doctors will be changed from a single type of experimental data analysis towards a holistic view, by using our *multi-aspect mining* approach.

1 Introduction

Multi-aspect mining in a multi-phase KDD (Knowledge Discovery and Data Mining) process is an important methodology for knowledge discovery from real-life data [5, 22, 26, 27]. There are two main reasons why a multi-aspect mining approach needs to be used for hepatitis data analysis.

The first reason is that we cannot expect to develop a single data mining algorithm for analyzing all main aspects of the hepatitis data towards a holistic view because of complexity of the real-world applications. Hence, various data mining agents need to be cooperatively used in the multi-phase data mining process for performing multi-aspect analysis as well as multi-level conceptual abstraction and learning.

The other reason is that when performing multi-aspect analysis for complex problems such as hepatitis data mining, a data mining task needs to be decomposed into sub-tasks. Thus these sub-tasks can be solved by using one or more data mining agents that are distributed over different computers. Thus the decomposition problem leads us to the problem of distributed cooperative system design.

More specifically, when therapy using IFN (interferon) medication for chronic hepatitis patients, various conceptual knowledge/rules will benefit for giving a

S. Tsumoto et al. (Eds.): AM 2003, LNAI 3430, pp. 210–235, 2005.

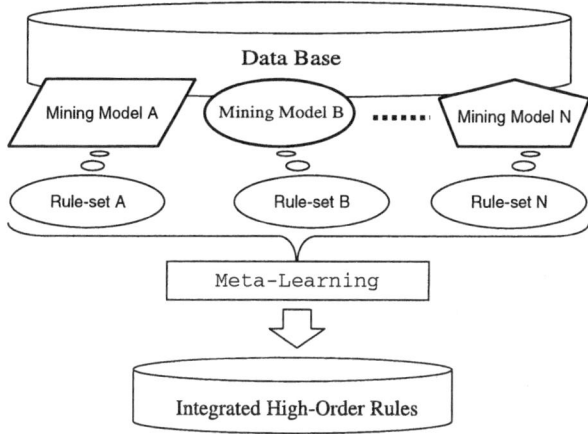

Fig. 1. A general model for multi-aspect mining and meta learning

treatment. The knowledge/rules, for instance, include (1) when the IFN should be used for a patient so that he/she will be able to be cured, (2) what kinds of inspections are important for a diagnosis, and (3) whether some peculiar data/patterns exist or not.

The paper describes our work on cooperatively using various data mining agents including the GDT-RS inductive learning system for discovering decision rules [23, 28], the LOI (learning with ordered information) for discovering ordering rules and important features [15, 29], as well as the POM (peculiarity oriented mining) for finding peculiarity data/rules [30], for multi-aspect analysis of the hepatitis data so that such rules mentioned above can be discovered automatically. Furthermore, by meta learning, the rules discovered by LOI and POM can be used to improve the quality of decision rules discovered by GDT-RS. Figure 1 gives a general model of our methodology for multi-aspect mining and meta learning.

We emphasize that both pre-processing/post-processing steps are important before/after using data mining agents. In particular, informed knowledge discovery, in general, uses background knowledge obtained from experts (e.g. medical doctors) about a domain (e.g. chronic hepatitis) to guide a spiral discovery process with multi-phase such as pre-processing, rule mining, and post-processing, towards finding interesting and novel rules/features hidden in data. Background knowledge may be of several forms including rules already found, taxonomic relationships, causal preconditions, ordered information, and semantic categories.

In our experiments, the result of the blood test of the patients, who received laboratory examinations before starting the INF treatment, is first pre-treated. After that, the pre-processed data are used for each data mining agent, respectively. By using the GDT-RS, the decision rules with respect to knowing whether a medical treatment is effective or not, can be found. And, by using the LOI, what attributes affect the medical treatment of hepatitis C greatly can be investigated. Furthermore, peculiar data/patterns with a positive/negative meaning can be checked out by using POM for finding interesting rules and/or data cleaning. Our methodology and experimental results show that the perspective of medical doctors will be changed from a single type of experimental data analysis towards a holistic view, by using our multi-aspect mining approach.

The rest of the paper is organized as follows. Section 2 describes how to preprocess the hepatitis data and decide the threshold values for condition attributes according to the background knowledge obtained from medical doctors. Section 3 gives an introduction to GDT-RS and discusses main results mined by using the GDT-RS and post-processing, which are based on a medical doctor's advice and comments. Then in Sections 4 and 5, we extend our system by adding the LOI (learning with ordered information) and POM (peculiarity oriented mining) data mining agents, respectively, for multi-aspect mining and meta learning. Finally, Section 6 gives concluding remarks.

2   Pre-processing

2.1   Selection of Inspection Data and Class Determination

We use the following conditions to extract inspection data.

- Patients of chronic hepatitis type C who may be medicated with IFN.
- Patients with the data of judging the IFN effect by using whether a hepatitis virus exists or not.
- Patients with inspection data that are collected in one year before IFN is used.

Thus, 197 patients with 11 condition attributes as shown in Table 1 are selected and will be used in our data mining agents.

Furthermore, the decision attribute (i.e. classes) is selected according to a result of judging the IFN effect by using whether a hepatitis virus exists or not. Hence, the 197 extracted patients can be classified into 3 classes as shown in Table 2.

2.2   Evaluation of Condition Attributes

As shown in Fig. 2, the condition attributes are evaluated as follows.

1. All the inspection values in one year before IFN is used for each patient are divided into two groups, the first half and the second half of the inspection values.

Table 1. Condition attributes selected

T-CHO	CHE	ALB	TP
T-BIL	D-BIL	I-BIL	PLT
WBC	HGB	GPT	

Table 2. The decision attribute (classes)

class	The condition of the patient after IFN	# of patients
R	Disappearance of the virus	58
N	Existence of virus	86
?	Reliability lack of data	53

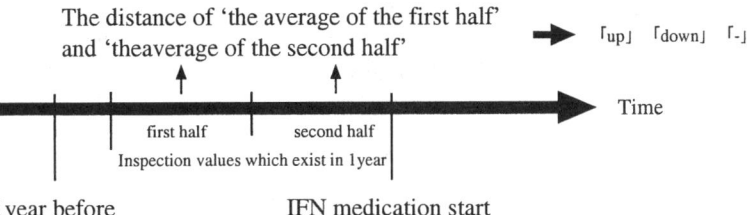

Fig. 2. The evaluation method of condition attributes

2. When the absolute value of the difference between average values of the first half and the second half of the inspection values exceeds the threshold, it is estimated as up or down. Otherwise, it is estimated as "–" (i.e. no change). Moreover, it is estimated as "?" in the case where not inspection data or only once (i.e. a patient is examined only once).

Furthermore, the threshold values can be decided as follows.

– **The threshold values for each attribute except GPT** are set up to 10% of the normal range of each inspection data. As the change of a hepatitis patient's GPT value will exceed the normal range greatly, the threshold value for the GPT needs to be calculated in a more complex method to be described below. The threshold values used for evaluating each condition attribute is shown in Table 3.

– **The threshold value for GPT** is calculated as follows. As shown in Fig. 3, the standard deviation of the difference of the adjacent test values of each hepatitis patient's GPT is first calculated, respectively; And then the standard deviation of such standard deviation is used as a threshold value.

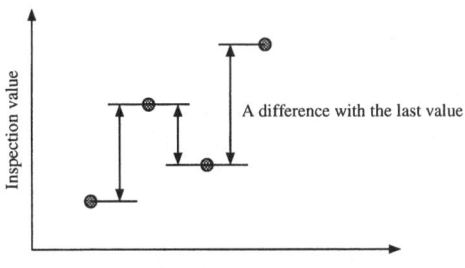

Fig. 3. Standard deviation of the difference of adjacent values

Table 3. The threshold values for evaluating condition attributes

T-CHO > 9.5	CHE > 25	ALB > 0.12	TP > 0.17
T-BIL > 0.1	D-BIL > 0.03	I-BIL > 0.07	PLT > 20
WBC > 0.5	HGB > 0.6	GPT > 54.56	

In the GPT test, let m be the number of patients, $t_m (1 \leq m \leq M)$ the time of test (that may be different for each patient), $d_{mi}(1 \leq i \leq t_m - 1)$ the difference of adjacent test values. Thus, the threshold value of GPT can be calculated in the following equation.

$$\text{threshold of GPT} = \sqrt{\frac{1}{M} \sum_{m=1}^{M} (s_m - \bar{s})^2} \qquad (1)$$

where $s_m (1 \leq m \leq M)$ is the standard deviation of the difference d_{mi} of the test value that is calculated for each patient, respectively, and $\bar{s}$ is the average value of s_m.

Finally, the threshold values are set up as shown in Table 3.

3   Miming by GDT-RS

3.1   GDT-RS

GDT-RS is a soft hybrid induction system for discovering decision rules from databases with uncertain and incomplete data [23, 28]. The system is based on a hybridization of the *Generalization Distribution Table (GDT)* and the *Rough Set* methodology. We recall some principles of GDT-RS to understand this application.

The main features of GDT-RS are the following:

- Biases for search control can be selected in a flexible way. Background knowledge can be used as a bias to control the initiation of GDT and in the rule discovery process.
- The rule discovery process is oriented toward inducing rules with high quality of classification of unseen instances. The rule uncertainty, including the ability to predict unseen instances, can be explicitly represented by the rule strength.
- A minimal set of rules with the minimal (semi-minimal) description length, having large strength, and covering of all instances can be generated.
- Interesting rules can be induced by selecting a discovery target and class transformation.

Generalization Distribution Table (GDT). We distinguish two kinds of attributes, namely: *condition* attributes and *decision* attributes (sometimes called class attributes) in a database. Condition attributes are used to describe possible instances in GDT while the decision attributes correspond to concepts (classes) described in a rule. Usually a single decision attribute is all what is required.

Any GDT consists of three components: *possible instances, possible generalizations* of instances, and *probabilistic relationships* between possible instances and possible generalizations.

Possible instances, represented at the top row of GDT, are defined by all possible combinations of attribute values from a database. *Possible generalizations* of instances, represented by the left column of a GDT, are all possible cases of generalization for all possible instances. A wild card "$*$" denotes the generalization for instances [1]. For example, the generalization $*b_0c_0$ means that the attribute a is superfluous (irrelevant) for the concept description. In other words, if an attribute a takes values from $\{a_0, a_1\}$ and both $a_0b_0c_0$ and $a_1b_0c_0$ describe the same concept, the attribute a is superfluous, i.e., the concept can be described by b_0c_0. Hence, we use the generalization $*b_0c_0$ to describe the set $\{a_0b_0c_0, a_1b_0c_0\}$.

The *probabilistic relationships* between possible instances and possible generalizations, represented by entries G_{ij} of a given GDT, are defined by means of a probabilistic distribution describing the strength of the relationship between any possible instance and any possible generalization. The prior distribution is assumed to be uniform, if background knowledge is not available. Thus, it is defined by Eq. (2)

$$G_{ij} = p(PI_j|PG_i) = \begin{cases} \dfrac{1}{N_{PG_i}} & \text{if } PI_j \in PG_i \\ \\ 0 & \text{otherwise} \end{cases} \tag{2}$$

where PI_j is the j-th possible instance, PG_i is the i-th possible generalization, and N_{PG_i} is the number of the possible instances satisfying the i-th possible generalization, i.e.,

$$N_{PG_i} = \prod_{k \in \{l|\ PG_i[l]=*\}} n_k \tag{3}$$

where $PG_i[l]$ is the value of the l-th attribute in the possible generalization PG_i and n_k is the number of values of k-th attribute. Certainly we have $\sum_j G_{ij} = 1$ for any i.

Assuming $E = \prod_{k=1}^m n_k$ the equation Eq. (2) can be rewritten in the following form:

$$G_{ij} = p(PI_j|PG_i) = \begin{cases} \dfrac{\displaystyle\prod_{k \in \{l|\ PG_i[l]\neq*\}} n_k}{E} & \text{if } PI_j \in PG_i \\ \\ 0 & \text{otherwise.} \end{cases} \tag{4}$$

Furthermore, rule discovery can be constrained by three types of biases corresponding to three components of the GDT so that a user can select more

---

[1] For simplicity, the wild card will be sometimes omitted in the paper.

general concept descriptions from an upper level or more specific ones from a lower level, adjust the strength of the relationship between instances and their generalizations, and define/select possible instances.

Rule Strength. Let us recall some basic notions for rule discovery from databases represented by decision tables [10]. A decision table (DT) is a tuple $T = (U, A, C, D)$, where U is a nonempty finite set of objects called the universe, A is a nonempty finite set of primitive attributes, and $C, D \subseteq A$ are two subsets of attributes that are called condition and decision attributes, respectively [14, 16]. By $IND(B)$ we denote the indiscernibility relation defined by $B \subseteq A$, $[x]_{IND(B)}$ denotes the indiscernibility (equivalence) class defined by x, and U/B the set of all indiscernibility classes of $IND(B)$. A descriptor over $B \subseteq A$ is any pair (a, v) where $a \in A$ and v is a value of a. If P is a conjunction of some descriptors over $B \subseteq A$ then by $[P]_B$ (or $[P]$) we denote the set of all objects in DT satisfying P.

In our approach, the rules are expressed in the following form:

$$P \rightarrow Q \text{ with } S$$

i.e., "**if** P **then** Q with the strength S" where P denotes a conjunction of descriptors over C (with non-empty set $[P]_{DT}$), Q denotes a concept that the rule describes, and S is a "measure of strength" of the rule defined by

$$S(P \rightarrow Q) = s(P) \times (1 - r(P \rightarrow Q)) \tag{5}$$

where $s(P)$ is the strength of the generalization P (i.e., the condition of the rule) and r is the noise rate function. The strength of a given rule reflects the incompleteness and uncertainty in the process of rule inducing influenced both by unseen instances and noise.

The strength of the generalization $P = PG$ is given by Eq. (6) under that assumption that the prior distribution is uniform

$$s(P) = \sum_l p(PI_l|P) = card([P]_{DT}) \times \frac{1}{N_P} \tag{6}$$

where $card([P]_{DT})$ is the number of observed instances satisfying the generalization P.

The strength of the generalization P represents explicitly the prediction for unseen instances. On the other hand, the noise rate is given by Eq. (7)

$$r(P \rightarrow Q) = 1 - \frac{card([P]_{DT}) \cap [Q]_{DT})}{card([P]_{DT})}. \tag{7}$$

It shows the quality of classification measured by the number of instances satisfying the generalization P which cannot be classified into class Q. The user can specify an allowed noise level as a threshold value. Thus, the rule candidates with the larger noise level than a given threshold value will be deleted.

One can observe that the rule strength we are proposing is equal to its confidence [1] modified by the strength of the generalization appearing on the left hand side of the rule. The reader can find in literature other criteria for rule strength estimation (see e.g., [3, 7, 13]).

Table 4. Rules with respect to class R

rule-ID	rule	accuracy
001	GPT(up)	(10/16)=62%
002	T-CHO(down) ∧ PLT(down)	(6/9)=66%
003	T-BIL(up) ∧ GPT(down)	(3/4)=75%
004	TP(down) ∧ GPT(down)	(3/4)=75%

Table 5. Rules with respect to class N

rule-ID	rule	accuracy
101	D-BIL(down)	(26/43)=60%
102	T-CHO(down) ∧ I-BIL(down)	(7/11)=63%
103	I-BIL(down) ∧ WBC(down)	(7/8)=87%
104	D-BIL(up) ∧ PLT(down)	(4/6)=66%
105	TP(up) ∧ I-BIL(down)	(5/6)=83%
106	TP(up) ∧ T-BIL(down)	(4/6)=66%
107	TP(up) ∧ PLT(down)	(4/5)=80%
108	CHE(up) ∧ T-BIL(down)	(2/4)=50%

Simplification of the Decision Table by GDT-RS. The process of rule discovery consists of decision table pre-processing including of selection and extraction of relevant attributes (features) and the relevant decision rule generation. The relevant decision rules can be induced from the minimal rules (i.e., with the minimal length of their left hand sides with respect to the discernibility between decisions) by tuning them (e.g., drooping some conditions to obtain more general rules better predisposed to classify new objects even if they not classify properly some objects from the training set). The relevant rules can be induced from the set of all minimal rules or its subset covering the set of objects of a given decision table [10, 16]. A representative approach for the problem of generation of the so called local relative reducts of condition attributes is the one to represent knowledge to be preserved about the discernibility between objects by means of the discernibility functions [14, 16].

It is obvious that by using the GDT one instance can be matched by several possible generalizations, and several instances can be generalized into one possible generalization. Simplifying a decision table by means of the GDT-RS system leads to a minimal (or sub-minimal) set of generalizations covering all instances. The main goal is to find a relevant (i.e., minimal or semi-minimal with respect to the description size) covering of instances still allowing to resolve conflicts between different decision rules recognizing new objects. The first step in the GDT-RS system for decision rules generation is based on computing of local relative reducts of condition attributes, by means of discernibility matrix method [14, 16]. Moreover, instead of searching for dispensable attributes we are rather searching for relevant attributes using a bottom-up method.

Any generalization matching instances with different decisions should be checked by means of Eq. (7). If the noise level is smaller than a threshold value,

Table 6. Patients covered by rules with respect to class R

rule-ID	Positive patient ID	Negative patient ID
001	158 351 534 547 778 801 909 923 940 942	35 188 273 452 623 712
002	91 351 650 703 732 913	169 712 952
003	431 592 700	122
004	37 71 730	122

such generalization is regarded as a reasonable one. Otherwise, the generalization is contradictory.

Furthermore, a rule, in GDT-RS, is selected according to its priority. The priority can be defined by the number of instances covered (matched) by a rule (i.e., the more instances are covered, the higher the priority is), by the number of attributes occurring on the left hand side of rule (i.e., the less the attribute number is, the higher the priority is), or by the rule strength.

We have developed two algorithms (called *"Optimal Set of Rules"* and *"Sub-Optimal Solution"*) for the GDT-RS implementation. The algorithms are not discussed since the page limitation. For such a discussion, see our papers [4, 28].

3.2   Results of Mining

In the experimental results at the accuracy 60%, only the rules with which the number of condition attributes is less than or equal to three are extracted. This is because the rules will become unclear if the number of condition attributes increases. Tables 4 and 5 show such rules that are divided into classes R and N, respectively. In the tables, *accuracy* denotes how many instances within all of instances covered by the rule are classified correctly.

Results of Post-processing. As a post-processing, we checked that each discovered rule covers what patient(s) related data. Tables 6 and 7 show the results, where the *Positive* (or *Negative*) *ID* means that the patient is covered by a rule as a *positive* (or *negative*) instance. From the tables, we can see it becomes clear that what patient group is covered by what rule. Hence it is useful for finding the main features of a patient group.

As an example of post-processing, Table 8 shows part of result of the post-processing about class R. Here "+" and "−" denote the patient covered by a rule as a positive or negative instance, respectively. For example, *rule-001* is covered by the patient IDs: {158, 778, 801, 909, 923, 940, 942}.

3.3   Analyses and Evaluations

The results derived by the GDT-RS and post-processing have been evaluated by a medical doctor based on acceptability and novelty of each rule. The evaluations of the rules are divided into five stages: 1 is the lowest and 5 is the highest evaluation for acceptability and novelty of each rule.

Table 7. Patients covered by rules with respect to class N

rule-ID	Positive patient ID	Negative patient ID
101	2 104 125 182 184 191 203 208 239 290 546 439 493 498 529 578 585 634 652 653 669 715 719 743 750 756	37 71 133 169 180 206 248 276 413 593 610 683 702 713 732 771 948
102	2 239 563 634 652 653 952	169 413 650 732
103	2 138 208 432 578 653 736	413
104	187 260 289 712	703 778
105	72 182 219 546 920	35
106	72 182 219 546	180 610
107	104 182 260 535	180
108	210 634	180 683

Evaluation of Rules. From the viewpoint of the rules with a higher support (e.g. *rule-001* and *rule-101*), we observed that

- It will heal up in many cases if a patient is medicated with IFN at the time when GPT is going up (hepatitis is getting worse);
- It does not heal up in many cases even if a patient is medicated with IFN at the time when D-BIL is descending.

Furthermore, the following two points on the effect of IFN are understood clearly.

- It is relevant to different types of hepatitis viruses;
- It is hard to be effective when there are large amounts of hepatitis virus.

Hence, we can see that *rule-001* and *rule-101* do not conflict with the existing medicine knowledge.

From the two rules, the hypothesis:

"IFN is more effective when the inflammation of hepatitis is stronger"

can be formed. Based on this hypothesis, we can evaluate the rules discovered as follows.

- In class R, the acceptability of the rules with respect to aggravation of the liver function will be good.
- In class N, the acceptability of the rules with respect to recovery of the liver function will be good.

Table 8. Post-processing about class R

Patient-ID	rule 001	rule 002	rule 003	rule 004
35	−			
37				+
71				+
78				
91		+		
122			−	−
158	+			
169	−			
⋮	⋮	⋮	⋮	⋮
778	+			
801	+			
909	+			
913		+		
923	+			
⋮	⋮	⋮	⋮	⋮
940	+			
942	+			
⋮	⋮	⋮	⋮	⋮

Table 9. Evaluation of rules with respect to class R

rule-ID	rule	accuracy	acceptability	novelty
001	GPT(up)	(10/16)=62%	4	5
002	T-CHO(down) ∧ PLT(down)	(6/9)=66%	3	5
003	T-BIL(up) ∧ GPT(down)	(3/4)=75%	4	5
004	TP(down) ∧ GPT(down)	(3/4)=75%	4	5

Table 10. Evaluation of rules with respect to class N

rule-ID	rule	accuracy	acceptability	novelty
101	D-BIL(down)	(26/43)=60%	4	5
102	T-CHO(down) ∧ I-BIL(down)	(7/11)=63%	2	3
103	I-BIL(down) ∧ WBC(down)	(7/8)=87%	2	3
104	D-BIL(up) ∧ PLT(down)	(4/6)=66%	1	1
105	TP(up) ∧ I-BIL(down)	(5/6)=83%	3	4
106	TP(up) ∧ T-BIL(down)	(4/6)=66%	3	4
107	TP(up) ∧ PLT(down)	(4/5)=80%	2	3
108	CHE(up) ∧ T-BIL(down)	(2/4)=50%	3	4

Hence, the evaluations as shown in Tables 9 and 10 can be obtained. In class N, we can see that the acceptability of some rules is 2. This is because both the recovery and aggravation of the liver function are included in the premise of the rules.

Evaluation of Post-processing. In the discovered rules, we can see there is some relevance among the patients supported by bilirubin (T-BIL, D-BIL, I-

Table 11. Category of discovered rules

	Recovery	Aggravation	Recovery and Aggravation
class R	rule 007 rule 008 rule 009 rule 011	rule 001 rule 002	rule 003 rule 004 rule 005 rule 006 rule 010
class N	rule 101 rule 105 rule 106 rule 108 rule 110	rule 104 rule 109	rule 102 rule 103 rule 107 rule 111

BIL) in class N. From the relation denoted in T-BIL = D-BIL + I-BIL, it is clear that the rules with respect to bilirubin are relevant. Hence the rules are supporting the same patients group.

Moreover, in order to examine the hypothesis, "the medical background which a rule shows is not contradictory to a patient's condition", the discovered rules are categorized, based on the liver function, into three categories: recovery, aggravation, or mixed recovery and aggravation, as shown in Table 11.

From Table 11, we observed that there are many rules with the same conditions in the rule group supported by a patients group, and it may conflict with unknown medical background that is not represented in the conditions of the rules. However, it does not mean that the rules are incorrect. The reason may be that the rules cannot be simply categorized by recovery and aggravation.

For example, although it can show the liver function aggravation, the lower values of WBC and ALB may not be the real reason of the liver function aggravation. On the other hand, since WBC and PLT are the same blood cell ingredient, and T-CHO and ALB are relevant to protein that makes liver, they may be relevant from this point of view. However, T-CHO and ALB do not only provide for liver, but also, for example, T-CHO is related to eating, and ALB is related to the kidney, respectively. Hence it cannot declare there is such correlation.

In summary, there is correlation if we are mentioning about mathematical relevance like BIL. However, it is difficult to find out correlation for others. We need the following methods to solve the issue.

- Finding out the rules which are significant from the statistical point of view, based on rough categorizing such as recovery and aggravation.
- Showing whether such rough categorizing is sufficient or not.

4   Rule Discovery by LOI

The LOI uses the background knowledge called *ordered relation* for discovering *ordering rules* and important attributes for an ordered decision class [15, 29].

In many information processing systems, objects are typically represented by their values on a finite set of attributes. Such information may be conveniently described in a tabular form [14]. The rows of the table correspond to objects of the universe, the columns correspond to a set of attributes, and each cell gives the value of an object with respect to an attribute.

Definition 1. *An information table is a quadruple:*

$$IT = (U, At, \{V_a \mid a \in At\}, \{I_a \mid a \in At\})$$

where U is a finite nonempty set of objects, At is a finite nonempty set of attributes, V_a is a nonempty set of values for $a \in At$ $I_a : U \rightarrow V_a$ is an information function.

For simplicity, we have considered only information tables characterized by a finite set of objects and a finite set of attributes. Each information function I_a is a total function that maps an object of U to exactly one value in V_a. An information table represents all available information and knowledge about the objects under consideration. Objects are only perceived, observed, or measured by using a finite number of properties.

However, such information table does not consider any semantic relationships between distinct values of a particular attribute. By incorporating semantics information, we may obtain different generalizations of information tables [6, 8, 15]. Generalized information tables may be viewed as information tables with added semantics.

Definition 2. *Let U be a nonempty set and $\succ$ be a binary relation on U. The relation $\succ$ is a weak order if it satisfies the two properties:*

$$\text{Asymmetry} : x \succ y \Longrightarrow \neg(y \succ x),$$
$$\text{Negative transitivity} : (\neg(x \succ y), \neg(y \succ z)) \Longrightarrow \neg(x \succ z).$$

An important implication of a weak order is that the following relation,

$$x \sim y \Longleftrightarrow (\neg(x \succ y), \neg(y \succ x)) \tag{8}$$

is an equivalence relation. For two elements, if $x \sim y$ we say x and y are indiscernible by $\succ$. The equivalence relation $\sim$ induces a partition $U/\sim$ on U, and an order relation $\succ^*$ on $U/\sim$ can be defined by:

$$[x]_\sim \succ^* [y]_\sim \Longleftrightarrow x \succ y \tag{9}$$

where $[x]_\sim$ is the equivalence class containing x. Moreover, $\succ^*$ is a linear order. Any two distinct equivalence classes of $U/\sim$ can be compared. It is therefore possible to arrange the objects into levels, with each level consisting of indiscernible elements defined by $\succ$. For a weak order, $\neg(x \succ y)$ can be written as $y \succeq x$ or $x \preceq y$, which means $y \succ x$ or $y \sim x$. For any two elements x and y, we have either $x \succ y$ or $y \succeq x$, but not both.

Definition 3. *An ordered information table is a pair:*

$$OIT = (IT, \{\succ_a \mid a \in At\})$$

where IT is a standard information table and $\succ_a$ is a weak order on V_a.

An ordering of values of a particular attribute a naturally induces an ordering of objects, namely, for $x, y \in U$:

$$x \succ_{\{a\}} y \Longleftrightarrow I_a(x) \succ_a I_a(y) \tag{10}$$

where $\succ_{\{a\}}$ denotes an order relation on U induced by the attribute a. An object x is ranked ahead of another object y if and only if the value of x on the attribute a is ranked ahead of the value of y on a. The relation $\succ_{\{a\}}$ has exactly the same properties as that of $\succ_a$. For a subset of attributes $A \subseteq At$, we define

$$x \succ_A y \Longleftrightarrow \forall a \in A[I_a(x) \succ_a I_a(y)]$$
$$\Longleftrightarrow \bigwedge_{a \in A} I_a(x) \succ_a I_a(y) \Longleftrightarrow \bigcap_{a \in A} \succ_{\{a\}} . \tag{11}$$

That is, x is ranked ahead of y if and only if x is ranked ahead of y according to all attributes in A. The above definition is a straightforward generalization of the standard definition of equivalence relations in rough set theory, where the equality relation $=$ is used [14].

For many real world applications, we also need a special attribute, called the decision attribute. The ordering of objects by the decision attribute is denoted by $\succ_{\{o\}}$ and is called the overall ordering of objects.

For example, since the larger the value of T-CHO is, the better, the order relation can be set to (VH $\succ$ H $\succ$ N $\succ$ L $\succ$ VL), where "$\succ$" denotes a weak order. Furthermore, if a decision attribute has two classes: R (response) and N (no response), the order relation can be set to $R \succ N$.

In order to mine ordering rules from an ordered information table, the ordered information needs to be merged into the ordered information table. There are many ways to do such a mergence. Here we mention a way by merging the ordered information into a binary information table. In the binary information table, we consider object pairs $(x, y) \in (U \times U)^+$. The information function is defined by:

$$I_a((x, y)) = \begin{cases} 1, & x \succ_{\{a\}} y \\ 0, & x \preceq_{\{a\}} y. \end{cases} \tag{12}$$

Statements in an ordered information table can be translated into equivalent statements in the binary information table. For example, $x \succ_{\{a\}} y$ can be translated into $I_a((x, y)) = 1$. In the translation process, we will not consider object pairs of the form (x, x), as we are not interested in them.

However, some useful information within original attribute-values may be lost in the binary information table. For example, the distance between the values, how better or worse cannot be represented in the binary information table. In order to meet the needs of real-world application, three extended methods have been developed for generating various ordered information tables, namely, *distance-based*, *standard-based* and *combination of distance and standard*, and their information functions are defined in Eqs. (13), (14) and (15), respectively. In Eq. (13), $d(x, y)$ denotes the distance between x and y.

$$I_a((x,y)) = \begin{cases} d(x,y), \; x \succ_{\{a\}} y, \\ 0, \; x \sim y, \\ -d(x,y), \; x \prec_{\{a\}} y. \end{cases} \quad (13)$$

$$I_a((x,y)) = \begin{cases} y \succ, \; x \succ_{\{a\}} y, \\ =, \; x \sim y, \\ y \prec, \; x \prec_{\{a\}} y. \end{cases} \quad (14)$$

$$I_a((x,y)) = \begin{cases} x \succ y, \; x \succ_{\{a\}} y, \\ x = y, \; x \sim y, \\ x \prec y, \; x \prec_{\{a\}} y. \end{cases} \quad (15)$$

By using the ordered information table, the issue of ordering rules mining can be regarded as a kind of classification. Hence, our GDT-RS rule mining system can be used to generate ordering rules from an ordered information table. The ordering rules can be used to predict the effect of IFN. Moreover, the most important attributes can be found when a rule with too many condition attributes.

In general, the large number of ordering rules may be generated. In order to give a ranking about what attributes are important, we use the following equation to analyse the frequency of each attribute in the generated ordering rules.

$$f = \frac{ca}{tc} \quad (16)$$

where f is the frequency of attribute, ca is the coverage of the attribute, and tc is the total coverage.

4.1   Experiment 1

In this experiment, we used the following 12 atrributes as condition attributes:
T-CHO, CHE, ALB, TP, T-BIL, D-BIL,
I-BIL, PLT, WBC, HGB, GPT, GOT
and use the same determination class as that used in GDT-RS (see Table 2). After the patients who have no data of whether the hepatitis virus exists or not are removed, the data of 142 patients was used.

For hepatitis C, it is possible to provide ordered relations in condition attributes and the decision class, respectively. First, the class (?) is removed from the dataset since we only consider the classes, R and N for mining by LOI. Then we use background knowledge for forming data granules by discretization of real-valued attributes as shown in Table 12, and the LOI will carry out on the transformed information table. Furthermore, we need to use ordered information between attribute values for making the ordered information table. In general, there exists background knowledge such as "if T-CHO lowers, then hepatitis generally gets worse" for each attribute. Hence we can define ordered information as shown in Table 13. From this table, we also can see that ordered

Table 12. Forming data granules by discretization in background knowledge

attribute	data granule
ALB	worse ← $UL \leq 2.5 < VL \leq 3.0 < L \leq 3.5 < M \leq 5.1 < H \rightarrow$ better
GPT	better ← $N \leq 40 < H \leq 100 < VH \leq 200 < UH \rightarrow$ worse
GOT	better ← $N \leq 40 < H \leq 100 < VH \leq 200 < UH \rightarrow$ worse
CHE	worse ← $VL \leq 100 < L \leq 180 < N \leq 430 < H \leq 510 < VH \rightarrow$ better
TP	worse ← $VL \leq 5.5 < L \leq 6.5 < N \leq 8.2 < H \leq 9.2 < VH \rightarrow$ better
T-BIL	better ← $L \leq 0.6 < M \leq 0.8 < H \leq 1.1 < VH \leq 1.5 < UH \rightarrow$ worse
PLT	worse ← $UL \leq 50 < VL \leq 100 < L \leq 150 < N \leq 350 < H \rightarrow$ better
WBC	worse ← $UL \leq 2 < VL \leq 3 < L \leq 4 < N \leq 9 < H \rightarrow$ better
T-CHO	worse ← $VL \leq 90 < L \leq 125 < N \leq 220 < H \leq 255 < VH \rightarrow$ better

Table 13. Ordered information for each attribute

attribute	ordered relationship
GOT	$N \succ H \succ VH \succ UH$
GPT	$N \succ H \succ VH \succ UH$
D-BIL	$0 \succ \infty$
T-BIL	$L \succ M \succ H \succ VH \succ UH$
T-CHO	$VH \succ H \succ N \succ L \succ VL$
I-BIL	$0 \succ \infty$
CHE	$VH \succ H \succ N \succ L \succ VL$
PLT	$H \succ N \succ L \succ VL \succ UL$
ALB	$H \succ M \succ L \succ VL \succ UL$
HGB	$\infty \succ 0$
TP	$VH \succ H \succ N \succ L \succ VL$
WBC	$H \succ N \succ L \succ VL \succ UL$
Class	$N \succ R$

information is directly given for the real-valued attributes, D-BIL, I-BIL, and HGB, without discretization, since no specific background knowledge is used for the discretization in this experiment.

The ordered information table is generated by using the *standard-based* method (i.e. Eq. (14) as shown in Fig. 4). The ordered information table may be viewed as an information table with added semantics (background knowledge). After such transformation, ordering rules can be discoverd from the ordered information table by using the GDT-RS rule mining system.

Results and Evaluation. The rules discovered by LOI are shown in Table 14, where the condition attributes in the rules denote the inspection value "go better" or "go worse".

The evaluation of acceptability and novelty for the rules heavily depends on the correctness of the ordered information. By investigating the values of each attribute in the ordered information table by using Eqs. (17) and (18), the correction rate of the background knowledge with respect to "go better" (or "go worse") can be obtained as shown in Table 15.

$$att_{\text{pos}} = \frac{\#ATT_{\succ,\succ}}{\#ATT_{\succ,\succ} + \#ATT_{\succ,\prec}} \qquad (17)$$

$$att_{\text{neg}} = \frac{\#ATT_{\prec,\prec}}{\#ATT_{\prec,\succ} + \#ATT_{\prec,\prec}} \qquad (18)$$

where $\#ATT$ is the number of different attribute values of attribute ATT in the ordered information table; $\succ, \succ$ denotes that the attribute value is "go better" and the patient is cured; $\succ, \prec$ denotes that the attribute value is "go better" but the patient is not cured; $\prec, \prec$ denotes that the attribute value is "go worse" and the patient is not cured; and $\prec, \succ$ denotes that the attribute value is "go worse" but the patient is cured.

The higher correction rate of the background knowledge (i.e. TP and HGB) can be explained that the background knowledge is consistent with the specific characteristics of the real collected data. On the contrary, the lower correction rate (i.e. WBC) may mean that the order relation given by an expert may not suitable for the specific data analysis. In this case, the order relation as common background knowledge needs to be adjusted according to specific characteristics of the real data such as the distribution and clusters of the real data. How to adjust the order relation is an important ongoing work.

4.2   Experiment 2

Although the data is the same as used in Experiment 1, the ordered relations used in Experiment 2 (see Table 16) is different. Furthermore, the ordered information

1. Change the attribute values to symbols.

	ALB	CHE	...	GOT	CLASS
p1	VH	VH	...	UH	R
p2	N	H	...	N	R
p3	L	L	...	VH	N
p4	H	VL	...	H	R
p5	H	H	...	VH	N
⋮			⋮		

2. Create the ordered information table by using the standard-based method.

Object	ALB	CHE	..	GOT	CLASS
(p1,p2)	N≻	H≻	...	N≺	=
(p1,p3)	L≻	L≻	...	VH≺	N≻
			⋮		
(p2,p1)	VH≺	VH≺	...	UH≻	=

Fig. 4. The creation of an ordered information table

Table 14. Rules of class N

Rules(SupportNUM > 10)	Support
PLT(N≺) ∧ D-BIL(H≻) ∧ GPT(VH≻)	27/30=90%
WBC(L≻) ∧ GOT(VH≻) ∧ GPT(VH≻)	20/22=90%
PLT(VL≻) ∧ GOT(VH≻) ∧ GPT(VH≻)	16/18=88%
PLT(L≻) ∧ TP(H≺) ∧ GOT(VH≺)	15/16=93%
D-BIL(H≻) ∧ GPT(VH≻)	14/17=82%
HGB(N≺) ∧ WBC(L≻) ∧ GOT(VH≻)	16/16=100%
D-BIL(H≻) ∧ GOT(H≻)	14/16=87%
D-BIL(H≻) ∧ GOT(H≻) ∧ GPT(VH≻)	12/15=80%
ALB(L≺) ∧ WBC(L≻) ∧ GPT(VH≻)	10/12=83%
...	...

Table 15. The correction rate of the background knowledge

Attribute	att_{pos}	att_{neg}
ALB	58.9%	67.2%
CHE	54.7%	70.6%
D-BIL	26.8%	35.3%
GOT	34.2%	47.3%
GPT	36.7%	47.8%
HGB	78.0%	81.4%
I-BIL	32.5%	53.1%
PLT	36.6%	49.5%
T-BIL	44.0%	47.1%
T-CHO	30.6%	48.3%
TP	62.7%	78.3%
WBC	9.5%	30.5%

Table 16. The ordered relations used in Experiment 2

T-CHO	104 ≺ 136 ≺ 151 ≺ 159 ≺ 182 ≺ 198 ≺ 260
CHE	3 ≺ 200 ≺ 250 ≺ 299 ≺ 373 ≺ 496
ALB	3.2 ≺ 3.8 ≺ 4.1 ≺ 4.4 ≺ 4.8
TP	5.7 ≺ 7.3 ≺ 7.5 ≺ 8.0 ≺ 9.0
T-BIL	0.40 ≺ 0.63 ≺ 0.86 ≺ 1.09 ≺ 2.7
D-BIL	0.03 ≺ 0.14 ≺ 0.31 ≺ 1.15
I-BIL	0.31 ≺ 0.50 ≺ 0.63 ≺ 1.60
PLT	56.3 ≺ 120 ≺ 167 ≺ 183 ≺ 215 ≺ 374
HGB	9.5 ≺ 13.2 ≺ 14.0 ≺ 14.3 ≺ 14.7 ≺ 15.8 ≺ 16.9
WBC	3.1 ≺ 4.0 ≺ 4.8 ≺ 5.4 ≺ 6.3 ≺ 6.9 ≺ 8.9
GPT	30 ≺ 88 ≺ 174 ≺ 231 ≺ 289 ≺ 605
GOT	24 ≺ 55 ≺ 101 ≺ 192 ≺ 330
Class	$N ≺ R$

table is generated by using the method of *combination of distance and standard* (i.e. Eq. (15)) in Experiment 2.

Table 17. Part of rules mined in Experiment 2

ID	rule	acceptability	novelty
001	ALB(3.8–4.1) ∧ D-BIL(0.31–1.15) ≻ ALB(4.1–4.4) ∧ D-BIL(0.14–0.31)	1	5
002	CHE(250–299) ∧ T-BIL(0.40–0.63) ≻ CHE(200–250) ∧ T-BIL(0.63–0.86)	4	3
003	T-CHO(136–151) ∧ I-BIL(0.31–0.50) ≻ T-CHO(198–260) ∧ I-BIL(0.50–0.63)	2	4
004	T-CHO(136–151) ∧ D-BIL(0.03–0.14) ≻ T-CHO(198–260) ∧ D-BIL(0.03–0.14)	2	3
005	TP(8.0–9.0) ∧ GPT(174–231) ≻ TP(5.7–7.3) ∧ GPT(30–88)	4	3
006	T-CHO(136–151) ∧ D-BIL(0.03–0.14) ≻ T-CHO(182–198) ∧ D-BIL(0.14–0.31)	3	4
007	TP(8.0–9.0) ∧ GOT(101–192) ≻ TP(5.7–7.3) ∧ GOT(24–55)	4	3
008	T-CHO(136–151) ∧ T-BIL(0.40–0.63) ≻ T-CHO(159–182) ∧ T-BIL(0.86–1.09)	3	4
009	T-CHO(136–151) ∧ D-BIL(0.03–0.14) ≻ T-CHO(104–136) ∧ D-BIL(0.14–0.31)	4	3
010	CHE(250–299) ∧ T-BIL(0.40–0.63) ≻ CHE(250–299) ∧ T-BIL(0.86–1.09)	3	2
011	TP(8.0–9.0) ∧ I-BIL(0.31–0.50) ≻ TP(8.0–9.0) ∧ I-BIL(0.50–0.63)	4	2
012	D-BIL(0.31–1.15) ∧ GPT(289–605) ≻ D-BIL(0.14–0.31) ∧ GPT(30–88)	2	4
013	TP(8.0–9.0) ∧ T-BIL(0.40–0.63) ≻ TP(7.3–7.5) ∧ T-BIL(0.86–1.09)	4	2
014	I-BIL(0.31–0.50) ∧ PLT(183–215) ≻ I-BIL(0.50–0.63) ∧ PLT(167–183)	5	2
015	I-BIL(0.31–0.50) ∧ WBC(3.1–4.0) ≻ I-BIL(0.50–0.63) ∧ WBC(4.0–4.8)	4	2
016	T-CHO(159–182) ∧ GPT(88–174) ≻ T-CHO(151–159) ∧ GPT(88–174)	4	2
017	ALB(4.4–4.8) ∧ GPT(289–605) ≻ ALB(4.1–4.4) ∧ GPT(30–88)	2	2
018	T-CHO(159–182) ∧ TP(8.0–9.0) ≻ T-CHO(198–260) ∧ TP(7.50–8.00)	3	3
019	ALB(4.4–4.8) ∧ WBC(6.3–6.9) ≻ ALB(4.1–4.4) ∧ WBC(5.4–6.3)	5	3
101	I-BIL((0.31–0.50) = (0.31–0.50)) ∧ PLT((183–215) = (183–215))	4	2
102	TP((8.0–9.0) = (8.0–9.0)) ∧ I-BIL((0.31–0.50) = (0.31–0.50))	4	3
103	T-CHO((136–151) = (136–151)) ∧ D-BIL((0.03–0.14) = (0.03–0.14))	3	2
104	PLT((56–120) = (56–120)) ∧ HGB((14.7–15.8) = (14.7–15.8)) ∧ WBC((4.8–5.4) = (4.8–5.4))	2	4
105	ALB((4.4–4.8) = (4.4–4.8)) ∧ WBC((6.9–8.9) = (6.9–8.9))	3	2
106	I-BIL((0.31–0.50) = (0.31–0.50)) ∧ WBC((3.1–4.0) = (3.1–4.0))	3	4
201	TP((5.7–7.3) = (5.6–7.3)) ∧ GOT((24–55) = (24–55))	3	4
202	T-CHO((198–260) = (198–260.4))	2	3
203	I-BIL((0.50–0.63) = (0.50–0.63)) ∧ GOT((24–55) – (24–55))	3	2
204	I-BIL((0.50–0.63) = (0.50–0.63)) ∧ GPT((30–88) = (30–88))	3	2
205	WBC((6.9–8.9) = (6.9–8.9))	4	2
206	PLT((167–183) = (167–183))	3	3
207	T-BIL((0.63–0.86) = (0.63–0.86)) ∧ D-BIL((0.03–0.14) = (0.03–0.14))	3	5
208	ALB((4.1–4.4) = (4.1–4.4)) ∧ TP((7.5–8.0) = (7.5–8.0))	4	1

Table 17 shows part of rules mined in Experiment 2. Here $ID0xx$ denotes the rules with $Class(N \succ R)$, $ID1xx$ with $Class(R = R)$, and $ID2xx$ with $Class(N = N)$, respectively. The results have been evaluated by a medical doctor based on acceptability and novelty of each rule. The evaluations of the rules are divided into five stages: 1 is the lowest and 5 is the highest evaluation for acceptability and novelty of each rule. For example, the rule $ID001$:

$$\text{ALB}((3.8, 4.1]) \wedge \text{D-BIL}((0.31, 1.15]) \succ \text{ALB}(4.1, 4.4]) \wedge \text{D-BIL}(0.14, 0.31])$$

is read that the use of INF for the patient with ALB(3.8, 4.1] and D-BIL(0.31, 1.15] is more effect than the patient with ALB(4.1, 4.4]) and D-BIL(0.14,0.31]), and the acceptability and novelty of the rule are 1 and 5, respectively. The rule with the "lowest" acceptability and the "highest" novelty can be explained that the novel knowledge may be discovered by refining and verifying such a hypothesis although it cannot be accepted by the existing medical knowledge.

5   Rule Discovery by POM

Peculiarity represents a new interpretation of interestingness, an important notion long identified in data mining [12, 25, 30]. Peculiarity, unexpected relationships/rules may be hidden in a relatively small number of data. *Peculiarity rules* are a typical regularity hidden in many scientific, statistical, medical, and transaction databases. They may be difficult to find by applying the standard association rule mining method [2], due to the requirement of large support. In contrast, the POM (peculiarity oriented mining) agent focuses on some interesting data (peculiar data) in order to find novel and interesting rules (peculiarity rules).

The main task of peculiarity oriented mining is the identification of peculiar data. An attribute-oriented method, which analyzes data from a new view and is different from traditional statistical methods, is recently proposed by Zhong *et al.* [30].

Peculiar data are a subset of objects in the database and are characterized by two features:

– very different from other objects in a dataset, and
– consisting of a relatively low number of objects.

The first property is related to the notion of distance or dissimilarity of objects. Institutively speaking, an object is different from other objects if it is far away from other objects based on certain distance functions. Its attribute values must be different from the values of other objects. One can define distance between objects based on the distance between their values. The second property is related to the notion of support. Peculiar data must have a low support.

At attribute level, the identification of peculiar data can be done by finding attribute values having properties 1) and 2). Table 18 shows a relation with attributes A_1, A_2, ..., A_m. Let x_{ij} be the value of A_j of the i-th tuple, and n the number of tuples. We suggested that the peculiarity of x_{ij} can be evaluated by a *Peculiarity Factor*, $PF(x_{ij})$,

Table 18. A sample table (relation)

A_1	A_2	...	A_j	...	A_m
x_{11}	x_{12}	...	x_{1j}	...	x_{1m}
x_{21}	x_{22}	...	x_{2j}	...	x_{2m}
$\vdots$	$\vdots$		$\vdots$		$\vdots$
x_{i1}	x_{i2}	...	x_{ij}	...	x_{im}
$\vdots$	$\vdots$		$\vdots$		$\vdots$
x_{n1}	x_{n2}	...	x_{nj}	...	x_{nm}

Table 19. Peculiarity rules with respect to class R

rule-ID	rule
p-1	CHE(329.5)
p-2	HGB(17.24)
p-3	T-BIL(1.586) ∧ I-BIL(0.943) ∧ D-BIL(0.643)
p-4	CHE(196) ∧ PLT(73.667)
p-5	PLT(176.5) ∧ T-CHO(117.75)
p-6	ALB(4.733) ∧ I-BIL(0.95)
p-7	TP(8.46) ∧ GOT(175.8) ∧ GPT(382.2)
p-8	ALB(3.9) ∧ T-CHO(120.667) ∧ TP(6.65) ∧ WBC(2.783)

$$PF(x_{ij}) = \sum_{k=1}^{n} N(x_{ij}, x_{kj})^{\alpha} \qquad (19)$$

where N denotes the conceptual distance, α is a parameter to denote the importance of the distance between x_{ij} and x_{kj}, which can be adjusted by a user, and $\alpha = 0.5$ as default.

With the introduction of conceptual distance, Eq. (19) provides a more flexible method to calculate peculiarity of an attribute value. It can handle both continuous and symbolic attributes based on a unified semantic interpretation. Background knowledge represented by binary neighborhoods can be used to evaluate the peculiarity if such background knowledge is provided by a user. If X is a continuous attribute and no background knowledge is available, we use the following distance:

$$N(x_{ij}, x_{kj}) = |x_{ij} - x_{kj}|. \qquad (20)$$

If X is a symbolic attribute and the background knowledge for representing the conceptual distances between x_{ij} and x_{kj} is provided by a user, the peculiarity factor is calculated by the conceptual distances [11, 20, 28]. The conceptual distances are assigned to 1 if no background knowledge is available.

Based on the peculiarity factor, the selection of peculiar data is simply carried out by using a threshold value. More specifically, an attribute value is peculiar if its peculiarity factor is above minimum peculiarity p, namely, $PF(x_{ij}) \geq p$.

Table 20. Peculiarity rules with respect to class N

rule-ID	rule
p-9	ALB(3.357) ∧ HGB(12.786) ∧ D-BIL(0.057) ∧ T-CHO(214.6) ∧ TP(5.671)
p-10	ALB(4.6) ∧ GPT(18.5)
p-11	HGB(12.24) ∧ I-BIL(0.783) ∧ GOT(143.167)
p-12	PLT(314) ∧ T-BIL(0.3) ∧ I-BIL(0.2) ∧ WBC(7.7)
p-13	CHE(361) ∧ PLT(253.5) ∧ WBC(8.5)
p-14	WBC(8.344)
p-15	ALB(3.514) ∧ CHE(133.714) ∧ T-BIL(1.229) ∧ I-BIL(0.814) ∧ D-BIL(0.414) ∧ GOT(160) ∧ GPT(146.857)
p-16	GOT(130.833) ∧ GPT(183.833)
p-17	T-CHO(127.5)
p-18	CHE(96.714) ∧ T-CHO(110.714) ∧ WBC(4.175)
p-19	PLT(243.429) ∧ WBC(7.957)

Table 21. Granulated peculiarity rules with respect to class R

rule-ID	rule
p-1'	CHE(N)
p-2'	HGB(N)
p-3'	T-BIL(H) ∧ I-BIL(H) ∧ D-BIL(VH)
p-4'	CHE(N) ∧ PLT(VL)
p-5'	PLT(N) ∧ T-CHO(L)
p-6'	ALB(N) ∧ I-BIL(H)
p-7'	TP(H) ∧ GOT(VH) ∧ GPT(UH)
p-8'	ALB(L) ∧ T-CHO(L) ∧ TP(N) ∧ WBC(VL)

The threshold value p may be computed by the distribution of PF as follows:

$$p = mean \ of \ PF(x_{ij}) + \beta \times standard \ deviation \ of \ PF(x_{ij}) \qquad (21)$$

where β can be adjusted by a user, and $\beta = 1$ is used as default. The threshold indicates that a data is a peculiar one if its PF value is much larger than the mean of the PF set. In other words, if $PF(x_{ij})$ is over the threshold value, x_{ij} is a peculiar data. By adjusting the parameter β, a user can control and adjust the threshold value.

Furthermore, a peculiarity rule is discovered by searching association among the peculiar data (or their granules).

5.1   Mining Results by POM

We have been applying the POM in the same hepatitis dataset as used in GDT-RS and LOI, and had some preliminary results [21]. Tables 19 and 20 show the peculiarity rules generated from the peculiar data without discretization, with respect to classes R and N, respectively. Furthermore, Tables 21 and 22

Table 22. Granulated peculiarity rules with respect to class N

rule-ID	rule
p-9'	ALB(L) ∧ HGB(N) ∧ D-BIL(N) ∧ T-CHO(N) ∧ TP(L)
p-10'	ALB(N) ∧ GPT(N)
p-11'	HGB(N) ∧ I-BIL(N) ∧ GOT(VH)
p-12'	PLT(N) ∧ T-BIL(N) ∧ I-BIL(N) ∧ WBC(N)
p-13'	CHE(N) ∧ PLT(N) ∧ WBC(N)
p-14'	WBC(N)
p-15'	ALB(L) ∧ CHE(L) ∧ T-BIL(H) ∧ I-BIL(N) ∧ D-BIL(H) ∧ GOT(VH) ∧ GPT(VH)
p-16'	GOT(VH) ∧ GPT(VH)
p-17'	T-CHO(N)
p-18'	CHE(VL) ∧ T-CHO(L) ∧ WBC(N)
p-19'	PLT(N) ∧ WBC(N)

Table 23. Some addition and change of data granules for Table 12

attribute	data granule
HGB	$L \leq 12 < N \leq 18 < H$
I-BIL	$N \leq 0.9 < H \leq 1.8 < VH \leq 2.7 < UH$
D-BIL	$N \leq 0.3 < H \leq 0.6 < VH \leq 0.9 < UH$
ALB	$VL \leq 3.0 < L \leq 3.9 < N \leq 5.1 < H \leq 6.0 < VH$
T-BIL	$N \leq 0.6 < H \leq 2.4 < VH \leq 3.6 < UH$

give the mined results with discretization and granulation by using background knowledge as shown in Tables 12 and 23.

We have also worked with Suzuki's group to integrate the Peculiarity Oriented Mining approach with the Exception Rules/Data Mining approach for discovering more refined LC (Liver Cirrhosis) and non-LC classification models [9, 19].

5.2   Meta Analysis and Learning

Based on the results mined by LOI and POM, the following meta rules can be used for learning more interesting decision rules and post-processing.

First, based on the attribute importance learned by LOI, the importance of the decision rules can be ranked. In other words, if there is a high-frequency attribute learned by LOI in a decision rule, the decision rule is regarded as a more important one than others.

Second, the attribute importance learned by LOI will be reflected in the heuristics for rule selection in GDT-RS. In other words, the rule candidates with a high-frequency attribute will be selected prior.

Third, the ordering rules are also used to check whether some decision rules mined by GDT-RS are inconsistent.

Fourth, if the peculiar data found by POM are with a negative meaning, then remove them from the dataset and the GDT-RS will be carried out again on the cleaned dataset.

Fifth, if the peculiar data found by POM are with a positive meaning, then the peculiarity rules will be generated by searching association among the peculiar data (or their granules).

6   Conclusions

We presented a multi-aspect mining approach in a multi-phase, multi-aspect hepatitis data analysis process. Both pre-processing and post-processing steps are important before/after using data mining agents. Informed knowledge discovery in real-life hepatitis data needs to use background knowledge obtained from medical doctors to guide the spiral discovery process with multi-phase such as pre-processing, rule mining, and post-processing, towards finding interesting and novel rules/features hidden in data.

Our methodology and experimental results show that the perspective of medical doctors will be changed from a single type of experimental data analysis towards a holistic view, by using our multi-aspect mining approach in which various data mining agents are used in a distributed cooperative mode.

Acknowledgements

This work was supported by the grant-in-aid for scientific research on priority area "Active Mining" from the Japanese Ministry of Education, Culture, Sports, Science and Technology.

References

1. Agrawal, R., Mannila, H., Srikant, R., Toivonen, H., Verkano, A., "Fast Discovery of Association Rules", in: Fayyad U.M., Piatetsky-Shapiro G., Smyth P., Uthurusamy R. (eds.) *Advances in Knowledge Discovery and Data Mining*, The MIT Press (1996) 307-328.
2. Agrawal R. et al. "Fast Discovery of Association Rules", *Advances in Knowledge Discovery and Data Mining*, AAAI Press (1996) 307-328.
3. Bazan, J. G. "A Comparison of Dynamic and Non-dynamic Rough Set Methods for Extracting Laws from Decision System" in: Polkowski, L., Skowron, A. (Eds.), *Rough Sets in Knowledge Discovery 1: Methodology and Applications*, Physica-Verlag (1998) 321-365.
4. Dong, J.Z., Zhong, N., and Ohsuga, S. "Probabilistic Rough Induction: The GDT-RS Methodology and Algorithms", in: Z.W. Ras and A. Skowron (eds.), *Foundations of Intelligent Systems*, LNAI 1609, Springer (1999) 621-629.
5. Fayyad, U.M., Piatetsky-Shapiro, G, and Smyth, P. "From Data Mining to Knowledge Discovery: an Overview", *Advances in Knowledge Discovery and Data Mining*, MIT Press (1996) 1-36.

6. Greco S., Matarazzo B., and Slowinski R. "Rough Approximation of a Preference Relation by Dominance Relations", *European Journal of Operational Research* Vol. 117 (1999) 63-83.
7. Grzymała-Busse, J.W. "Applications of Rule Induction System LERS", in: L. Polkowski, A. Skowron (Eds.) *Rough Sets in Knowledge Discovery 1: Methodology and Applications*, Physica-Verlag (1998) 366-375.
8. Iwinski, T.B. "Ordinal Information System", *Bulletin of the Polish Academy of Sciences, Mathematics*, Vol. 36 (1998) 467-475.
9. Jumi, M., Suzuki, E., Ohshima, M., Zhong, N., Yokoi, H., Takabayashi, K. "Spiral Discovery of a Separate Prediction Model from Chronic Hepatitis Data", *Proc. Third International Workshop on Active Mining (AM)* (2004) 1-10.
10. Komorowski, J., Pawlak, Z., Polkowski, L. and Skowron, A. *Rough Sets: A Tutorial*, S. K. Pal and A. Skowron (eds.) *Rough Fuzzy Hybridization: A New Trend in Decision Making*, Springer (1999) 3-98.
11. Lin, T.Y. "Granular Computing on Binary Relations 1: Data Mining and Neighborhood Systems", L. Polkowski and A. Skowron (eds.) *Rough Sets in Knowledge Discovery*, Vol. 1, Physica-Verlag (1998) 107-121.
12. Liu, B., Hsu W., Chen, S., and Ma, Y. "Analyzing the Subjective Interestingness of Association Rules", *IEEE Intelligent Systems*, Vol.15, No.5 (2000) 47-55.
13. Mitchell, T.,M. *Machine Learning*, Mc Graw-Hill (1997).
14. Pawlak, Z. *Rough Sets, Theoretical Aspects of Reasoning about Data*, Kluwer (1991).
15. Sai, Y., Yao, Y.Y., and Zhong, N. "Data Analysis and Mining in Ordered Information Tables", *Proc. 2001 IEEE International Conference on Data Mining (ICDM'01)*, IEEE Computer Society Press (2001) 497-504.
16. Skowron, A. and Rauszer, C. "The Discernibility Matrixes and Functions in Information Systems", R. Slowinski (ed.) *Intelligent Decision Support*, Kluwer (1992) 331-362.
17. Slowinski, R., Greco, S., Matarazzo, B. "Rough Set Analysis of Preference-Ordered Data", J.J. Alpigini, et al (eds.) *Rough Sets and Current Trends in Computing*, LNAI 2475, Springer (2002) 44-59.
18. Suzuki, E. Undirected Discovery of Interesting Exception Rules, *International Journal of Pattern Recognition and Artificial Intelligence*, World Scientific, Vol.16, No.8 (2002) 1065-1086.
19. Suzuki, E., Zhong, N., Yokoi, H., and Takabayashi, K. "Spiral Mining of Chronic Hepatitis Data", *Proc. ECML/PKDD-2004 Discovery Challenge* (2004) 185-196.
20. Yao, Y.Y. "Granular Computing using Neighborhood Systems", Roy, R., Furuhashi, T., Chawdhry, P.K. (eds.) *Advances in Soft Computing: Engineering Design and Manufacturing*, Springer (1999) 539-553.
21. Yokoi, H., Hirano, S., Takabayashi, K., Tsumoto, S., and Satomura, Y. "Active Mining in Medicine: A Chronic Hepatitis Case – Towards Knowledge Discovery in Hospital Information Systems", *Journal of Japanese Society for Artificial Intelligence*, Vol.17, No.5 (2002) 622-628 (in Japanese).
22. Zhong, N. and Ohsuga, S. "Toward A Multi-Strategy and Cooperative Discovery System", *Proc. First Int. Conf. on Knowledge Discovery and Data Mining (KDD-95)*, AAAI Press (1995) 337-342.
23. Zhong, N., Dong, J.Z., and Ohsuga, S., "Rule Discovery in Medical Data by GDT-RS", Special Issue on Comparison and Evaluation of KDD Methods with Common Medical Datasets, *Journal of Japanese Society for Artificial Intelligence*, Vol.15, No.5 (2000) 774-781 (in Japanese).

24. Zhong, N. "Knowledge Discovery and Data Mining", *the Encyclopedia of Micro-computers*, Volume 27 (Supplement 6) Marcel Dekker (2001) 93-122.
25. Zhong, N., Yao, Y.Y., Ohshima, M., and Ohsuga, S. "Interestingness, Peculiarity, and Multi-Database Mining", *Proc. 2001 IEEE International Conference on Data Mining (ICDM'01)*, IEEE Computer Society Press (2001) 566-573.
26. Zhong, N. and Ohsuga, S. "Automatic Knowledge Discovery in Larger Scale Knowledge-Data Bases", C. Leondes (ed.) *The Handbook of Expert Systems*, Vol.4: Chapter 29, Academic Press (2001) 1015-1070.
27. Zhong, N., Liu, C., and Ohsuga, S. "Dynamically Organizing KDD Process", *International Journal of Pattern Recognition and Artificial Intelligence*, Vol. 15, No. 3, World Scientific (2001) 451-473.
28. Zhong, N., Dong, J.Z., and Ohsuga, S. "Rule Discovery by Soft Induction Techniques", *Neurocomputing*, An International Journal, Vol. 36 (1-4) Elsevier (2001) 171-204.
29. Zhong, N., Yao, Y.Y., Dong, J.Z., Ohsuga, S., "Gastric Cancer Data Mining with Ordered Information", J.J. Alpigini et al (eds.) *Rough Sets and Current Trends in Computing*, LNAI 2475, Springer (2002) 467-478.
30. Zhong, N., Yao, Y.Y., Ohshima M., "Peculiarity Oriented Multidatabase Mining", *IEEE Transactions on Knowledge and Data Engineering*, Vol.15, No.4 (2003) 952-960.

Sentence Role Identification in Medline Abstracts: Training Classifier with Structured Abstracts

Masashi Shimbo, Takahiro Yamasaki, and Yuji Matsumoto

Graduate School of Information Science,
Nara Institute of Science and Technology,
8916-5 Takayama, Ikoma, Nara 630-0192, Japan
{shimbo, takah-ya, matsu}@is.naist.jp

Abstract. The abstract of a scientific paper typically consists of sentences describing the background of study, its objective, experimental method and results, and conclusions. We discuss the task of identifying which of these "structural roles" each sentence in abstracts plays, with a particular focus on its application in building a literature retrieval system. By annotating sentences in an abstract collection with role labels, we can build a literature retrieval system in which users can specify the roles of the sentences in which query terms should be sought. We argue that this facility enables more goal-oriented search, and also makes it easier to narrow down search results when adding extra query terms does not work. To build such a system, two issues need to be addressed: (1) how we should determine the set of structural roles presented to users from which they can choose the target search area, and (2) how we should classify each sentence in abstracts by their structural roles, without relying too much on human supervision. We view the task of role identification as that of text classification based on supervised machine learning. Our approach is characterized by the use of *structured abstracts* for building training data. In structured abstracts, which is a format of abstracts popular in biomedical domains, sections are explicitly marked with headings indicating their structural roles, and hence they provide us with an inexpensive way to collect training data for sentence classifiers. Statistics on the structured abstracts contained in Medline give an insight on determining the set of sections to be presented to users as well.

Keywords: Medline, structured abstracts, information retrieval, text classification.

1 Introduction

With the rapid increase in the volume of scientific literature, there has been growing interest in systems with which researchers can find relevant pieces of literature with less effort. Online literature retrieval services, including PubMed [11] and CiteSeer [7], are gaining popularity, as they provide users with access to large database of abstracts or full papers.

PubMed helps researchers in medicine and biology by enabling search in the Medline abstracts [9]. It also supports a number of auxiliary ways to filter search results. For example, users can limit search with the content of the title and journal fields, or by specifying the range of publication dates. All these additional facilities, however, rely

S. Tsumoto et al. (Eds.): AM 2003, LNAI 3430, pp. 236–254, 2005.

on information external to the content of abstract text. This paper exploit information inherent in abstracts, in order to make retrieval process more goal-oriented.

The information we exploit is the structure underlying abstract text. The literature search system we implemented allows search to be limited within portions of an abstract, where 'portions' are selected from the typical structural roles within an abstract, such as Background, Objective, (Experimental) Methods, (Experimental) Results, and Conclusions. We expect such a system to substantially reduce users' effort to narrow down search results, which may be huge with only one or two query terms. This expectation is based on the postulate that some of these 'portions' are more relevant to the goal of users compared with the rest. For example, a clinician, trying to find whether an effect of a chemical substance on a disease is known or not, can ask the search engine for passages in which the names of the substance and the disease both occur, but only in the sentences describing results and conclusions. And if a user wants to browse through what is addressed in each paper, listing only sentences describing study objective (and possibly conclusions) should be convenient.

With conventional search systems in which adding extra query terms is the only measure of narrowing down, it is not easy (if not possible) to achieve the same effect as the role-restricted search. Moreover, it is not always evident to users what extra query terms are effective for narrowing down. Specifying the target roles of sentences may be helpful in this case, providing an alternative way for limiting search.

An issue in building such a system is how to infer the roles of sentences in the abstract collection. Because of the volume of the collection is often huge, manually labeling sentences is not a viable option; it is therefore desirable to automate this process. To automate this task, it is natural to formulate the task as that of supervised text classification, in which sentences are classified into one of the predefined set of structural roles. The main topics of this paper are (1) how to reduce reliance on human supervision in making training data for the sentence classifiers, and (2) what classes, or sections, should be presented to users so that they can effectively restrict search. This last decision must be made on account of a trade-off between usability and accuracy of sentence classification. We also examine (3) what types of features are effective for classification.

The rest of this paper is organized as follows. We first present some statistics on structured abstracts in Medline and state the set of classes used in the subsequent discussions (Section 2). Section 3 describes the techniques used for building classifier and computing features used for classification. These features are described in Section 4. We then present experimental results showing the effect of various features used for classification (Section 5), followed by a summary of the Medline search system we implemented (Section 6). Finally we conclude in Section 7.

2   Structured Abstracts in Medline

Our method of classifying sentences into their structural roles relies on 'structured abstracts' contained in Medline. The abstracts of this type have explicit sections marked in text, and hence are usable for training sentence classifiers which assign a section label to each sentence in the remaining 'unstructured' abstracts having no explicit sectioning information.

Table 1. Ratio of structured and unstructured abstracts in Medline 2002

	# of abstracts /	%
Structured	374,585 /	6.0%
Unstructured	5,912,271 /	94.0%
Total	11,299,108 / 100.0%	

Table 2. Frequency of individual sections in structured abstracts from Medline 2002

Sections	# of abstracts	# of sentences
CONCLUSION	352,153	246,607
RESULT	324,479	1,378,785
METHOD	209,910	540,415
BACKGROUND	120,877	264,589
OBJECTIVE	165,972	166,890
⋮	⋮	⋮

This section present and analyze some statistics on the structured abstracts contained in Medline, which may affect the quality of training data and, in effect, the performance of resulting sentence classifiers. We also determine the set of classes presented to users on the basis of analysis in this section.

2.1 Structured Abstracts

Since its proposal in 1987, a growing number of biological and medical journals have begun to adopt so-called 'structured abstracts' [1]. These journals require abstract text to be divided into sections reflecting the structure of the abstract. Sectioning schemes are sometimes regulated by journals, and sometimes left to the choice of authors. The commonly used section names include BACKGROUND, OBJECTIVE, and CONCLU-SIONS. Each section in structured abstracts are explicitly marked with a heading (usually written in all upper-case letters, and followed by a colon). Therefore, a heading indicates the structural role (i.e., class) of the sentences following them. Unfortunately, the number of unstructured abstracts in Medline far exceeds that of structured abstracts (Table 1). Tables 2 and 3 respectively show the frequencies of individual headings and sectioning schemes.

2.2 Section Headings = Classes?

The fact that unstructured abstracts form a majority leads to the idea of automatically assigning a section label to each sentence in unstructured abstracts. This labeling process can be formulated as a sentence classification task if we fix a set of sections (classes) into which sentences should be classified[1]. An issue here is what classes, or sections, must be

---

[1] It is possible that a sentence belongs to two or more sections, such as when it consists of a clause describing research background and another clause describing research objective. However, since this is relatively rare, we assume a sentence is the minimum unit of role assignment throughout the paper.

Table 3. Frequency of sectioning schemes (# of abstracts)

Rank	# /	%	Section sequence
1	61,603 /	16.6%	BACKGROUND / METHOD(S) / RESULTS / CONCLUSION(S)
*2	54,997 /	14.7%	OBJECTIVE / METHOD(S) / RESULTS / CONCLUSION(S)
*3	25,008 /	6.6%	PURPOSE / METHOD(S) / RESULTS / CONCLUSION(S)
4	11,412 /	3.0%	PURPOSE / MATERIALS AND METHOD(S) / RESULTS / CONCLUSION(S)
5	8,706 /	2.3%	BACKGROUND / OBJECTIVE / METHOD(S) / RESULTS / CONCLUSION(S)
6	8,321 /	2.2%	OBJECTIVE / STUDY DESIGN / RESULTS / CONCLUSION(S)
7	7,833 /	2.1%	BACKGROUND / METHOD(S) AND RESULTS / CONCLUSION(S)
*8	7,074 /	1.9%	AIM(S) / METHOD(S) / RESULTS / CONCLUSION(S)
9	6,095 /	1.6%	PURPOSE / PATIENTS AND METHOD(S) / RESULTS / CONCLUSION(S)
10	4,087 /	1.1%	BACKGROUND AND PURPOSE / METHOD(S) / RESULTS / CONCLUSION(S)
⋮	⋮	⋮	⋮
Total	374,585 / 100.0%		

presented to users so that they can specify the portion of abstract texts to which search should be limited. It is natural to choose these classes from section headings occurring in structured abstracts, because they reflect the conventional wisdom and it will allow us to use those abstracts to train sentence classifiers used for labeling unstructured abstracts. The problem is that there are more than 6,000 distinct headings in Medline 2002.

To maintain usability, the number of sections offered to users must be kept as small as possible, but not so small as to impair the usefulness of role-limited search. But then, if we restrict the number of classes, how should a section in a structured abstract be treated when its heading does not match any of the restricted classes? In most cases, translating a section into the classes of similar roles is straightforward, unless the selection of the classes is unreasonable. For instance, identifying PURPOSE section with OBJECTIVE section should generally be admissible. In practice, however, there are section headings such as "BACKGROUND AND PURPOSES." If BACKGROUND and PURPOSES are two distinct classes presented to users, which we believe is a reasonable decision, we need to determine which of these two classes each sentence in the section belongs to. Therefore, at least some of the sentences in structured abstracts need to go through the same labeling process as the unstructured abstracts.

Even when the section they belong to has a heading that seems straightforward to assign a class, there are cases in which we have to classify sentences in a structured abstract. The above mentioned OBJECTIVE (or PURPOSE) class is actually one such class that needs sentence-wise classification. Below, we will analyze this case further.

As Table 3 shows, the most frequent *sequences* of headings are

1. BACKGROUND, METHOD(S), RESULTS, and CONCLUSION(S), followed by
2. OBJECTIVE, METHOD(S), RESULTS, and CONCLUSION(S).

Both of the above formats have only one of the two sections, BACKGROUND and OB-JECTIVE, but not both. Inspecting abstracts conforming to these formats we found that most of these two sections actually contain both the sentences describing research background, and those describing research objective; sentences describing research background occurred frequently in OBJECTIVE, and a large number of sentences describing research objective were found in BACKGROUND as well.

This observation suggests that when an abstract contains only one BACKGROUND or OBJECTIVE section, we should not take these headings as class labels for granted. We should instead apply a sentence classifier to each sentence under these headings.

To verify this claim, we computed Sibson's information radius (Jensen-Shannon divergence) [8] for each section. Information radius D_{JS} between two probability distributions $p(x)$ and $q(x)$ is defined as follows, using Kullback-Leibler divergence D_{KL}.

$$D_{JS}(p\|q) = \frac{1}{2}\left[D_{KL}\left(p\|\frac{p+q}{2}\right) + D_{KL}\left(q\|\frac{p+q}{2}\right)\right]$$
$$= \frac{1}{2}\left[\sum_x p(x)\log\frac{p(x)}{(p(x)+q(x))/2} + \sum_x q(x)\log\frac{q(x)}{(p(x)+q(x))/2}\right].$$

Hence, information radius is a measure of dissimilarity between distributions. It is symmetric in p and q, and is always well-defined; these properties do not hold with D_{KL}.

Table 4 shows that the sentences under the BACKGROUND and OBJECTIVE sections have similar distributions of word bigrams (a sequence of consecutive words of length 2) and the combination of words and word bigrams. Also note the smaller divergence between these classes (bold faced figures), compared with those for the other class pairs. The implication is that these two headings are probably unreliable as separate class labels.

Table 4. Information radius between the sections

Class	BACKGROUND	OBJECTIVE	METHOD	RESULT	CONCLUSION
	(a) Word bigrams				
BACKGROUND	0	**0.1809**	0.3064	0.3152	0.2023
OBJECTIVE	**0.1809**	0	0.2916	0.3256	0.2370
METHOD	0.3064	0.2916	0	0.2168	0.3201
RESULT	0.3152	0.3256	0.2168	0	0.2703
CONCLUSION	0.2023	0.2370	0.3201	0.2703	0
	(b) Word unigrams and bigrams				
Class	BACKGROUND	OBJECTIVE	METHOD	RESULT	CONCLUSION
BACKGROUND	0	**0.1099**	0.2114	0.2171	0.1202
OBJECTIVE	**0.1099**	0	0.1965	0.2221	0.1465
METHOD	0.2114	0.1965	0	0.1397	0.2201
RESULT	0.2171	0.2221	0.1397	0	0.1847
CONCLUSION	0.1202	0.1465	0.2201	0.1847	0

2.3   Structural Role Identification as Text Classification

The task of sentence role identification can be cast as that of text classification in which sentences are classified into one of the classes representing structural roles. As mentioned earlier, this formulation requires the set of classes to be fixed. With the statistics presented in the previous subsections, and the frequency of individual headings (Table 2) in particular, we adopt the most frequent five headings as the classes representing sentence roles, namely, BACKGROUND, OBJECTIVE, METHOD, RESULT, and CONCLUSION. In the subsequent sections, we will examine the performance of classifiers trained with structured abstracts, mostly under this five-class setting.

The inclusion of BACKGROUND and OBJECTIVE as individual classes may sound contradictory to the analysis in Section 2.2, namely, that BACKGROUND and OBJEC-TIVE headings are unreliable to be taken as the class labels because these sections typically consist of sentences describing both background and objective. It is however not acceptable to merge them as a single class, even though doing so might make classification easier. Merging them would deteriorate the usefulness of the system, since they are quite different in their structural roles, and, as a result, they have different utility depending on the users' search objective. We will address the problem of mixture of sentences describing background and objective in the experiment of Section 5.2.

3   Technical Background

This section reviews the techniques used in designing sentence role classifiers.

3.1   Support Vector Machines

The Support Vector Machine (SVM) is a supervised machine learning method for binary classification. Let the training data of size m be

$$(x_1, y_1), \ldots, (x_m, y_m), \quad x_i \in \mathbb{R}^n, \ y_i \in \{+1, -1\}$$

such that x_i is the n-dimensional vector representation for the i-th datum (example), and y_i is the label indicating whether the example is positive $(+1)$ or negative (-1).

Given these data, SVM computes a hyperplane

$$f(x) = w \cdot x + b = 0 \quad w \in \mathbb{R}^n, \ b \in \mathbb{R}$$

in the n-dimensional space that separates positive examples from negative ones, i.e., for any $i \in \{1, \ldots, l\}$,

$$y_i f(x_i) = y_i(w \cdot x + b) > 0. \tag{1}$$

Generally, if given data is indeed linearly separable, there exist infinitely many separating hyperplanes that satisfy eq. (1). Among these, SVM chooses the one that maximizes the *margin*, which is the distance from the nearest examples to the hyperplane. This margin-maximization feature of SVM makes it less prone to over-fitting in a higher dimensional feature space, as it has been proven that such "optimal" separating hyperplanes minimize the expected error on test data [15]. The nearest example vectors to the separating hyperplane are called *support vectors*, reflecting the fact that the optimal hyperplane (or vector w) is a linear combination of these vectors.

Finding the optimal hyperplane reduces to solving a quadratic optimization problem. After this hyperplane (namely, w and b) is obtained, SVM predicts label y for a given test example x with the following decision function.

$$y = \text{sgn}(f(x)) = \text{sgn}(w \cdot x + b).$$

Even if the examples are not linearly separable, the problem is still solvable with a variation of SVMs, called soft-margin SVMs [4, 15], which allow a small amount of exceptional examples (called bounded support vectors) to violate separability condition (1). Acceptable range of exceptions is controllable through soft-margin parameter $C \in [0, \infty)$, where smaller C tolerates a larger number of bounded support vectors.

It is also possible to first map the examples into higher-dimensional feature space and find separating hyperplane in this space, with the help of the kernel trick [12].

3.2 Multi-class Classification with Support Vector Machines

SVM is a binary classifier while the task of sentence role identification is a multi-class classification involving five classes. For this reason, SVM cannot be applied to this task directly, and instead we construct multiple SVMs and combine their output. There are two simple ways to combine multiple SVMs to obtain multi-class classification, namely, the (i) one-versus-the-rest and (ii) pairwise methods. We will use both of these methods in Section 5 and compare their performance.

One-Versus-the-Rest. In the one-versus-the-rest method, we first construct five SVM classifiers, each one designed to distinguish sentence belonging to a class from the rest; BACKGROUND, OBJECTIVE, METHOD, RESULT, and CONCLUSION. In training these SVMs, we use the sentences in one class as the positive examples, and those in the other classes as the negative examples.

Given a test example, we apply the five trained SVM classifiers to this example independently and combine the results as follows. For ease of exposition, first assume that we are using linear kernels and thus the input space is identical to the feature space. For each class index $i = 1, \dots 5$, let $f_i(x) = w_i \cdot x + b_i = 0$ be the separating hyperplane of the SVM designed to separate the i-th class from the rest. We determine the class assigned to a given test example x to be the one represented by the SVM with the largest $d_i(x)$ among $i = 1, \dots, 5$, where $d_i(x)$ is the signed distance of an example x from the hyperplane $f_i(x) = 0$; i.e.,

$$d_i(x) = \frac{f_i(x)}{|w_i|} = \frac{w_i \cdot x + b_i}{|w_i|}. \tag{2}$$

When we use non-linear kernels, we essentially follow the same rule, except that in this case x in equation (2) represents not the example itself but its image in the kernel-induced feature space. Although the image x and the vector w_i are generally not available due to high or infinite dimensionality of the induced feature space (which, in turn, is the dimensionality of x and w_i), the kernel trick allows us to compute the value of $|w_i|$ as well as $f_i(x)$. It follows that the signed distance from the image x in the feature space to the separating hyperplane $f_i(x) = 0$ (also in the feature space) is still computable with equation (2) even in the case of non-linear kernels.

Pairwise Combination. In the pairwise method, we build a total of $C(5,2) = 10$ SVMs. Each SVM corresponds to a pair of distinct classes, and is trained to distinguish between the classes participating in the pair. The final class of a given test example is determined by counting the vote each class receives from the 10 SVMs. Although the number of SVMs needed is higher than the one-versus-the-rest method, component SVM classifiers in the pairwise method are trained only with the examples belonging to the classes in the pair, and hence training them usually takes much less time than those of the one-versus-the-rest classifiers.

4   Feature Set

In Section 5, we will examine various types of features for sentence role identification and evaluate their performance. The types of features examined are described in this section. These features can be categorized into those which represent the information internal to the sentence in question, and those representing textual context surrounding the sentence. We refer to the former as 'non-contextual' features and the latter as 'contextual' features.

4.1   Words and Word Bigrams

As the most basic types of non-contextual features, we use words and contiguous word bigrams contained in sentences. To be specific, a sentence is represented as a binary vector in which each coordinate corresponds to a word (or word bigram), and has a value of 1 if the word (word bigram) occurs in a sentence at least once; Otherwise, the vector has 0 at the coordinate.

4.2   Tense

Another type of non-contextual feature we examine is base on the tense of sentences. A majority of authors seem to prefer changing tense depending on the structural role; some of them write the background of study in the past perfect tense, and others write objective in the present tense. To verify this claim, we examined the distribution of the tense of 135489 sentences in 11898 structured abstracts in Medline 2002, all of which have the section sequence of BACKGROUND, OBJECTIVE, METHOD, RESULTS and CONCLUSION.

We obtained the tense information of each sentence as follows. Given a sentence as input, we applied Charniak parser [2] to it, to obtain its phrase structure tree. We then recursively applied the Collins head rules [3] to this phrase structure tree, which yields the dependency structure tree of the sentence. From the dependency tree, we identify the head verb of a sentence, which is the verb located nearest to the root of the tree. The process so far is illustrated in Figures 1–3. Finally, the information on the tense of a head verb can be obtained from the part-of-speech tag Charniak parser associates to it. Table 5 lists the Penn Treebank tags for verbs output by Charniak parser. We incorporate each of these as a feature as well. A problem here is that the Penn Treebank tag associated with head verb alone does not allow us to distinguish the verbs 'have', 'has' and 'had' used as a normal verb (as in 'I had a good time.') from those used as a auxiliary verb introducing present or past perfect tense (as in 'I have been to Europe.'). Hence, we not

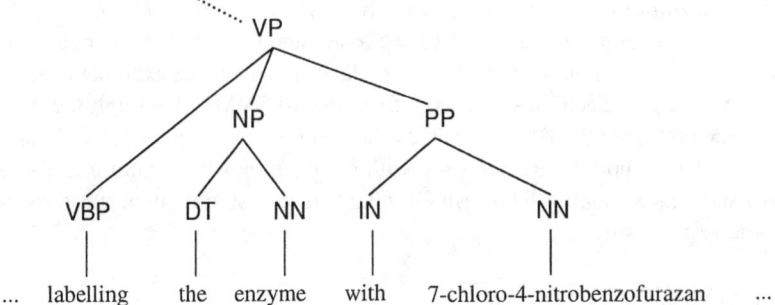

Fig. 1. Phrase structure subtree. Leaf nodes correspond to surface words, and each non-leaf node is labeled with a syntax category

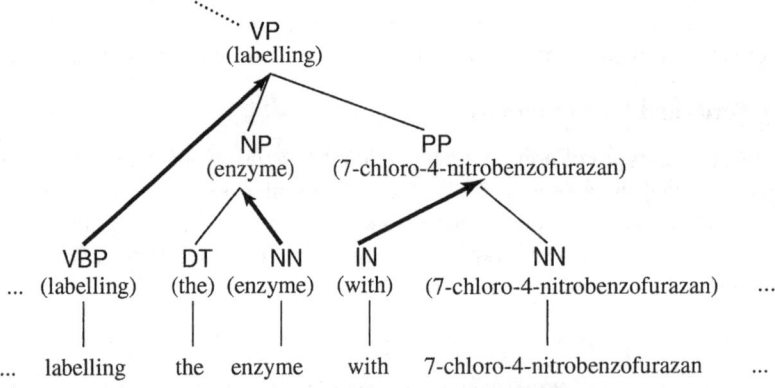

Fig. 2. Phrase structure subtree labeled with headwords. Bold arrows depicts the inheritance of head words by the head rules, and inherited head words are shown in parentheses

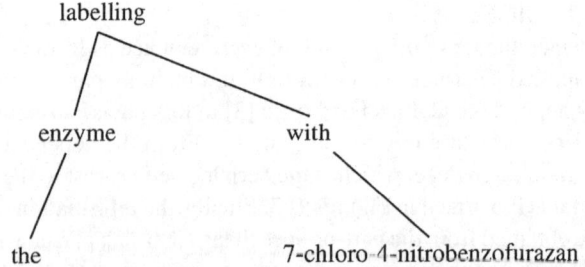

Fig. 3. Dependency tree. This tree is obtained from Figure 2, by first colescing the leaf nodes with their parents, and then recursively coalescing the nodes connected with the bold arrows

Table 5. The tags used in our experiment: Penn Treebank tags for verbs

Tag	Meaning	Example
VB	verb, base form	To *determine* the nature …
VBG	verb, present participle or gerund	patients *receiving* …
VBP	verb, present tense, not third person singular	results *suggest* that …
VBZ	verb, present tense, third person singular	This study *shows* that …
VBD	verb, past tense	We *analyzed* the …
VBN	verb, past participle	photographs *taken* for …
MD	modal auxiliary	We *can* make …

Table 6. Distribution of the tense of head verbs included in each class (%)

Tense	BACKGROUND	OBJECTIVE	METHOD	RESULT	CONCLUSION
VB	1.2	27.9	0.6	0.7	1.7
VBG	0.1	0.5	0.3	0.3	0.0
VBP	20.2	3.9	1.6	2.4	25.4
VBZ	38.2	53.4	1.8	3.2	33.8
VBD	6.9	3.5	91.0	86.0	16.6
VBN	0.7	3.5	2.5	3.2	0.7
MD	9.0	1.0	0.1	1.1	19.5
Present perfect	22.8	0.9	0.3	0.6	1.4
Past perfect	0.1	0.0	0.3	1.2	0.7
Others	0.7	2.0	1.2	1.4	0.6
Total	100	100	100	100	100

Table 7. Distribution of the class given the tense of head verbs (%)

Tense	BACKGROUND	OBJECTIVE	METHOD	RESULT	CONCLUSION	Total
VB	5.8	75.3	3.9	7.0	8.1	100
VBG	8.2	19.6	29.9	37.2	5.1	100
VBP	36.5	4.0	4.1	9.4	46.0	100
VBZ	44.8	4.6	3.0	8.1	39.6	100
VBD	1.9	8.3	34.3	50.9	4.5	100
VBN	5.6	14.4	25.1	49.8	5.1	100
MD	28.2	1.8	0.7	8.8	61.4	100
Present perfect	86.2	2.1	1.7	4.5	5.4	100
Past perfect	9.3	15.8	23.8	42.7	8.4	100

only use the tags of Table 5 as the features, but also introduce the features indicating 'present perfect tense' and 'past perfect tense.' The coordinate in a feature vector for present perfect tense has 1 if the sentence has 'have' or 'has' as its head verb, and also has another past participle verb depending on the head verb in its dependency structure tree. The feature for 'past perfect tense' is defined likewise when a sentence has the head verb of 'had.'

Tables 6 and 7 respectively show the distribution of the tense of head verbs in each class, and the distribution of classes given a tense. As we see from these tables, some tense exhibits a strongly correlated with the class of the sentence. For example, if we know that a sentence is written in present perfect tense, there is more than 85% of a chance that the sentence is speaking about the background of the study. In addition, the distribution of tense of the head verb is significantly different from one class to another.

In Section 5.3, we examine the effectiveness of the tense of the head verb of each sentence as the feature for classification.

4.3   Contextual Information

Since we are interested in labeling a *series* of sentences, we can expect that classification performance to be improved by incorporating information gained from textual context into the feature set. Context features should allow us to capture the following tendency, among others.

- It is unlikely that experimental results (RESULT) are presented before the description of experimental design (METHOD). Thus, whether the preceding sentences have been labeled as METHOD conditions the probability of the present sentence being classified as RESULT.
- The sentences of the same class have a good chance of occurring consecutively; we would not expect authors to interleave sentences describing experimental results (RESULT) with those in CONCLUSION and OBJECTIVE classes.

There are several conceivable ways to represent contextual information. Because it is not clear which representation is most effective, we examine the following types of context representation in an experiment of Section 5.1.

1. Class label of the previous sentence in the present abstract.
2. Class labels of the previous two sentences.
3. Class label of the next sentence.
4. Class labels of the next two sentences.
5. Relative location of the current sentence within an abstract.
6. Non-contextual features (word and word bigram features) of the previous sentence.
7. Non-contextual features of the next sentence.
8. Non-contextual features of the previous and the next sentences.

5   Experiments

This section reports the results of the experiments we conducted to examine the performance of sentence classifiers.

5.1   Contextual Information

In the first experiment, we evaluated the performance of different context feature representations. In this experiment, structured abstracts from Medline 2002 were used. The classes we considered (or, sections into which sentences are classified) are OBJECTIVE, METHOD(S), RESULTS, and CONCLUSION(S). Note that this set does not coincide with the five classes we employed in the final system. According to Table 3, the section sequence consisting of these sections are only second after the sequence BACKGROUND / METHOD(S) / RESULTS / CONCLUSION. However, identifying the sentences with headings PURPOSE and AIM with those with OBJECTIVE makes the corresponding sectioning scheme the most frequent. Hence, we collected structured abstracts whose heading sequences match one of the following patterns:

1. OBJECTIVE / METHOD(S) / RESULTS / CONCLUSION(S),
2. PURPOSE / METHOD(S) / RESULTS / CONCLUSION(S),
3. AIM(S) / METHOD(S) / RESULTS / CONCLUSION(S).

After removing all symbols and replacing every contiguous sequence of numbers with a single symbol '#', we split each of these abstracts into sentences using the UIUC sentence splitter. [14], We then filtered out the abstracts that produced a sentence with less than three words, regarding it as a possible error in sentence splitting. This yielded a total of 82,936 abstracts.

To reduce the number of features, we only took into account word bigrams occurring in at least 0.05% of the sentences, which amounts to 9,078 distinct bigrams. On the other hand, we used all words as the features to avoid null feature vectors. The number of unigram word features was 104,733, and this makes a total of 113,811 features excluding the number context features.

We obtained 103,962 training examples (sentences) from 10,000 abstracts randomly sampled from the set of the 82,936 structured abstracts, and 10,356 test examples (sentences) from 1,000 abstracts randomly sampled from the rest of the set.

For each of the nine context feature representations listed in Section 4.3, a set of four soft-margin SVMs, one for each class, was built using the one-versus-the-rest configuration, yielding a total of $4 \cdot 9 = 36$ SVMs. The quadratic kernel was used with SVMs, and the soft margin (or capacity) parameter C was tuned independently for each SVM to achieve best performance. The performance of different context features are shown in Table 8.

In training SVMs with Features (1)–(4), the classes of surrounding sentences are the correct labels obtained in the training data. In the test phase, because training data are

Table 8. Performance of context features (one-versus-the-rest)

Feature types	Accuracy (%)	
	sentence	abstract
(0) Non-contextual features alone (No context features)	83.6	25.0
(1) (0) + Class label of the previous sentence	88.9	48.9
(2) (0) + Class labels of the previous two sentences	89.9	50.6
(3) (0) + Class label of the next sentence	88.9	50.9
(4) (0) + Class labels of the next two sentences	89.3	51.2
(5) (0) + Relative location of the current sentence	91.9	50.7
(6) (0) + Non-contextual features of the previous sentence	87.3	37.5
(7) (0) + Non-contextual features of the next sentence	88.1	39.0
(8) (0) + Non-contextual features of the previous and the next sentences	89.7	46.4

not labeled, we first applied SVMs to the surrounding sentences, and used the induced labels as their classes; thus, these context features are not necessarily correct.

There was not much difference in the performance of contextual features as far as accuracy was measured on a per-sentence basis. All contextual features (1)–(8) obtained about 90% accuracy, which is an improvement of 4 to 8% over the baseline (0) in which no context features were used. By contrast, the accuracy on a per-abstract basis, in which a classification of an abstract is judged to be correct only if all the constituent sentences are correctly classified, varied between 37% and 51%. The maximum accuracy of 51%, a 26% improvement over the baseline (0), was obtained for features (3), (4), and (5).

5.2   Pairwise Classification Performance

The analysis of Section 2.2 suggests that it is unreliable to regard the section headings BACKGROUND and OBJECTIVE as the labels of sentences in these sections. The BACKGROUND sections frequently contain sentences that should rather be classified as OBJECTIVE, and vice versa. Yet, it is not acceptable to merge them as a single class, because they are quite different in their structural roles; doing so would severely impair the utility of the system.

A solution to this and similar situations is to build a specialized SVM classifier that distinguish between the pair of classes involved, in a manner similar to the pairwise method for multi-class classification of Section 3.2. The next experiment assessed the feasibility of this approach.

This time, we collected 11,898 abstracts consisting of either one of the following heading sequences:

1. BACKGROUND, OBJECTIVE, METHOD(S), RESULTS, CONCLUSION(S),
2. OBJECTIVE, BACKGROUND, METHOD(S), RESULTS, CONCLUSION(S).

Thus, the abstracts having only one of BACKGROUND and OBJECTIVE are not included in this experiment, in order to avoid the mixture of sentences of different roles in these classes; such mixture was observed only when exactly one of these sections occurred in an abstract.

Table 9. Pairwise classification performance (F-measure) using no context features

Class pair	F-measure
BACKGROUND / OBJECTIVE	96.1
BACKGROUND / METHOD	96.1
BACKGROUND / RESULT	92.2
BACKGROUND / CONCLUSION	81.3
OBJECTIVE / METHOD	92.3
OBJECTIVE / RESULT	95.1
OBJECTIVE / CONCLUSION	94.5
METHOD / RESULT	91.3
METHOD / CONCLUSION	96.9
RESULT / CONCLUSION	93.9

Table 10. Performance of context features (pairwise combination)

Feature types	Accuracy (%) sentence	abstract
(0) Non-contextual features alone (No context features)	83.5	19.5
(1) (0) + Class label of the previous sentence	90.0	50.2
(2) (0) + Class labels of the previous two sentences	91.1	53.2
(3) (0) + Class label of the next sentence	89.3	53.1
(4) (0) + Class labels of the next two sentences	90.1	54.4
(5) (0) + Relative location of the current sentence	92.4	47.9
(6) (0) + Non-contextual features of the previous sentence	86.9	32.0
(7) (0) + Non-contextual features of the next sentence	87.2	31.0
(8) (0) + Non-contextual features of the previous and the next sentences	89.9	43.2

The abstracts in this collection went through the same preprocessing as in Section 5.1, and the number of sentences that survived preprocessing was 135,489. We randomly sampled 90% of the collected abstracts as training data, and retained the rest for testing. For each of the 10 $(= C(5,2))$ pairs of section labels, an SVM was trained only with the sentences belonging to that specific pair of sections, using one section as positive examples and the other as negative examples. Again, we used quadratic kernels and the bag-of-words and word-bigrams features. No context features were used this time.

The result is shown in Table 9. Note that an F-measure of 96.1 was observed in discriminating BACKGROUND from OBJECTIVE, which is a specific example discussed in Section 2.2. This result implies the feasibility of the pairwise classification approach in this task.

For reference, we present in Table 10 the performance of the multi-class classification with pairwise combination using various context features. This experiment was conducted under the same setting as Section 5.1. The difference in performance appears to be marginal between the one-versus-the-rest (cf. Table 8) and pairwise combination methods.

5.3 Tense Information

In this experiment, we used the tense information in addition to the word and word-bigrams, in the pairwise multi-class classification setting. The result is listed in Table 11. From this table, we see that the improvement in multi-class classification performance brought about by the tense features were marginal. However, turning our eyes to the classification of individual class pairs (Table 12), we see a modest improvement in performance in class pairs such as OBJECTIVE vs. METHOD, and BACKGROUND vs.

Table 11. Multi-class classification using tense information (Accuracy: %)

Features	Sentence	Abstract
Without tense information	83.5	19.5
With tense information	83.7	20.9

Table 12. Performance for individual class pair using the word, word bigrams and tense features

Class pair	F-measure
BACKGROUND / OBJECTIVE	96.3
BACKGROUND / METHOD	96.1
BACKGROUND / RESULTS	92.8
BACKGROUND / CONCLUSION	81.7
OBJECTIVE / METHOD	93.1
OBJECTIVE / RESULTS	95.2
OBJECTIVE / CONCLUSION	94.9
METHOD / RESULTS	91.3
METHOD / CONCLUSION	97.2
RESULTS / CONCLUSION	94.2

RESULTS. We note that these pairs coincide with those having quite distinct distribution of tense (cf. Table 6).

5.4   Evaluation with Unstructured Abstracts

The result presented so far is evaluated with the structured abstracts. However, our final goal is to label unstructured abstracts with these data. This subsection reports the result of applying the sentence role classifier trained with structured abstracts, to a small amount of manually labeled unstructured abstracts. The labeled test data consists of 14,153 sentences from 1,731 abstracts. The distribution of the five role classes is shown in Table 13, and that of the class sequence in Table 14. As seen from Table 13, the distribution of classes is quite similar between the structured abstracts used for training and unstructured abstracts used for testing.

The result of this experiment is shown in Table 15. Without context features, the sentence-wise accuracy drops from 83% to 75%, and abstract-wise accuracy from 25% to 15%. Among the context features, Features (7) (non-context features of surrounding sentences) and (8) (relative location of the sentences within an abstract) performed best. The types of context features using class labels, namely, Features (1)–(4), performed poorly in this experiment; they often exhibited a classification accuracy worse than the case where no context features were used. The reason for this poor performance should

Table 13. Frequency of sentence role classes in unstructured and structured abstracts

class	unstructured abstracts # sentences / %	structured abstracts # sentences / %
BACKGROUND	2,207 / 15.6	22,095 / 16.3
OBJECTIVE	1,286 / 9.1	12,666 / 9.3
METHOD	2,320 / 16.4	30,564 / 22.6
RESULTS	6,184 / 43.7	48,064 / 35.5
CONCLUSION	2,254 / 15.9	22.100 / 16.3
Total	14,153 / 100	135,489 / 100

Table 14. Frequency of class sequences in unstructured abstracts

# abstracts / %	class sequence
236 / 13.6	BACKGROUND / OBJECTIVE / METHOD / RESULTS / CONCLUSION
222 / 12.8	BACKGROUND / METHOD / RESULTS / CONCLUSION
182 / 10.5	OBJECTIVE / METHOD / RESULTS / CONCLUSION
150 / 8.7	BACKGROUND / OBJECTIVE / RESULTS / CONCLUSION
107 / 6.1	METHOD / RESULTS / CONCLUSION
⋮ ⋮	⋮
Total 1,731 / 100.0	

Table 15. Classification accuracy of unstructured abstracts using SVMs trained with structured abstracts

Feature types	Accuracy (%) Sentence	Abstract
(0) Words and word bigrams	75.4	15.0
(1) (0) + Class of the next sentence	68.1	16.3
(2) (0) + Classes of the next two sentences	64.2	10.7
(3) (0) + Class of the next sentence	71.7	15.7
(4) (0) + Classes of the next two sentences	72.2	15.6
(5) (0) + Non-contextual features of the previous sentence	76.2	17.3
(6) (0) + Non-contextual features of the next sentence	76.2	16.9
(7) (0) + Non-contextual features of the previous and next sentences	78.3	20.1
(8) (0) + Relative location	78.6	19.4

be that we trained the classifier using only structured abstracts with a fixed heading sequence.

6 A Prototype Implementation

Using the feature set described in Section 3.1 together with the context feature (5) of Section 4.3, we constructed five SVM classifiers, one for each of the five sections: BACKGROUND, OBJECTIVE, METHOD, RESULT, and CONCLUSION. With these SVMs, we labeled the sentences in the unstructured abstracts in Medline 2003 whose publication year is either 2001 or 2002. The same labeling process was also applied to the sentences in structured abstracts when correspondence was not evident between their section headings and one of the above five sections. For instance, when the heading was 'MATERIALS AND METHODS,' we did not apply the labeling process, but regarded it as 'METHOD'; when it was 'METHODS AND RESULTS,' the classifiers were applied in order to tell which of the two classes, METHOD and RESULT, each constituent sentence belongs to.

As an exception, when a structured abstract contained either one of BACKGROUND or OBJECTIVE (or equivalent) sections but not both, we also classified the sentences in these sections into one of the BACKGROUND and the OBJECTIVE classes, using the pairwise classifier described in Section 5.2 for discriminating these two classes. This exception reflects the observation made in Section 2.2.

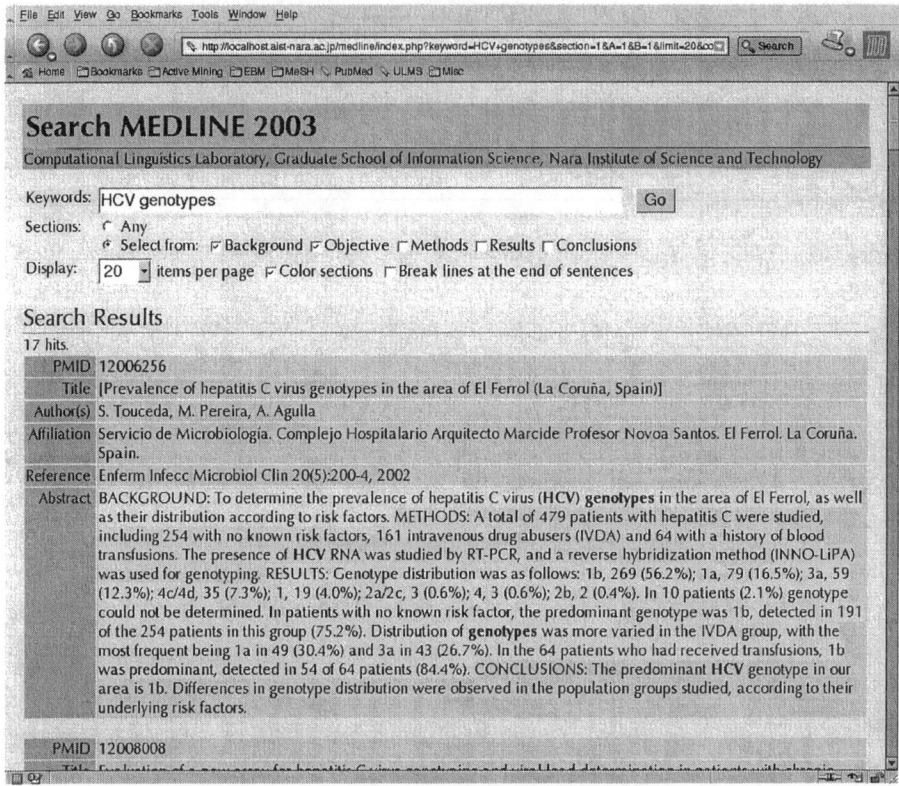

Fig. 4. Screen shot of the prototype search system

An experimental literature retrieval system was implemented using PHP on top of the Apache web server. The full-text retrieval engine Namazu [10] was used as a back-end search engine[2]. A screenshot is shown in Figure 4. The form on the page contains a field for entering query terms, a 'Go' button and radio buttons marked 'Any' and 'Select from' for choosing whether the keyword search should be performed on the whole abstract texts, or on limited sections. If the user chooses 'Select from' button rather than 'Any,' the check boxes on its right are activated. These boxes corresponds to the five target sections, BACKGROUND, OBJECTIVE, METHOD, RESULT, and CONCLUSION.

In the search result section in the lower half of the screen, the query terms found in a specified section are highlighted in bold face letters, and the sections are shown in different background colors.

---

[2] We are currently re-implementing the system so that it uses a plain relational database as the back-end, instead of Namazu.

7   Conclusions and Future Work

We have reported our first attempt to exploit the underlying structure of abstract text for searching through Medline. We have proposed to use structured abstracts in Medline for building such a system, in particular, to train sentence classifier for the remaining unstructured abstracts. We have discussed the feasibility of using section headings in structured abstracts as class indicators, and identified some cases in which they are not reliable.

By fixing sequence of labels to the most frequent five, namely, BACKGROUND, OBJECTIVE, METHOD, RESULT, and CONCLUSION, we obtained an approximately 78% classification accuracy in classifying unstructured abstracts with a classifier trained with structured abstracts and context information.

The implemented system is only experimental, requiring further elaboration both in terms of user interface design and classification performance.

On the user-interface side, the adequacy of five sections presented to users needs evaluation. In particular, OBJECTIVE and CONCLUSION are different as they respectively describe what is sought and what is really achieved in a paper, but they are similar in the sense that they provide a summary of what the paper deals with. These sections do not describe the details of experiments (METHOD and RESULT), nor what has been done elsewhere (BACKGROUND). Thus grouping them into one class might be sufficient for most users.

As to improving classification performance, we plan to pursue a different (yet in a sense more natural) use of structured abstracts for more robust classification. To be specific, we will formulate the problem of sentence classification as a form of semi-supervised classification, in which a small volume of hand-labeled unstructured abstracts is combined with a large volume of structured abstracts. In this setting, each section heading in structured abstracts is not an indicator of the section label but merely a feature which is not always present. As a result, the sentences in structured abstracts are treated as unlabeled examples.

Another avenue of future work is to incorporate a re-ranking procedure of label sequences based on the overall consistency of sequences. Here, by 'consistency' we mean the constraint on label sequences mentioned in Section 4.3, such as conclusions never appear in the beginning of an abstract, and the sections hardly occur interleaved with each other. Although some of these constraints can be captured through the context features of Section 4.3, a more elaborate mechanism is desirable; the context features only affect local decisions performed sequentially, but does not take into account the 'global' consistency of a label sequence as a whole. The similar lines of research [6, 13] have been reported recently in machine learning and natural language processing communities, in which the sequence of classification results is optimized over all possible sequences.

We also plan to incorporate features that reflect cohesion or coherence between sentences [5].

Acknowledgment

This research was supported in part by MEXT under Grant-in-Aid for Scientific Research on Priority Areas (B) no. 759. The first author was also supported in part by MEXT under Grant-in-Aid for Young Scientists (B) no. 15700098.

References

[1] Ad Hoc Working Group for Critical Appraisal of Medical Literature. A proposal for more informative abstracts of clinical articles. *Annals of Internal Medicine*, 106(4):598–604, 1987.

[2] Eugene Charniak. A maximum-entropy-inspired parser. In *Proceedings of the Second Meeting of North American Chapter of Association for Computational Linguistics (NAACL-2000)*, pages 132–139, 2000.

[3] Michael Collins. *Head-Driven Statistical Models for Natural Language Processing*. PhD dissertation, University of Pennsylvania, 1999.

[4] Corinna Cortes and Vladimir Vapnik. Support-vector networks. *Machine Learning*, 20:273–297, 1995.

[5] M. A. K. Halliday and Ruqaiya Hasan. *Cohesion in English*. Longman, London, 1976.

[6] John Lafferty, Andrew McCallum, and Fernando Pereira. Conditional random fields: probabilistic models for segmenting and labeling sequence data. In *Proceedings of the 18th International Conference on Machine Learning (ICML-2001)*, pages 282–289. Morgan Kaufmann, 2001.

[7] Steve Lawrence, C. Lee Giles, and Kurt Bollacker. Digital libraries and autonomous citation indexing. *IEEE Computer*, 32(6):67–71, 1999.

[8] Lillian Lee and Fernando Pereira. Measures of distributional similarity. In *Proceedings of the 37th Annual Meeting of the Association for Comutational Linguistics (ACL-99)*, pages 25–32, 1999.

[9] MEDLINE. http://www.nlm.nih.gov/databases/databases_medline.html, 2002–2003. U.S. National Library of Medicine.

[10] Namazu. http://www.namazu.org/, 2000.

[11] PubMed. http://www.ncbi.nlm.nih.gov/PubMed/, 2003. U.S. National Library of Medicine.

[12] Bernhard Schölkopf and Alex J. Smola. *Learning with Kernels*. MIT Press, 2002.

[13] Fei Sha and Fernando Pereira. Shallow parsing with conditional random fields. In *Proceedings of the Human Language Technology Conference North American Chapter of Association for Computational Linguistics (HLT-NAACL 2003)*, pages 213–220, Edmonton, Alberta, Canada, 2003. Association for Computational Linguistics.

[14] UIUC sentence splitter software. http://l2r.cs.uiuc.edu/~cogcomp/cc-software.htm, 2001. University of Illinois at Urbana-Champaign.

[15] Vladimir Vapnik. *Statistical Learning Theory*. John Wiley & Sons, 1998.

$CHASE_2$ – Rule Based Chase Algorithm for Information Systems of Type λ

Agnieszka Dardzińska[1,2] and Zbigniew W. Raś[1,3]

[1] UNC-Charlotte, Department of Computer Science, Charlotte, N.C. 28223, USA
[2] Bialystok Technical University, Dept. of Mathematics, ul. Wiejska 45A,
15-351 Bialystok, Poland
[3] Polish Academy of Sciences, Institute of Computer Science, Ordona 21,
01-237 Warsaw, Poland

Abstract. A rule-based chase algorithm (called $Chase_2$), presented in this paper, provides a strategy for predicting what values should replace the null values in a relational database. When information about an object is partially incomplete (a set of weighted values of the same attribute can be treated as an allowed attribute value), $Chase_2$ is decreasing that incompleteness. In other words, when several weighted values of the same attribute are assigned to an object, $Chase_2$ will increase their standard deviation. To make the presentation clear and simple, we take an incomplete information system S of type λ as the model of data. To begin $Chase_2$ process, each attribute in S that has either unknown or incomplete values for some objects in S is set, one by one, as a decision attribute and all other attributes in S are treated as condition attributes. Assuming that d is the decision attribute, we take a subsystem S_1 of S by selecting from S any object x such that $d(x) \neq NULL$. Now, the subsystem S_1 is used for extracting rules describing values of attribute d. In the next step, each incomplete slot in S which is in the column corresponding to attribute d is chased by previously extracted rules from S_1, describing d. All other incomplete attributes in a database are processed the same way. This concludes the first loop of $Chase_2$. The whole process is recursively repeated till no more new values can be predicted by $Chase_2$. In this case, we say that a fixed point in values prediction was reached.

1 Introduction

Common problems encountered by Query Answering Systems (QAS), introduced by Raś in [15], [18], either for Information Systems or for Distributed Autonomous Information Systems ($DAIS$) include the handling of incomplete attributes when answering a query. One plausible solution to answer a query involves the generation of rules describing all incomplete attributes used in a query and then chasing the unknown values in the local database with respect to the generated rules. These rules can be given by domain experts and also can be discovered either locally or at remote sites of $DAIS$. Since all unknown

S. Tsumoto et al. (Eds.): AM 2003, LNAI 3430, pp. 255–267, 2005.

values would not necessarily be found, the process is repeated on the enhanced database until all unknowns are found or no new information is generated. When the fixed point is reached, QAS will run the original query against the enhanced database. The results of the query run on three versions of the information system have been compared by Dardzińska and Raś in [5]: $DAIS$ with a complete local database, $DAIS$ with incomplete local database (where incomplete information can be represented only in terms of null values), and $DAIS$ with a local incomplete database enhanced by rule-based chase algorithm. The chase algorithm presented in [5] was based only on consistent set of rules. The notion of a tableaux system and the chase algorithm based on functional dependencies F is presented for instance in [1]. Chase algorithm based on functional dependencies always terminates if applied to a finite tableaux system. It was shown that, if one execution of the algorithm generates a tableaux system that satisfies F, then every execution of the algorithm generates the same tableaux system.

There are many methods to replace missing values with predicted values or estimates [23], [19], [11], [7]. Some of them are given below:

- **Most Common Attribute Value.** It is one of the simplest methods to deal with missing attribute values. The value of the attribute that occurs most often is selected to be the value for all the unknown values of the attribute.
- **Concept Most Common Attribute Value.** This method is a restriction of the first method to the concept, i.e., to all examples with the same value of the decision. The value of the attribute, which occurs the most common within the concept is selected to be the value for all the unknown values of the attribute within that concept. This method is also called maximum relative frequency method, or maximum conditional probability method.
- **C4.5.** This method is based on entropy and splitting the example with missing attribute values to all concepts [14].
- **Method of Assigning all Possible Values of the Attribute.** In this method, an example with a missing attribute value is replaced by a set of new examples, in which the missing attribute value is replaced by all possible values of the attribute.
- **Method of Assigning all Possible Values of the Attribute Restricted to the Given Concept.** This method is a restriction of the previous method to the concept, indicated by an example with a missing attribute value.
- **Event-Covering Method.** This method is also a probabilistic approach to fill in the unknown attribute values by event-covering. Event covering is defined as a strategy of selecting a subset of statistically independent events in the outcome space of variable-pairs, disregarding whether or not the variables are statistically independent.

To impute categorical dimension missing values, two types of approaches can be used:

- **Rule Based Techniques** (e.g., association rule, rule induction techniques, etc.)
- **Statistical Modelling** (e.g., multinomial, log-linear modelling, etc.)

Two main rule based models have been considered: rule induction techniques and association rules. For categorical attributes with low cardinality domains (few values), rule induction techniques such as decision tree [14] and decision systems [10] can be used to derive the missing values. However, for categorical attributes with large cardinality domains (many values), the rule induction techniques may suffer due to too many predicted classes. In this case, the combination of association relationships among categorical attributes and statistical features of possible attribute values can be used to predict the best possible values of missing data. The discovered association relationships among different attributes can be thought as constraint information of their possible values and can then be used to predict the true values of missing attributes.

Algorithm, presented in this paper, for predicting what attribute value should replace an incomplete value of a categorical attribute in a given dataset has a clear advantage over many other methods for predicting incomplete values mainly because of the use of existing associations between values of attributes, in a chase strategy, repeatedly for each newly generated dataset till some fixpoint is reached. To find these associations we can use either any association rule mining algorithm or any rule discovery algorithm like $LERS$ (see [8]), or Rosetta (see [20]). Unfortunately, these algorithms, including Chase algorithm presented by us in [5], do not handle partially incomplete data, where $a(x)$ is equal, for instance, to $\{(a_1, 1/4), (a_2, 1/4), (a_3, 1/2)\}$.

We assume here that a is an attribute, x is an object, and $\{a_1, a_2, a_3\} \subseteq V_a$. By V_a we mean the set of values of attribute a. The weights assigned to these three attribute values should be read as:

- the confidence that $a(x) = a_1$ is $1/4$,
- the confidence that $a(x) = a_2$ is $1/4$,
- the confidence that $a(x) = a_3$ is $1/2$.

In this paper we present a new chase algorithm (called $Chase_2$) which can be used for chasing incomplete information systems with rules which do not have to be consistent (this assumption was required in $Chase_1$ presented in [5]). We propose how to compute the confidence of inconsistent rules and next we show how these rules are used by Chase2.

So, the assumption placed on incompleteness of data in this paper allows to have a set of weighted attribute values as a value of an attribute. Additionally, we assume that the sum of these weights has to be equal 1. The definition of an information system of type λ given in this paper is a modification of definitions given by Dardzińska and Raś in [5],[4] and used later by Raś and Dardzińska in [17] to talk about semantic inconsistencies among sites of DIS from the query answering point of view. Type λ is introduced mainly to monitor the weights assigned to values of attributes by $Chase_2$ algorithm (the algorithm checks if they are greater than or equal to λ). If the weight assigned by $Chase_2$ to one of the attribute values describing object x is below the acceptable threshold, then this attribute value is no longer considered as a value which describes x.

2 Handling Incomplete Values Using Chase Algorithms

There is a relationship between interpretation of queries and the way incomplete information in an information system is seen. Assume that we are concerned with identifying all objects in the system satisfying a given description. For example, an information system might contain information about students in a class and classify them using four attributes of *hair color, eye color, gender* and *size*. A simple query might be to find all students with *brown hair* and *blue eyes*. When the information system is incomplete, students having *brown hair* and unknown *eye color* can be handled by either including or excluding them from the answer to the query. In the first case we talk about optimistic approach to query interpretation while in the second one we talk about pessimistic approach. Another option to handle such a query is to discover rules for *eye color* in terms of the attributes *hair color, gender,* and *size*. Then, these rules can be applied to students with unknown *eye color* to discover that color and possibly the same to identify more objects satisfying the query. Consider that in our example one of the generated rules said:

$$(hair, brown) \wedge (size, medium) \rightarrow (eye, brown)$$

Thus, if one of the students having *brown hair* and *medium size* has no value for *eye color*, then this student should not be included in the list of students with *brown hair* and *blue eyes*. Attributes *hair color* and *size* are classification attributes and *eye color* is the decision attribute.

Now, let us give an example showing the relationship between incomplete information about objects in an information system and the way queries (attribute values) are interpreted. Namely, the confidence in object x that he has *brown hair* is 1/3 can be either written as $(brown, 1/3) \in hair(x)$ or $(x, 1/3) \in I(brown)$, where I is an interpretation of queries (the term *brown* is treated here as a query).

In [5] we presented $Chase_1$ strategy based on the assumption that only consistent subsets of rules extracted from an incomplete information system S can be used for replacing Null values by new less incomplete values in S. Clearly, rules discovered from S do not have to be consistent in S. Taking this fact into consideration, the algorithm $Chase_2$ proposed in this paper has less restrictions and it allows chasing information system S with inconsistent rules as well.

Assume that $S = (X, A, V)$, where $V = \bigcup \{V_a : a \in A\}$ and each $a \in A$ is a partial function from X into $2^{V_a} - \{\emptyset\}$. In the first step of $Chase$ algorithms, we identify all incomplete attributes used in S. An attribute is incomplete if there is an object in S with incomplete information on this attribute. The values of all incomplete attributes in S are treated as concepts to be learned (in a form of rules) either only from S or from S and its remote sites (if S is a part of a distributed autonomous information system).

The second step of $Chase$ algorithms is to extract rules describing these concepts. These rules are stored in a knowledge base D for S ([15],[18],[17]). Algorithm $Chase_1$ presented in [5] assumes that all inconsistencies in D have to be repaired before they are used in the chase process. To get rules from S

describing attribute value v_a of attribute a we extract them from the subsystem $S_1 = (X_1, A, V)$ of S where $X_1 = \{x \in X : card(a(x)) = 1\}$. $Chase_2$ does not have such restrictions.

The final step of $Chase$ algorithms is to replace incomplete information in S by values provided by rules in D.

3   Partially Incomplete Information Systems

We say that $S = (X, A, V)$ is a partially incomplete information system of type λ, if S is an incomplete information system and the following three conditions hold:

- $a_S(x)$ is defined for any $x \in X$, $a \in A$,

- $(\forall x \in X)(\forall a \in A)[(a_S(x) = \{(a_i, p_i) : 1 \leq i \leq m\}) \to \sum_{i=1}^{m} p_i = 1]$,

- $(\forall x \in X)(\forall a \in A)[(a_S(x) = \{(a_i, p_i) : 1 \leq i \leq m\}) \to (\forall i)(p_i \geq \lambda)]$.

Now, let us assume that S_1, S_2 are partially incomplete information systems, both of type λ. Both systems are classifying the same set of objects X using the same set of attributes A. The meaning and granularity of values of attributes from A in both systems S_1, S_2 is also the same. Additionally, we assume that $a_{S_1}(x) = \{(a_{1i}, p_{1i}) : 1 \leq m_1\}$ and $a_{S_2}(x) = \{(a_{2i}, p_{2i}) : 1 \leq m_2\}$.

We say that containment relation Ψ holds between S_1 and S_2, if the following two conditions hold:

- $(\forall x \in X)(\forall a \in A)[card(a_{S_1(x)}) \geq card(a_{S_2(x)})]$,

- $(\forall x \in X)(\forall a \in A)[[card(a_{S_1}(x)) = card(a_{S_2}(x))] \to$
$$[\textstyle\sum_{i \neq j} |p_{2i} - p_{2j}| > \sum_{i \neq j} |p_{1i} - p_{1j}|]].$$

Instead of saying that containment relation holds between S_1 and S_2, we can equivalently say that S_1 was transformed into S_2 by containment mapping Ψ. This fact can be presented as a statement $\Psi(S_1) = S_2$ or $(\forall x \in X)(\forall a \in A)[\Psi(a_{S_1}(x)) = \Psi(a_{S_2}(x))]$. Similarly, we can either say that $a_{S_1}(x)$ was transformed into $a_{S_2}(x)$ by Ψ or that containment relation Ψ holds between $a_{S_1}(x)$ and $a_{S_2}(x)$. In other words, the containment mapping Ψ transforms any partially incomplete value $a_{S_1(x)}$ of any attribute a, describing object x, into a new value $a_{S_2(x)}$ which is more complete. We can easily agree that the condition $card(a_{S_1(x)}) > card(a_{S_2(x)})$ guarantees that. The intuitive explanation of the condition $[\sum_{i \neq j} |p_{2i} - p_{2j}| > \sum_{i \neq j} |p_{1i} - p_{1j}|]$ is the following: larger average distance between weights assigned to all possible values of attribute a describing x guarantees more precise knowledge about x with respect to attribute a. In other words, if $a_{S_1(x)} = \{(a_1, \frac{1}{2}), (a_2, \frac{1}{2})\}$, then there is no preference between a_1 or a_2. Now, if $a_{S_2(x)} = \{(a_1, \frac{1}{3}), (a_2, \frac{2}{3})\}$, then our believe in the value a_2 is higher than in the value a_1. It means that our knowledge about x with respect to a is improved because the new uncertainty is lower.

Table 1. Information System S_1

X	a	b	c	d	e
x_1	$\{(a_1,\frac{1}{3}),(a_2,\frac{2}{3})\}$	$\{(b_1,\frac{2}{3}),(b_2,\frac{1}{3})\}$	c_1	d_1	$\{(e_1,\frac{1}{2}),(e_2,\frac{1}{2})\}$
x_2	$\{(a_2,\frac{1}{4}),(a_3,\frac{3}{4})\}$	$\{(b_1,\frac{1}{3}),(b_2,\frac{2}{3})\}$		d_2	e_1
x_3		b_2	$\{(c_1,\frac{1}{2}),(c_3,\frac{1}{2})\}$	d_2	e_3
x_4	a_3		c_2	d_1	$\{(e_1,\frac{2}{3}),(e_2,\frac{1}{3})\}$
x_5	$\{(a_1,\frac{2}{3}),(a_2,\frac{1}{3})\}$	b_1	c_2		e_1
x_6	a_2	b_2	c_3	d_2	$\{(e_2,\frac{1}{3}),(e_3,\frac{2}{3})\}$
x_7	a_2	$\{(b_1,\frac{1}{4}),(b_2,\frac{3}{4})\}$	$\{(c_1,\frac{1}{3}),(c_2,\frac{2}{3})\}$	d_2	e_2
x_8		b_2	c_1	d_1	e_3

Table 2. Information System S_2

X	a	b	c	d	e
x_1	$\{(a_1,\frac{1}{3}),(a_2,\frac{2}{3})\}$	$\{(b_1,\frac{2}{3}),(b_2,\frac{1}{3})\}$	c_1	d_1	$\{(e_1,\frac{1}{3}),(e_2,\frac{2}{3})\}$
x_2	$\{(a_2,\frac{1}{4}),(a_3,\frac{3}{4})\}$	b_1	$\{(c_1,\frac{1}{3}),(c_2,\frac{2}{3})\}$	d_2	e_1
x_3	a_1	b_2	$\{(c_1,\frac{1}{2}),(c_3,\frac{1}{2})\}$	d_2	e_3
x_4	a_3		c_2	d_1	e_2
x_5	$\{(a_1,\frac{3}{4}),(a_2,\frac{1}{4})\}$	b_1	c_2		e_1
x_6	a_2	b_2	c_3	d_2	$\{(e_2,\frac{1}{3}),(e_3,\frac{2}{3})\}$
x_7	a_2	$\{(b_1,\frac{1}{4}),(b_2,\frac{3}{4})\}$	c_1	d_2	e_2
x_8	$\{(a_1,\frac{2}{3}),(a_2,\frac{1}{3})\}$	b_2	c_1	d_1	e_3

So, if containment mapping Ψ converts an information system S to S', then S' is more complete than S. In other words, it has to be a pair $(a,x) \in A \times X$ such that either Ψ has to decrease the number of attribute values in $a_S(x)$ or the average difference between confidences assigned to attribute values in $a_S(x)$ has to be increased by Ψ (their standard deviation is increasing).

To give an example of a containment mapping Ψ, let us take two information systems S_1, S_2 both of the type λ, represented as Table 1 and Table 2, respectively.

It can be easily checked that the values assigned to $e(x_1)$, $b(x_2)$, $c(x_2)$, $a(x_3)$, $e(x_4)$, $a(x_5)$, $c(x_7)$, and $a(x_8)$ in S_1 are different from the corresponding values in S_2. In each of these eight cases, an attribute value assigned to an object in S_2 is less general than the value assigned to the same object in S_1. It means that $\Psi(S_1) = S_2$.

Assume now that $L(D) = \{(t \to v_c) \in D : c \in In(A)\}$ (called a knowledge-base) is a set of all rules extracted initially from $S = (X, A, V)$ by $ERID(S, \lambda_1, \lambda_2)$, where $In(A)$ is the set of incomplete attributes in S and λ_1, λ_2 are thresholds for minimum support and minimum confidence, correspondingly. $ERID$ is the algorithm for discovering rules from incomplete information systems, presented by Dardzińska and Raś in [4].

The type of incompleteness in [4] is the same as in this paper but we did not provide a threshold value λ for the minimal confidence of attribute values assigned to objects. The algorithm $ERID$ works the same way for incomplete information systems of type λ, since the knowledge discovery process in $ERID$ is independent from the largeness of parameter λ.

Now, let us assume that $S = (X, A, V)$ is an information system of type λ and t is a term constructed in a standard way (for predicate calculus expressions) from values of attributes in V seen as *constants* and from two functors $+$ and $*$. By $N_S(t)$, we mean the standard interpretation of a term t in S defined as (see [18]):

- $N_S(v) = \{(x, p) : (v, p) \in a(x)\}$, for any $v \in V_a$,
- $N_S(t_1 + t_2) = N_S(t_1) \oplus N_S(t_2)$,
- $N_S(t_1 * t_2) = N_S(t_1) \otimes N_S(t_2)$,

where, for any $N_S(t_1) = \{(x_i, p_i)\}_{i \in I}$, $N_S(t_2) = \{(x_j, q_j)\}_{j \in J}$, we have:

- $N_S(t_1) \oplus N_S(t_2) =$
    $$\{(x_i, p_i)\}_{i \in (I-J)} \cup \{(x_j, p_j)\}_{j \in (J-I)} \cup \{(x_i, max(p_i, q_i))\}_{i \in I \cap J},$$
- $N_S(t_1) \otimes N_S(t_2) = \{(x_i, p_i \cdot q_i)\}_{i \in (I \cap J)}.$

The interpretation N_S was proposed by Raś & Joshi in [18]. It preserves a number of properties required for the transformation process of terms including the distributive property: $t_1 * (t_2 + t_3) = (t_1 * t_2) + (t_1 * t_3)$. This property is used in the incomplete value imputation algorithm $Chase_2$, presented in this paper, to compute correctly the confidence of rules approximating incomplete values in S.

Assume that $N_S(t_1) = \{(x_i, p_i) : i \in K\}$ and $N_S(t_2) = \{(x_i, q_i) : i \in K\}$. This notation allows to have weights p_i, q_i equal to zero. There is a number of well known options available to interpret $N_S(t_1) * N_S(t_2)$ and $N_S(t_1) + N_S(t_2)$. Some of them are listed below (see [16]).

Interpretations T_0, T_1, T_2, T_3, T_4, T_5 for the functor $*$:

- Interpretation T_0: $N_S(t_1) * N_S(t_2) = \{(x_i, S_1(p_i, q_i)) : i \in K\}$, where $S_1(p_i, q_i)$ = [if $max(p_i, q_i) = 1$, then $min(p_i, q_i)$, else 0].
- Interpretation T_1: $N_S(t_1) * N_S(t_2) = \{(x_i, max\{0, p_i + q_i - 1\}) : i \in K\}$.
- Interpretation T_2: $N_S(t_1) * N_S(t_2) = \{(x_i, \frac{[p_i \cdot q_i]}{[2 - (p_i + q_i - p_i \cdot q_i)]}) : i \in K\}$.
- Interpretation T_3: $N_S(t_1) * N_S(t_2) = \{(x_i, p_i \cdot q_i) : i \in K\}$.
- Interpretation T_4: $N_S(t_1) * N_S(t_2) = \{(x_i, \frac{[p_i \cdot q_i]}{[p_i + q_i - p_i \cdot q_i]}) : i \in K\}$.
- Interpretation T_5: $N_S(t_1) * N_S(t_2) = \{(x_i, min\{p_i, q_i\}) : i \in K\}$.

Interpretations S_0, S_1, S_2, S_3, S_4, S_5 for the functor $+$:

- Interpretation S_0: $N_S(t_1) + N_S(t_2) = \{(x_i, S_2(p_i, q_i)) : i \in K\}$, where $S_2(p_i, q_i) = [$ if $min(p_i, q_i) = 0$, then $max(p_i, q_i)$, else 1].
- Interpretation S_1: $N_S(t_1) + N_S(t_2) = \{(x_i, min\{1, p_i + q_i\}) : i \in K\}$.
- Interpretation S_2: $N_S(t_1) + N_S(t_2) = \{(x_i, \frac{[p_i + q_i]}{[1 + p_i \cdot q_i]}) : i \in K\}$.
- Interpretation S_3: $N_S(t_1) + N_S(t_2) = \{(x_i, p_i + q_i - p_i \cdot q_i) : i \in K\}$.
- Interpretation S_4: $N_S(t_1) + N_S(t_2) = \{(x_i, \frac{[p_i + q_i - 2 \cdot p_i \cdot q_i]}{[1 - p_i \cdot q_i]}) : i \in K\}$.
- Interpretation S_5: $N_S(t_1) + N_S(t_2) = \{(x_i, max\{p_i, q_i\}) : i \in K\}$.

So, by taking all combinations of (T_i, S_j), we can consider 36 possible interpretations for the pair of functors $(\cdot, +)$. Only 7 of them satisfy the distributivity law $t \cdot (t_1 + t_2) = (t \cdot t_1) + (t \cdot t_2)$. Here they are: (T_0, S_5), (T_0, S_0), (T_2, S_5), (T_3, S_5), (T_4, S_5), (T_5, S_5), (T_5, S_0). It can be easily checked that for any conjunct term t, $T_0(t) < T_1(t) < T_2(t) < T_3(t) < T_4(t) < T_5(t)$. So, T_0 is the most pessimistic whereas T_5 is the most optimistic interpretation of the operator $\cdot$. Similarly, for any disjunct term t, $S_5(t) < S_4(t) < S_3(t) < S_2(t) < S_1(t) < S_0(t)$. So, S_5 is the most pessimistic whereas S_0 is the most optimistic interpretation of the operator $+$. The choice of (T_3, S_5) for the interpretation of $(\cdot, +)$ is easily justified assuming that terms in the form of conjuncts are built only from values of different attributes.

Now, let us go back to $Chase_2$ converting information system S of type λ to a new and more complete information system $Chase_2(S)$ of the same type. This algorithm is new in comparison to known strategies for chasing incomplete data in relational tables because of the assumption concerning partial incompleteness of data (sets of weighted attribute values can be assigned to an object as its value). This assumption forced us to develop a new discovery algorithm, called $ERID$, for extracting rules from tables similar to incomplete systems of type λ (see [4]) so it can be applied in $Chase_2$ algorithm given below.

Algorithm $Chase_2(S, In(A), L(D))$;
   Input   System $S = (X, A, V)$,
                 set of incomplete attributes $In(A) = \{a_1, a_2, ..., a_k\}$ in S,
                 set of rules $L(D)$ discovered from S by $ERID$.
   Output System $Chase(S)$
    begin
    S':= S;
    $j := 1$;
    while $j \leq k$ **do**
    begin
    $S_j := S$;
    for all $x \in X$ **do**
      $q_j := 0$;
      begin
      $b_j(x) := \emptyset$;
      $n_j := 0$;
      for all $v \in V_{a_j}$

begin
if $card(a_j(x)) \neq 1$ and $\{(t_i \rightarrow v) : i \in I\}$
    is a maximal subset of rules from $L(D)$
    such that $(x, p_i) \in N_{S_j}(t_i)$ **then**
    if $\sum_{i \in I} [p_i \cdot conf(t_i \rightarrow v) \cdot sup(t_i \rightarrow v)] \geq \lambda$ **then**
    begin
        $b_j(x) := b_j(x) \cup \{(v, \sum_{i \in I}[p_i \cdot conf(t_i \rightarrow v) \cdot sup(t_i \rightarrow v)])\};$
        $n_j := n_j + \sum_{i \in I}[p_i \cdot conf(t_i \rightarrow v) \cdot sup(t_i \rightarrow v)]$
    end
end
    $q_j := q_j + n_j;$
end
if $\Psi(a_j(x)) = [b_j(x)/q_j]$ **then** $a_j(x) := [b_j(x)/q_j];$
$j := j + 1;$
end
$S := \bigcap\{S_j : 1 \leq j \leq k\};$ /definition of $\bigcap\{S_j : 1 \leq j \leq k\}$ is given below/
if $S \neq S'$ **then** $Chase_2(S, In(A), L(D))$ **else** $Chase(S) := S$
end

Information system $S = \bigcap\{S_j : 1 \leq j \leq k\}$ is defined as:

$a_S(x) = \{a_{S_j}(x): if\ a = a_j\ for\ any\ j \in \{1, 2, ..., k\}\}$

for any attribute a and object x.

Still, one more definition is needed to complete the presentation of algorithm *Chase*. Namely, we say that:

$[b_j(x)/p] = \{(v_i, p_i/p)\}_{i \in I}$, if $b_j(x) = \{(v_i, p_i)\}_{i \in I}$.

Algorithm $Chase_2$ converts any incomplete or partially incomplete information system S to a new information system which is more complete. At each recursive call of $Chase_2$, its input data including S, $L(D)$, and from time to time $In(A)$ are changing. So, before any recursive call is executed, these new data have to be computed first.

Now, we give the time complexity $(T - Comp)$ of algorithm *Chase*. Assume first that $S = S(0) = (X, A, V)$, $card(In(A)) = k$, and $n = card(X)$. We also assume that $S(i) = Chase^i(S)$ and

$n(i) = card\{x \in X : (\exists a \in A)[a_{S(i)}(x) \neq 1]\}$, both for $i \geq 0$.

Clearly, $n(0) > n(1) > n(2) > ... > n(p) = n(p + 1)$, because information system $Chase^{i+1}(S)$ is more complete than information system $Chase^i(S)$, for any $i \geq 0$.

$T - Comp(Chase) = \bigcirc[\sum_{i=0}^{p}[k \cdot [n + n(i) \cdot card(L(D)) \cdot n] + n(i)]] =$
$\bigcirc[\sum_{i=0}^{p}[k \cdot [n(i) \cdot card(L(D)) \cdot n]]] = \bigcirc[k^2 \cdot n^3 \cdot m].$

The final worst case complexity of *Chase* is based on the observation that p can not be larger than $k \cdot n$. We also assume here that $m = card(L(D))$.

To explain the algorithm, we apply $Chase_2$ to information system S_3 presented by Table 3. We assume that $L(D)$ contains the following rules (listed

Table 3. Information System S_3

X	a	b	c	d	e
x_1	$\{(a_1,\frac{1}{3}),(a_2,\frac{2}{3})\}$	$\{(b_1,\frac{2}{3}),(b_2,\frac{1}{3})\}$	c_1	d_1	$\{(e_1,\frac{1}{2}),(e_2,\frac{1}{2})\}$
x_2	$\{(a_2,\frac{1}{4}),(a_3,\frac{3}{4})\}$	$\{(b_1,\frac{1}{3}),(b_2,\frac{2}{3})\}$		d_2	e_1
x_3	a_1	b_2	$\{(c_1,\frac{1}{2}),(c_3,\frac{1}{2})\}$	d_2	e_3
x_4	a_3		c_2	d_1	$\{(e_1,\frac{2}{3}),(e_2,\frac{1}{3})\}$
x_5	$\{(a_1,\frac{2}{3}),(a_2,\frac{1}{3})\}$	b_1	c_2		e_1
x_6	a_2	b_2	c_3	d_2	$\{(e_2,\frac{1}{3}),(e_3,\frac{2}{3})\}$
x_7	a_2	$\{(b_1,\frac{1}{4}),(b_2,\frac{3}{4})\}$	$\{(c_1,\frac{1}{3}),(c_2,\frac{2}{3})\}$	d_2	e_2
x_8		b_2	c_1	d_1	e_3

Table 4. Information System S_4

X	a	b	c	d	e
x_1	$\{(a_1,\frac{1}{3}),(a_2,\frac{2}{3})\}$	$\{(b_1,\frac{2}{3}),(b_2,\frac{1}{3})\}$	c_1	d_1	$\{(e_3,\frac{41}{100}),(e_2,\frac{59}{100})\}$
x_2	$\{(a_2,\frac{1}{4}),(a_3,\frac{3}{4})\}$	$\{(b_1,\frac{1}{3}),(b_2,\frac{2}{3})\}$		d_2	e_1
x_3	a_1	b_2	$\{(c_1,\frac{1}{2}),(c_3,\frac{1}{2})\}$	d_2	e_3
x_4	a_3		c_2	d_1	$\{(e_1,\frac{2}{3}),(e_2,\frac{1}{3})\}$
x_5	$\{(a_1,\frac{2}{3}),(a_2,\frac{1}{3})\}$	b_1	c_2		e_1
x_6	a_2	b_2	c_3	d_2	e_3
x_7	a_2	$\{(b_1,\frac{1}{4}),(b_2,\frac{3}{4})\}$	$\{(c_1,\frac{1}{3}),(c_2,\frac{2}{3})\}$	d_2	e_2
x_8	a_3	b_2	c_1	d_1	e_3

with their support and confidence) defining attribute e and extracted from S_3 by $ERID$:

$r_1 = [a_1 \rightarrow e_3]$ $(sup(r_1) = 1,\ conf(r_1) = 0.5)$
$r_2 = [a_2 \rightarrow e_2]$ $(sup(r_2) = 5/3,\ conf(r_2) = 0.51)$
$r_3 = [a_3 \rightarrow e_1]$ $(sup(r_3) = 17/12,\ conf(r_3) = 0.51)$
$r_4 = [b_1 \rightarrow e_1]$ $(sup(r_4) = 2,\ conf(r_4) = 0.72)$
$r_5 = [b_2 \rightarrow e_3]$ $(sup(r_5) = 8/3,\ conf(r_5) = 0.51)$
$r_6 = [c_2 \rightarrow e_1]$ $(sup(r_6) = 2,\ conf(r_6) = 0.66)$
$r_7 = [c_3 \rightarrow e_3]$ $(sup(r_7) = 7/6,\ conf(r_7) = 0.64)$
$r_8 = [a_3 \cdot c_1 \rightarrow e_3]$ $(sup(r_8) = 1,\ conf(r_8) = 0.8)$
$r_9 = [a_3 \cdot d_1 \rightarrow e_3]$ $(sup(r_9) = 1,\ conf(r_9) = 0.5)$
$r_{10} = [c_1 \cdot d_1 \rightarrow e_3]$ $(sup(r_{10}) = 1,\ conf(r_{10}) = 0.5)$

It can be noticed that values $e(x_1)$, $e(x_4)$, $e(x_6)$ of the attribute e are changed in S_3 by $Chase_2$ algorithm. The next section shows how to compute these three values and how to convert them, if needed, to a new set of values satisfying the constraints required by system S_4 to remain its λ status. Similar process is applied to all incomplete attributes in S_3. After all changes corresponding to all incomplete attributes are recorded, system S_3 is replaced by $\Psi(S_3)$ and the whole process is recursively repeated till a fix point is reached.

Algorithm $Chase_2$ will compute new value for $e(x_1) = \{(e_1, 1/2), (e_2, 1/2)\}$ denoted by $e_{new}(x_1) = \{(e_1, ?), (e_2, ?), (e_3, ?)\}$. To do that $Chase_2$ identifies all rules in $L(D)$ supported by x_1. It can be easily checked that r_1, r_2, r_4, r_5, and r_{10} are the rules supported by x_1. To calculate support of x_1 for r_1, we take: $1 \cdot \frac{1}{2} \cdot \frac{1}{3}$. In a similar way we calculate the support of x_1 for the remaining rules. As the result, we get the list of weighted values of attribute e supported by $L(D)$ for x_1, as follows:

$(e_3, \frac{1}{3} \cdot 1 \cdot \frac{1}{2} + \frac{1}{3} \cdot \frac{8}{3} \cdot \frac{51}{100} + 1 \cdot 1 \cdot \frac{1}{2}) = (e_3, 1.119)$

$(e_2, \frac{2}{3} \cdot \frac{5}{3} \cdot \frac{51}{100}) = (e_2, 1.621)$

$(e_1, \frac{2}{3} \cdot 2 \cdot \frac{72}{100}) = (e_1, 0.96)$.

So the value of attribute e for x_1 supported by $L(D)$ will be:

$e_{new}(x_1) = \{(e_1, \frac{0.96}{0.96+1.621+1.119}), (e_2, \frac{1.621}{0.96+1.621+1.119}), (e_3, \frac{1.119}{0.96+1.621+1.119})$
$= \{(e_1, 0.26), (e_2, 0.44), (e_3, 0.302)\}$

In a similar way we compute the value of e for x_4:

$(e_3, 1 \cdot 1 \cdot \frac{1}{2}) = (e_3, 0.5)$

$(e_2, 0)$

$(e_1, 1 \cdot \frac{17}{12} \cdot \frac{51}{100}) = (e_1, 0.722)$

we have:

$e_{new}(x_4) = \{(e_1, \frac{0.722}{0.5+0.722}), (e_3, \frac{0.5}{0.5+0.722})\} = \{(e_1, 0.59), (e_3, 0.41)\}$

And finally, for x_6:

$(e_3, \frac{8}{3} \cdot 1 \cdot \frac{51}{100} + 1 \cdot \frac{7}{6} \cdot \frac{64}{100}) = (e_3, 2.11)$

$(e_2, 1 \cdot \frac{5}{3} \cdot \frac{51}{100}) = (e_2, 0.85)$

$(e_1, 0)$

we have:

$e_{new}(x_6) = \{(e_2, \frac{0.85}{2.11+0.85}), (e_3, \frac{2.11}{2.11+0.85})\} = \{(e_2, 0.29), (e_3, 0.713)\}$

For $\lambda = 0.3$ the values of $e(x_1)$ and $e(x_6)$ will change to:
$e(x_1) = \{(e_2, 0.59), (e_3, 0.41)\}$, $e(x_6) = \{(e_3, 1)\}$.

Table 4 shows the resulting table.

Initial testing performed on several incomplete tables of the size $50 \times 2,000$ with randomly generated data gave us quite promising results concerning the precision of $Chase_2$. We started with a complete table S and removed from it 10 percent of its values randomly. This new table is denoted by S'. For each incomplete column in S', let's say d, we use $ERID$ to extract rules defining d in terms of other attributes in S'. These rules are stored in $L(D)$. In the following step, we apply $Chase_2$, making d maximally complete. Independently, the same procedure is applied to all other incomplete columns. As the result, we obtain a new table S'. Now, the whole procedure is repeated again on S'. The process continues till the fix point is reached. Now, we compare the new values stored in the empty slots of the initial table S' with the corresponding values in S. Based on this comparison, we easily compute the precision of $Chase_2$.

4   Conclusion

We expect much better results if a single information system is replaced by distributed autonomous information systems investigated in [15], [17], [18]. This is justified by experimental results showing higher confidence in rules extracted through distributed data mining than in rules extracted through local mining.

References

1. Atzeni, P., DeAntonellis, V. (1992) Relational database theory, The Benjamin Cummings Publishing Company
2. Benjamins, V. R., Fensel, D., Prez, A. G. (1998) Knowledge management through ontologies, in *Proceedings of the 2nd International Conference on Practical Aspects of Knowledge Management (PAKM-98)*, Basel, Switzerland.
3. Chandrasekaran, B., Josephson, J. R., Benjamins, V. R. (1998) The ontology of tasks and methods, in *Proceedings of the 11th Workshop on Knowledge Acquisition, Modeling and Management*, Banff, Alberta, Canada
4. Dardzińska, A., Raś, Z.W. (2003) On Rules Discovery from Incomplete Information Systems, in **Proceedings of ICDM'03 Workshop on Foundations and New Directions of Data Mining**, (Eds: T.Y. Lin, X. Hu, S. Ohsuga, C. Liau), Melbourne, Florida, IEEE Computer Society, 2003, 31-35
5. Dardzińska, A., Raś, Z.W. (2003) Chasing Unknown Values in Incomplete Information Systems, in **Proceedings of ICDM'03 Workshop on Foundations and New Directions of Data Mining**, (Eds: T.Y. Lin, X. Hu, S. Ohsuga, C. Liau), Melbourne, Florida, IEEE Computer Society, 2003, 24-30
6. Fensel, D., (1998), *Ontologies: a silver bullet for knowledge management and electronic commerce*, Springer-Verlag, 1998
7. Giudici, P. (2003) Applied Data Mining, Statistical Methods for Business and Industry, Wiley, West Sussex, England
8. Grzymala-Busse, J. (1991) On the unknown attribute values in learning from examples, in *Proceedings of ISMIS'91*, LNCS/LNAI, Springer-Verlag, Vol. 542, 1991, 368-377
9. Grzymala-Busse, J. (1997) A new version of the rule induction system *LERS*, in *Fundamenta Informaticae*, IOS Press, Vol. 31, No. 1, 1997, 27-39
10. Grzymala-Busse, J., Hu, M. (2000) A Comparison of several approaches to missing attribute values in data mining, in *Proceedings of the Second International Conference on Rough Sets and Current Trends in Computing*, RSCTC'00, Banff, Canada, 340-347
11. Little, R., Rubin, D.B. (1987) Statistical analysis with missing data, New York, John Wiley and Sons
12. Pawlak, Z. (1991) Rough sets-theoretical aspects of reasoning about data, Kluwer, Dordrecht

13. Pawlak, Z. (1991) Information systems - theoretical foundations, in **Information Systems Journal**, Vol. 6, 1981, 205-218
14. Quinlan, J. (1989) Unknown attribute values in induction, in *Proceedings of the Sixth International Machine Learning Workshop*, 164-168
15. Raś, Z.W. (1997) Resolving queries through cooperation in multi-agent systems, in **Rough Sets and Data Mining**, (Eds. T.Y. Lin, N. Cercone), Kluwer Academic Publishers, 1997, 239-258
16. Raś, Z.W., Arramreddy, S. (2004) Rough sets approach for handling inconsistencies in semantics of queries, PPT presentation on http://www.cs.uncc.edu/~ras/KDD-02/1
17. Raś, Z.W., Dardzińska, A. (2004) Ontology Based Distributed Autonomous Knowledge Systems, in **Information Systems International Journal**, Elsevier, Vol. 29, No. 1, 2004, 47-58
18. Raś, Z.W., Joshi, S. Query approximate answering system for an incomplete DKBS, in **Fundamenta Informaticae Journal**, IOS Press, Vol. 30, No. 3/4, 1997, 313-324
19. Schafer, J.L. (1997) Analysis of incomplete multivariate data, Book 72, Chapman and Hall series Monographs on Statistics and Applied Probability, Chapman and Hall, London
20. Skowron, A (1993) Boolean reasoning for decision rules generation, in J. Komorowski & Z. W. Raś, eds., *Proceedings of the 7th International Symposium on Methodologies for Intelligent Systems*, LNAI, Springer Verlag, No. 689, 1993, 295-305
21. Sowa, J.F. (2000b) Knowledge Representation: Logical, Philosophical, and Computational Foundations, Brooks/Cole Publishing Co., Pacific Grove, CA.
22. Sowa, J.F. (1999a) Ontological categories, in L. Albertazzi, ed., *Shapes of Forms: From Gestalt Psychology and Phenomenology to Ontology and Mathematics*, Kluwer Academic Publishers, Dordrecht, 1999, pp. 307-340.
23. Wu, X., Barbara, D. (2002) Learning missing values from summary constraints, in *KDD Explorations*, Vol. 4, No. 1
24. Van Heijst, G., Schreiber, A., Wielinga, B. (1997) Using explicit ontologies in KBS development, in *International Journal of Human and Computer Studies*, Vol. 46, No. 2/3, 183-292.

Empirical Comparison of Clustering Methods for Long Time-Series Databases

Shoji Hirano and Shusaku Tsumoto

Department of Medical Informatics,
Shimane University School of Medicine,
89-1 Enya-cho, Izumo, Shimane 693-8501, Japan
hirano@ieee.org
tsumoto@computer.org

Abstract. In this paper we report some characteristics of time-series comparison methods and clustering methods found empirically using a real-world medical database. First, we examined basic characteristics of two sequence comparison methods, multiscale matching (MSM) and dynamic time warping (DTW), using a simple sine wave and its variants. Next, we examined the characteristics of various combinations of sequence comparison methods and clustering methods, in terms of interpretability of generating clusters, using a time-series medical database. Although the subjects for comparison were limited, the results demonstrated that (1) shape representation parameters in MSM could capture the structural feature of time series; for example, the difference of amplitude was successfully captured using rotation term, and that differences on phases and trends were also successfully reflected in the dissimilarity. (2) However, the dissimilarity induced by MSM lacks linearity compared with DTW. It was also demonstrated that (1) complete-linkage criterion (CL-AHC) outperforms average-linkage (AL-AHC) criterion in terms of the interpret-ability of a dendrogram and clustering results, (2) combination of DTW and CL-AHC constantly produced interpretable results, (3) combination of DTW and RC would be used to find core sequences of the clusters. MSM may suffer from the problem of 'no-match' pairs, however, the problem may be eluded by using RC as a subsequent grouping method.

1 Introduction

Clustering of time-series data [1] has been receiving considerable interests as a promising method for discovering interesting features shared commonly by a set of sequences. One of the most important issues in time-series clustering is determination of (dis-)similarity between the sequences. Basically, the similarity of two sequences is calculated by accumulating distances of two data points that are located at the same time position, because such a distance-based similarity has preferable mathematical properties that extend the choice of subsequent grouping algorithms. However instead, this method requires that the lengths of

S. Tsumoto et al. (Eds.): AM 2003, LNAI 3430, pp. 268–286, 2005.

all sequences be the same. Additionally, it cannot compare structural similarity of the sequences; for example, if two sequences contain the same number of peaks, but at slightly different phases, their 'difference' is emphasized rather than their structural similarity [2].

These drawbacks are serious in the analysis of time-series data collected over long time. The long time-series data have the following features. First, the lengths and sampling intervals of the data are not uniform. Starting point of data acquisition would be several years ago or even a few decades ago. Arrangement of the data should be performed, however, shortening a time-series may cause the loss of precious information. Second, long-time series contains both long-term and short-term events, and their lengths and phases are not the same. Additionally, the sampling interval of the data would be variant due to the change of acquisition strategy over long time.

Some methods are considered to be applicable for clustering long time series. For example, dynamic time warping (DTW) [3] can be used to compare the two sequences of different lengths since it seeks the closest pairs of points allowing one-to-many point matching. This feature also enable us to capture similar events that have time shifts. Another approach, multiscale structure matching [6, 5, 4], can also be used to do this work, since it compares two sequences according to the structural similarity of partial segments derived based on the inflection points of the original sequences. However, there are few studies that empirically evaluate usefulness of these methods on real-world long time-series data sets.

This paper reports the results of empirical comparison of similarity measures and grouping methods on the hepatitis data set [7], in addition to a synthetic dataset. The hepatitis dataset is the unique, long time-series medical dataset that involves the following features: irregular sequence length, irregular sampling interval and co-existence of clinically interesting events that have various length (for example acute events and chronic events). We split a clustering procedure into two processes: similarity computation and grouping. For similarity computation, we employed DTW and multiscale matching. For grouping, we employed conventional agglomerative hierarchical clustering [8] and rough sets-based clustering [9], based on the feature that they can take a proximity matrix as an input and do not require direct access to the data values; thus they are suitable for handling relative similarity produced by multiscale matching. For every combination of the similarity computation methods and grouping methods, we performed clustering experiments and visually evaluated validity and interpretability of the results.

The rest of this paper is organized as follows. Section 2 briefly describes the methodologies of the comparison methods and clustering methods used in the experiment. Section 3 presents the characteristics of time-series comparison methods observed on a synthetic dataset. Section 4 presents the characteristics of various combinations of time-series comparison methods and clustering methods obtained empirically on the hepatitis dataset. Finally Section 5 concludes the technical results.

2   Methods

We implemented two clustering algorithms, agglomerative hierarchical clustering (AHC) in [8] and rough sets-based clustering (RC) in [9]. For AHC we employed two linkage criteria, average-linkage AHC (CL-AHC) and complete-linkage AHC (AL-AHC). We also implemented algorithms of symmetrical time warping described briefly in [2] and one-dimensional multiscale matching described in [4]. In the following subsections we briefly explain their methodologies.

2.1   Agglomerative Hierarchical Clustering (AHC)

Hierarchical clustering (HC) has been widely applied to cluster analysis since it can visualize hierarchical structure of clusters using a dendrogram. Basically, there are two types of algorithms for HC: agglomerative HC (AHC) and divisive HC (DHC). AHC initially assigns an independent cluster to each object. Then it seeks the most similar pair of clusters and merges it into one cluster. This process is repeated until all of the initial clusters are merged into single cluster. DHC is an inverse procedure of AHC. It starts from single cluster and finally divides it into object number of clusters. Practically, in both methods, merge or spilt is terminated when the step of similarity to merge/split the next clusters is remarkably large.

AHC has several options in determining the strategy of merging clusters. Some of them are listed below.

Single Linkage. One way to select a cluster is to take the intergroup dissimilarity to be that of the closest pair:

$$d_{SL}(G, H) = \min_{x_i \in G, x_j \in H} d(x_i, x_j),$$

where G and H are clusters to be merged in the next step, x_i and x_j are objects in G and H respectively, $d(x_i, x_j)$ is the dissimilarity between x_i and x_j. If $d_{SL}(G, H)$ is the smallest among possible pairs of clusters, G and H will be merged in the next step. The clustering based on this distance is called single linkage agglomerative hierarchical clustering (SL-AHC), also called nearest-neighbor technique.

Complete Linkage. Another way to select a cluster is to take the intergroup dissimilarity to be that of the furthest pair:

$$d_{CL}(G, H) = \max_{x_i \in G, x_j \in H} d(x_i, x_j)$$

where G and H are clusters to be merged in the next step. The clustering based on this distance is called complete linkage agglomerative hierarchical clustering (CL-AHC), also called furthest-neighbor technique.

Average Linkage. Another way to select a cluster is to take the intergroup dissimilarity to be that of the average dissimilarities between all pairs of objects. Every pair is made up of two objects; one object from each cluster:

$$d_{AL}(G, H) = \frac{1}{n_G + n_H} \sum_{i=1}^{n_G} \sum_{j=1}^{n_H} d(x_i, x_j)$$

where G and H are clusters to be merged in the next step, n_G and n_H respectively represent the numbers of objects in G and H. This is called the average linkage agglomerative hierarchical clustering (AL-AHC), also called the unweighted pair-group method using the average approach (UPGMA).

2.2   Rough-Sets Based Clustering

Generally, if similarity of objects is represented only as a relative similarity, it is not an easy task to construct interpretable clusters because some of important measures such as inter- and intra-cluster variances are hard to be defined. The rough-set based clustering method is a clustering method that clusters objects according to the indiscernibility of objects. It represents denseness of objects according to the *indiscernibility degree*, and produces interpretable clusters even for the objects mentioned above.

The clustering method lies its basis on the indiscernibility of objects, which forms basic property of knowledge in rough sets [11]. Let us first introduce some fundamental definitions of rough sets related to our work. Let $U \neq \phi$ be a universe of discourse and X be a subset of U. An equivalence relation, R, classifies U into a set of subsets $U/R = \{X_1, X_2, ...X_m\}$ in which following conditions are satisfied:

$(1) X_i \subseteq U, X_i \neq \phi$ for any i,
$(2) X_i \cap X_j = \phi$ for any i, j,
$(3) \cup_{i=1,2,...n} X_i = U$.

Any subset X_i, called a category, represents an equivalence class of R. A category in R containing an object $x \in U$ is denoted by $[x]_R$. For a family of equivalence relations $\mathbf{P} \subseteq \mathbf{R}$, an indiscernibility relation over $\mathbf{P}$ is denoted by $IND(\mathbf{P})$ and defined as follows

$$IND(\mathbf{P}) = \bigcap_{R \in \mathbf{P}} IND(R).$$

The clustering method consists of two steps: (1)assignment of initial equivalence relations and (2)iterative refinement of initial equivalence relations. In the first step, we assign an initial equivalence relation to every object. An initial equivalence relation classifies the objects into two sets: one is a set of objects similar to the corresponding objects and another is a set of dissimilar objects. Let $U = \{x_1, x_2, ..., x_n\}$ be the entire set of n objects. An initial equivalence relation R_i for object x_i is defined as

$$U/R_i = \{P_i, \ U - P_i\}, \tag{1}$$

where

$$P_i = \{x_j|\ d(x_i, x_j) \le Th_{di}\}, \quad \forall x_j \in U. \tag{2}$$

$d(x_i, x_j)$ denotes dissimilarity between objects x_i and x_j, and Th_{di} denotes an upper threshold value of dissimilarity for object x_i. The equivalence relation, R_i classifies U into two categories: P_i, which contains objects similar to x_i and $U - P_i$, which contains objects dissimilar to x_i. When $d(x_i, x_j)$ is smaller than Th_{di}, object x_j is considered to be indiscernible to x_i. The threshold value Th_{di} can be determined automatically according to the denseness of objects on the dissimilarity plane [9]. Indiscernible objects under all equivalence relations form a cluster. In other words, a cluster corresponds to a category X_i of $U/IND(\mathbf{R})$.

In the second step, we refine the initial equivalence relations according to their global relationships. First, we define an *indiscernibility degree*, $\gamma(x_i, x_j)$, for two objects x_i and x_j as follows.

$$\gamma(x_i, x_j) = \frac{\sum_{k=1}^{|U|} \delta_k^{indis}(x_i, x_j)}{\sum_{k=1}^{|U|} \delta_k^{indis}(x_i, x_j) + \sum_{k=1}^{|U|} \delta_k^{dis}(x_i, x_j)}, \tag{3}$$

where

$$\delta_k^{indis}(x_i, x_j) = \begin{cases} 1, \text{if} \ (x_i \in [x_k]_{R_k} \wedge x_j \in [x_k]_{R_k}) \\ 0, \text{otherwise.} \end{cases} \tag{4}$$

and

$$\delta_k^{dis}(x_i, x_j) = \begin{cases} 1, \text{if} \ (x_i \in [x_k]_{R_k} \wedge x_j \notin [x_k]_{R_k}) \ \text{or} \\ \quad \ \text{if} \ (x_i \notin [x_k]_{R_k} \wedge x_j \in [x_k]_{R_k}) \\ 0, \text{otherwise.} \end{cases} \tag{5}$$

Equation (4) shows that $\delta_k^{indis}(x_i, x_j)$ takes 1 only when the equivalence relation R_k regards both x_i and x_j as indiscernible objects, under the condition that both of them are in the same equivalence class as x_k. Equation (5) shows that $\delta_k^{dis}(x_i, x_j)$ takes 1 only when R_k regards x_i and x_j as discernible objects, under the condition that either of them is in the same class as x_k. By summing $\delta_k^{indis}(x_i, x_j)$ and $\delta_k^{dis}(x_i, x_j)$ for all $k(1 \le k \le |U|)$ as in Equation (3), we obtain the percentage of equivalence relations that regard x_i and x_j as indiscernible objects.

Objects with high indiscernibility degree can be interpreted as similar objects. Therefore, they should be classified into the same cluster. Thus we modify an equivalence relation if it has ability to discern objects with high γ as follows:

$$R_i' = \{\{P_i'\}, \{U - P_i'\}\}$$

$$P_i' = \{x_j|\gamma(x_i, x_j) \ge T_h\}, \quad \forall x_j \in U.$$

This prevents generation of small clusters formed due to the too fine classification knowledge. T_h is a threshold value that determines indiscernibility of objects. Therefore, we associate T_h with roughness of knowledge and perform iterative refinement of equivalence relations by constantly decreasing Th. Consequently, coarsely classified set of sequences are obtained as $U/IND(\mathbf{R'})$. Note that each refinement process is performed using the previously 'refined' set of equivalence relations, as the state of the indiscernibility degree may change after refinement.

2.3   Multiscale Matching

Multiscale matching is a structural comparison method for planar curves. It observes curve's features at various levels, from detail to gross, and finds their structural correspondence throughout all scales. There are many ways of representing multi-level features of planar curves, for example frequency-based filtering. Among them, description based on scale-space filtering [12, 6] has been widely used because curvature is a primary feature that represents the structure of a planar curve, and this method guarantees monotonicity of structural changes induced by scale changes. Ueda et al. [5] developed, based on the scale-space filtering, a segment-based structural comparison method that enables the use of discrete scales and comparison of largely distorted planar curves. We have extended this method so that it can be applied to the comparison of time series. For details, see ref. [4].

We modified segment difference in multiscale matching as follows.

$$d(a_i^{(k)}, b_j^{(h)}) = \max(\theta, l, \phi, g), \tag{6}$$

where θ, l, ϕ, g respectively represent differences on rotation angle, length, phase and gradient of segments $a_i^{(k)}$ and $b_j^{(h)}$ at scales k and h. These differences are defined as follows:

$$\theta(a_i^{(k)}, b_j^{(h)}) = |\theta_{a_i}^{(k)} - \theta_{b_j}^{(h)}| / 2\pi, \tag{7}$$

$$l(a_i^{(k)}, b_j^{(h)}) = \left| \frac{l_{a_i}^{(k)}}{L_A^{(k)}} - \frac{l_{b_j}^{(h)}}{L_B^{(h)}} \right|, \tag{8}$$

$$\phi(a_i^{(k)}, b_j^{(h)}) = \left| \frac{\phi_{a_i}^{(k)}}{\Phi_A^{(k)}} - \frac{\phi_{b_j}^{(h)}}{\Phi_B^{(h)}} \right|, \tag{9}$$

$$g(a_i^{(k)}, b_j^{(h)}) = |g_{a_i}^{(k)} - g_{b_j}^{(h)}|. \tag{10}$$

We have selected the maximum operation with four parameters as the result of empirical comparison with other operators such as minimum and weighted average. Figure 1 provides an illustrative explanation of these terms. Multiscale matching usually suffers from the shrinkage of curves at high scales caused by excessive smoothing with a Gaussian kernel. On one-dimensional time-series data, shrinkage makes all sequences flat at high scales. In order to elude this problem, we applied shrinkage correction proposed by Lowe [10].

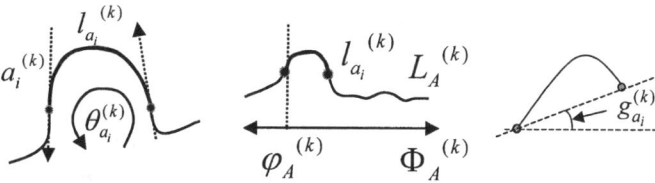

Fig. 1. Segment difference

3   Experiment 1: Characteristics of the Dissimilarity Measures

First, for the purpose of recognizing fundamental characteristics of the dissimilarity measure presented in the previous section, we applied MSM and DTW to some fundamental sequences and compared the produced dissimilarities. Mathematical representations of the sequences we employed were listed below.

$$
\begin{aligned}
w_1 &: \quad y(t) = \sin(2.5t) & w_5 &: \quad y(t) = \sin(2.5t) + 0.2(t - 9.0) \\
w_2 &: \quad y(t) = 2\sin(2.5t) & w_6 &: \quad y(t) = \sin(2.5t) - 0.2(t - 9.0) \\
w_3 &: \quad y(t) = 0.5\sin(2.5t) & w_7 &: \quad y(t) = 0.5e^{0.1t}\sin(2.5t) \\
w_4 &: \quad y(t) = \sin(2.5t + 0.5\pi) & w_8 &: \quad y(t) = 0.5e^{-0.1t+0.6\pi}\sin(2.5t) \\
& & w_9 &: \quad y(t) = 2 \times \sin(2 * 2.5t)
\end{aligned}
$$

The range of $t(= \Phi)$ was set to $0 \leq t < 6\pi$. The sampling interval was $1/500\Phi$. Thus each data consisted of 500 points. The scale σ for MSM was changed for 30 levels, starting from 1.0 to 30.0 with the interval of 1.0. Note that the replacement of segments would theoretically never occur because all of the eight sequences were generated from single sine wave. Practically, some minor replacement occurred because implementation of the algorithm required exceptional treatment at the both ends of the sequences. However, since they affected all the sequences commonly, we simply ignored the influence.

Figures 2–5 provide the shapes of nine test sequences: w_1 to w_9. Sequence w_1 was a simple sine wave which was also the basis for generating other eight sequences. For references, w_1 is superimposed on each of the figures. Sequences w_2 and w_3 were generated by changing amplitude of w_1 to twice and half respectively. These two sequences and w_1 had inflection points at the same places and their corresponding subsequences had the same lengths, phases, and gradients. Thus we used these sequences for evaluation of contribution of rotation angles to representing difference on amplitude. Sequence w_4 was generated by adding -0.5π delay to w_1 and used for evaluation of contribution of the phase term. Sequence w_5 and w_6 were generated by adding long-term increasing and decreasing trends to w_1. We used them for evaluating the contribution of the gradient term. Sequences w_7 and w_8 were generated by exponentially changing amplitude of w_1. They were used for testing how the dissimilarity behaves for nonlinear change of amplitude. Sequence w_9 was generated by changing frequency and amplitude of w_1 to twice. It was used to test sensitivity to compression in time domain. As we describe in Section 4.1, time-series medical data may contain sequences of unequal length. Thus it becomes important to demonstrate how the dissimilarity measure deals with such cases. Note that we did not directly evaluated the length term because it was hard to create a wave such that only length of a subsequence changes while preserving other factors.

Tables 1 and 2 provide the dissimilarity matrices obtained by applying multiscale matching and DTW to each pairs of the nine sequences, respectively. In order to evaluate the basic topological property of the dissimilarity, we here listed all elements in the matrix. From Table 1, it can be confirmed that the

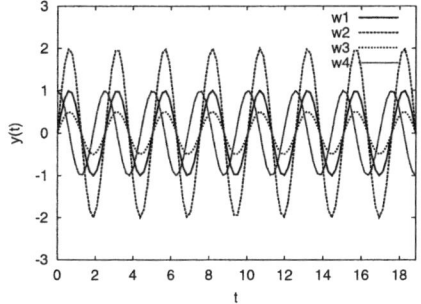

Fig. 2. Test sequences w_1–w_4

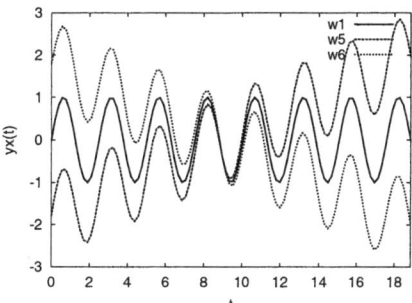

Fig. 3. Test sequences w_5 and w_6

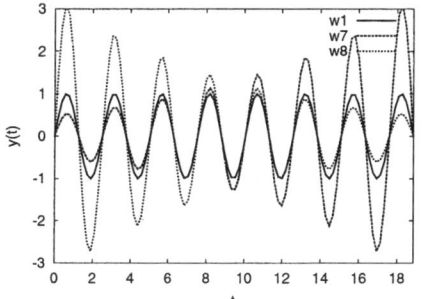

Fig. 4. Test sequences w_7 and w_8

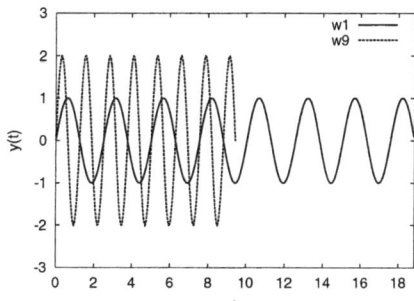

Fig. 5. Test sequence w_9

dissimilarity is non-negative ($d(w_i, w_j) \geq 0$), and satisfies both of reflectivity ($d(w_i, w_i) = 0$) and symmetry ($d(w_i, w_j) = d(w_j, w_i)$). These three properties are empirically known to be preserved for other types of data including real-life ones. However, triangular inequality is known to be violated in some cases, because the best observation scales can be different if sequences being compared are different. Dissimilarity is derived independently for each pairs. Additionally,

Table 1. Dissimilarity matrix produced by multiscale matching (normalized by the maximum value)

	w_1	w_2	w_3	w_4	w_5	w_6	w_7	w_8	w_9
w_1	0.000	0.574	0.455	0.644	0.541	0.611	0.591	0.662	0.782
w_2	0.574	0.000	0.774	0.749	0.736	0.675	0.641	0.575	0.451
w_3	0.455	0.774	0.000	0.834	0.720	0.666	0.586	0.736	0.950
w_4	0.644	0.749	0.834	0.000	0.816	0.698	0.799	0.635	0.745
w_5	0.541	0.736	0.720	0.816	0.000	0.917	0.723	0.624	0.843
w_6	0.611	0.675	0.666	0.698	0.917	0.000	0.624	0.726	0.806
w_7	0.591	0.641	0.586	0.799	0.723	0.624	0.000	1.000	0.765
w_8	0.662	0.575	0.736	0.635	0.624	0.726	1.000	0.000	0.683
w_9	0.782	0.451	0.950	0.745	0.843	0.806	0.765	0.683	0.000

Table 2. Dissimilarity matrix produced by DTW (normalized by the maximum value)

	w_1	w_2	w_3	w_4	w_5	w_6	w_7	w_8	w_9
w_1	0.000	0.268	0.134	0.030	0.399	0.400	0.187	0.187	0.164
w_2	0.268	0.000	0.480	0.283	0.447	0.445	0.224	0.224	0.033
w_3	0.134	0.480	0.000	0.146	0.470	0.472	0.307	0.307	0.268
w_4	0.030	0.283	0.146	0.000	0.407	0.379	0.199	0.201	0.184
w_5	0.399	0.447	0.470	0.407	0.000	1.000	0.384	0.477	0.264
w_6	0.400	0.445	0.472	0.379	1.000	0.000	0.450	0.411	0.262
w_7	0.187	0.224	0.307	0.199	0.384	0.450	0.000	0.372	0.151
w_8	0.187	0.224	0.307	0.201	0.477	0.411	0.372	0.000	0.151
w_9	0.164	0.033	0.268	0.184	0.264	0.262	0.151	0.151	0.000

it is possible that matching failure occurs. For example, a sine waves containing n periods and another sine wave containing $n + 1$ periods never matches; thus we are basically unable to represent their dissimilarity in a reasonable manner. More generally, if there is no possible set of segment pairs that satisfies complete match criterion – original sequence should be formed completely without any gaps or overlaps by concatenating the segments– within the given universe of segments, matching will fail and triangular inequality will not be satisfied.

Comparison of w_2 and w_3 with w_1 yielded $d(w_2, w_3) > d(w_1, w_2) > d(w_1, w_3)$, meaning that the large amplitude induced large dissimilarity. The order was the same as that of DTW. As mentioned above, these three sequences had completely the same factors except for rotation angle. Thus rotation angle successfully captured difference of amplitudes as that difference of shapes. Comparison of w_4 with w_1 showed that difference of phase was successfully translated to the dissimilarity. Taking w_2 and w_3 into account, one may argue that the order of dissimilarities does not follow the order of dissimilarities produced by DTW. We consider that this occurred because, due to phase shift, the shape of w_4 at the edge became different from those of w_1, w_2 and w_3. Therefore matching was performed accompanying replacement of segments at higher scale and thus cost for segment replacement might be added to the dissimilarity.

Comparison of w_5 and w_6 with w_1 yielded $d(w_5, w_6) >> d(w_1, w_6) > d(w_1, w_5)$. This represents that dissimilarity between w_5 and w_6 that have completely different trends was far larger than the dissimilarity to w_1 that has flat trend. Dissimilarities $d(w_1, w_5)$ and $d(w_1, w_6)$ were not the same due to the characteristics of the test sequences; since w_5 had increasing trends and first diverged towards the vertical origin, it reached to the first inflection points in shorter route than that in w_6. The order of dissimilarities was the same as that of DTW. Comparison of w_7 and w_8 with w_1 yielded $d(w_7, w_8) >> d(w_1, w_7) > d(w_1, w_8)$, meaning that difference on amplitude was accumulated and far larger dissimilarity was assigned to $d(w_7, w_8)$ than $d(w_1, w_7)$ or $d(w_1, w_8)$. Finally, comparison of w_9 with w_1 and w_2 yielded $d(w_1, w_9) >> d(w_1, w_2)$. This represents that the change of sharpness was captured as rotation angle. DTW produced quite small dissimilarities between w_1 and w_9 because of its one-to-many matching property.

4   Experiment 2: Characteristics of the Combination of Dissimilarity Measures and Clustering Methods

In this experiment, we investigated, using the real-world time-series medical data, the characteristics of various combinations of similarity calculation methods and grouping methods.

4.1   Materials

We employed the chronic hepatitis dataset [7], which were provided as a common dataset for ECML/PKDD Discovery Challenge 2002 and 2003. The dataset contained long time-series data on laboratory examinations, which were collected at Chiba University Hospital in Japan. The subjects were 771 patients of hepatitis B and C who received examinations during 1982 and 2001. We manually removed sequences for 268 patients because biopsy information was not provided for them and thus their virus types were not clearly specified. According to the biopsy information, the expected constitution of the remaining 503 patients were B / C-noIFN / C-IFN = 206 / 100 / 197, where B, C-noIFN, C-IFN respectively represent the patients of type B hepatitis, patients of type C hepatitis who did not receive the interferon therapy, and those of type C hepatitis who received the interferon therapy. Due to existence of missing examinations, the numbers of available sequences could be less than 503. The dataset contained a total of 983 laboratory examinations. In order to simplify our experiments, we selected 13 blood tests that are relevant to the liver function: ALB, ALP, G-GL, G-GTP, GOT, GPT, HGB, LDH, PLT, RBC, T-BIL, T-CHO and TTT. Details of each examination are available at the URL [7].

Each sequence originally had different sampling intervals from one day to several years. Figure 6 provides an example, showing a histogram of sampling intervals of PLT sequences. From preliminary analysis we found that majority of intervals ranged from one week to one month, and most of the patients received examinations on a fixed day of a week. According to this observation, we

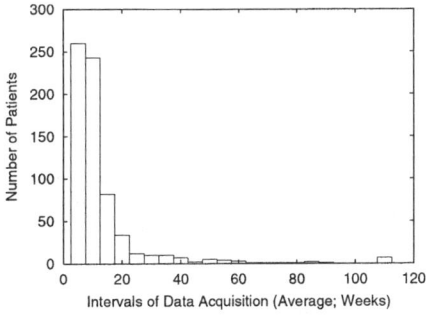

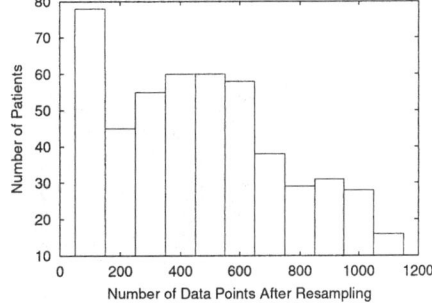

Fig. 6. Histogram of the average sampling intervals of PLT sequences

Fig. 7. Histogram of the number of data points in resampled PLT sequences

determined re-sampling interval to seven days. A simple summary showing the number of data points after re-sampling was as follows (item=PLT, $n = 498$) : mean=441.0, sd=295.1, median=427.0, maximum=1079, minimum=1. Note that one point equals to one week; therefore, 441.0 points equals to 441.0 weeks, namely, about 8.5 years. Figure 7 provides a histogram of the number of data point in the resampled PLT sequences.

4.2   Experimental Procedure

We investigated the usefulness of various combinations of similarity calculation methods and grouping methods in terms of the interpretability of the clustering results. Figure 8 shows a snapshot of the system that we have developed for interpreting clustering results. The system can visualize dendrograms for the time-series data, generated by using AHCs, as shown in the left window of the figure. When a user specifies a cutting point on the dendrogram, corresponding cluster contents is visualized on the right window. For RC, cluster constitution first appears on the right window. When a user specifies a cluster, time-series belonging to the cluster are visualized.

Procedures of experiments are shown in Figure 9. First, we selected one examination, for example ALB, and split the corresponding sequences into three subsets, B, C-noIFN and C-IFN, according to the virus type and administration of interferon therapy. Next, for each of the three subgroups, we computed dissimilarity of each pair of sequences by using DTW. After repeating the same process with multiscale matching, we obtained 2×3 sets of dissimilarities: one obtained by DTW, and another obtained by multiscale matching.

Then we applied grouping methods AL-AHC, CL-AHC and RC to each of the three dissimilarity sets obtained by DTW. This yielded 3×3=9 sets of clusters. After applying the same process to the sets obtained by multiscale-matching, we obtained the total of 18 sets of clusters. The above process is repeated with the remaining 12 examination items. Consequently, we constructed 12×18 clustering results. Note that in this experiments we did not perform cross-examination comparison, for example comparison of an ALB sequence with a GPT sequence.

We used the following parameters for rough clustering: $\sigma = 5.0$, $T_h = 0.3$. In AHC, cluster linkage was terminated when increase of dissimilarity firstly exceeded mean+SD of the set of all increase values.

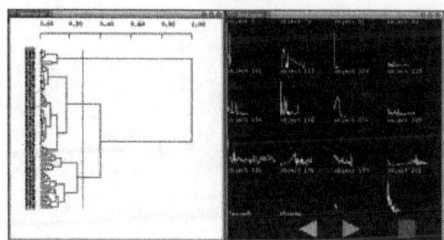   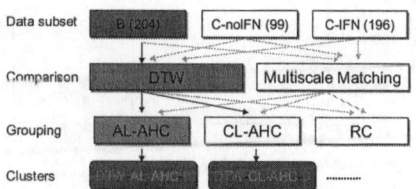

Fig. 8. System for visualizing dendrograms and cluster constitutions

Fig. 9. Scheme of experiments

4.3   Experimental Results

Table 3 provides the numbers of generated clusters for each combination. Let us explain the table using the raw whose first column is marked ALB. The second column "Number of Instances" represents the number of patients who received the ALB examination. Its value 204/99/196 represents that 204 patients of Hepatitis B, 99 patients of Hepatitis C (who did not take IFN therapy) and 196 patients of Hepatitis C (who received IFN therapy) received this examination. Since one patient has one time-series examination result, the number of patients corresponds to the number of sequences. The third column represents the method used for sequence comparison (DTW or MSM). The fourth, fifth and sixth columns include the number of clusters generated respectively by using AL-AHC, CL-AHC and RC. Numbers separated by a slash mark represent the number of clusters for B/C-noIFN/C-IFN cases. For example, using DTW and AL-AHC, 204 hepatitis B sequences were grouped into 8 clusters. 99 C-

Table 3. Comparison of the number of generated clusters. Each item represents clusters for Hepatitis B / C-noIFN / C-IFN cases

Exam	Number of Instances	Comparison Method	Number of Generated Clusters		
			AL-AHC	CL-AHC	RC
ALB	204 / 99 / 196	DTW	8 / 3 / 3	10 / 6 / 5	38 / 22 / 32
		MSM	19 / 11 / 12	22 / 21 / 27	6 / 14 / 31
ALP	204 / 99 / 196	DTW	6 / 4 / 6	7 / 7 / 10	21 / 12 / 29
		MSM	10 / 18 / 14	32 / 16 / 14	36 / 12 / 46
G-GL	204 / 97 / 195	DTW	2 / 2 / 5	2 / 2 / 11	1 / 1 / 21
		MSM	15 / 16 / 194	16 / 24 / 194	24 / 3 / 49
G-GTP	204 / 99 / 196	DTW	2 / 4 / 11	2 / 6 / 7	1 / 17 / 4
		MSM	38 / 14 / 194	65 / 14 / 19	35 / 8 / 51
GOT	204 / 99 / 196	DTW	8 / 10 / 25	8 / 4 / 7	50 / 18 / 60
		MSM	19 / 12 / 24	35 / 19 / 19	13 / 14 / 15
GPT	204 / 99 / 196	DTW	3 / 17 / 7	7 / 4 / 7	55 / 29 / 51
		MSM	23 / 30 / 8	24 / 16 / 16	11 / 7 / 25
HGB	204 / 99 / 196	DTW	3 / 4 / 13	2 / 3 / 9	1 / 16 / 37
		MSM	43 / 15 / 15	55 / 19 / 22	1 / 12 / 78
LDH	204 / 99 / 196	DTW	7 / 7 / 9	15 / 10 / 8	15 / 15 / 15
		MSM	20 / 25 / 195	24 / 9 / 195	32 / 16 / 18
PLT	203 / 99 / 196	DTW	2 / 13 / 9	2 / 7 / 6	1 / 15 / 19
		MSM	33 / 5 / 12	34 / 15 / 17	1 / 11 / 25
RBC	204 / 99 / 196	DTW	3 / 4 / 6	3 / 4 / 7	1 / 14 / 26
		MSM	32 / 16 / 13	40 / 23 / 17	1 / 6 / 17
T-BIL	204 / 99 / 196	DTW	6 / 5 / 5	9 / 5 / 4	203 / 20 / 30
		MSM	17 / 25 / 6	20 / 30 / 195	11 / 23 / 48
T-CHO	204 / 99 / 196	DTW	2 / 2 / 7	5 / 2 / 5	20 / 1 / 27
		MSM	12 / 13 / 13	17 / 23 / 19	12 / 5 / 23
TTT	204 / 99 / 196	DTW	7 / 2 / 5	8 / 2 / 6	25 / 1 / 32
		MSM	29 / 10 / 6	39 / 16 / 16	25 / 16 / 23

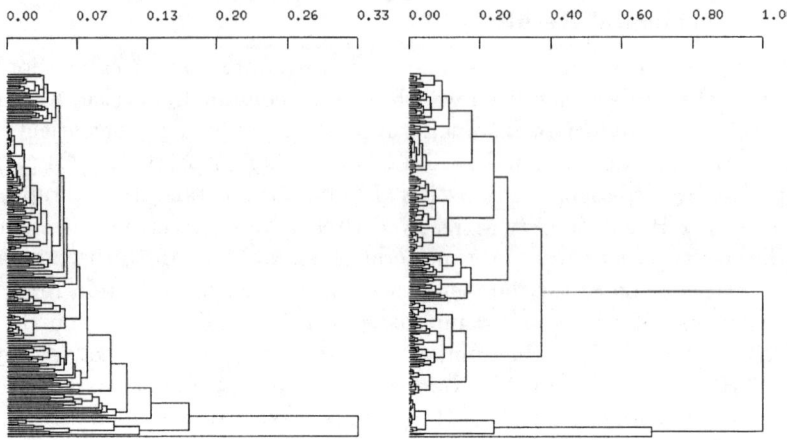

Fig. 10. Dendrograms for the GPT sequences of type B hepatitis patients. Comparison Method=DTW. Grouping method = AL-AHC (left), CL-AHC (right)

noIFN sequences were grouped into 3 clusters, and 196 C-IFN sequences were also grouped into 3 clusters.

DTW and AHCs. Let us first investigate the case of DTW-AHC. Comparison of DTW-AL-AHC and DTW-CL-AHC implies that the results can be different if we use different linkage criterion. Figure 10 left image shows a dendrogram generated from the GTP sequences of type B hepatitis patients using DTW-AL-AHC. It can be observed that the dendrogram of AL-AHC has an ill-formed structure like 'chaining', which is usually observed with single-linkage AHC. For such an ill-formed structure, it is difficult to find a good point to terminate merging of the clusters. In this case, the method produced three clusters containing 193, 9 and 1 sequences respectively. Almost all types of sequences were included in the first, largest cluster and thus no interesting information was obtained.

On the contrary, the dendrogram of CL-AHC shown in the right of Figure 10 demonstrates a well formed hierarchy of the sequences. With this dendrogram the method produced 7 clusters containing 27, 21, 52, 57, 43, 2, and 1 sequences each. Figure 11 shows examples of the sequences grouped into the first four clusters. One can observe interesting features for each cluster. The first cluster contains sequences that involve continuous vibration of the GPT values. These patterns may imply that the virus continues to attack the patient's body periodically. The second cluster contains very short, meaningless sequences, which may represent the cases that patients stop or cancel receiving the treatment quickly. The third cluster contains another interesting pattern: vibrations followed by the flat, low values. There are two possible cases that represent this pattern. The first case is that the patients were cured by some treatments or naturally. The second case is that the patients entered into the terminal stage and there remains no matters producing GPT. It is difficult to know which of the two cases a sequence belongs

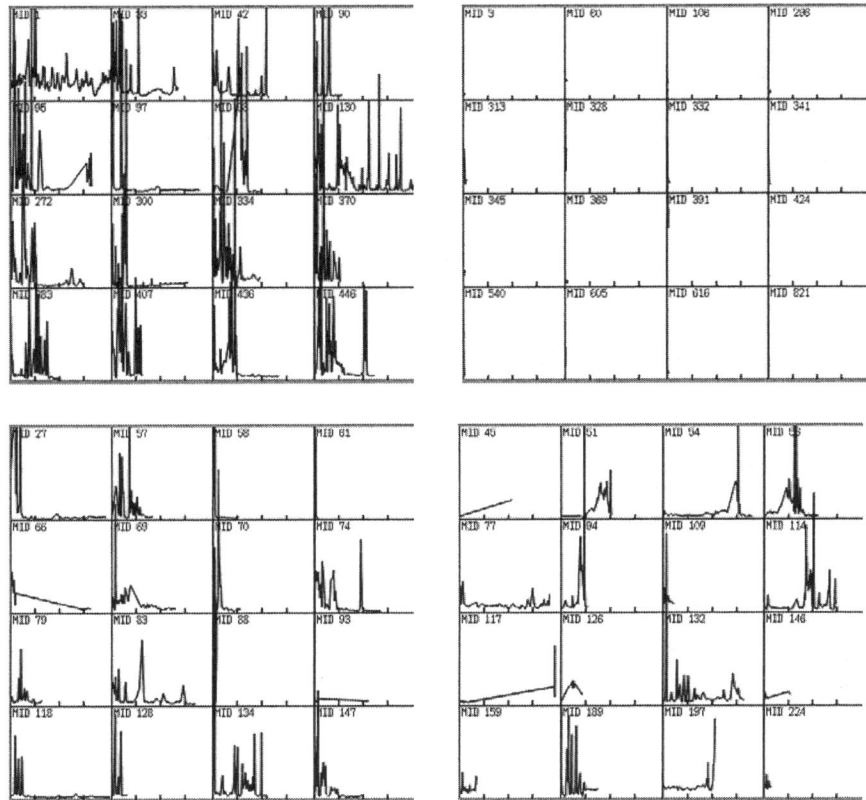

Fig. 11. Examples of the clustered GPT sequence for type B hepatitis patients. Comparison Method=DTW. Grouping method=CL-AHC. Top Left: 1st cluster (27 cases), Top Right: 2nd cluster (21 cases), Bottom Left: 3rd cluster (52 cases), Bottom Right; 4th cluster (57 cases). Sequences are selected according to MID order

to, until other types of information such as PLT and CHE level are taken into account. The fourth cluster contains sequence that have mostly triangular shape.

DTW and RC. For the same data, rough set-based clustering method produced 55 clusters. Fifty five clusters were too many for 204 objects, however, 41 of 55 clusters contained less than 3 sequences, and furthermore, 31 of them contained only one sequence. This was because of the rough set-based clustering tends to produce independent, small clusters for objects being intermediate of the large clusters. Ignoring small ones, we obtained a total of 14 clusters containing 53, 16, 10, 9, 9 ... objects each. The largest cluster contained short sequences quite similarly to the case of DTW-CL-AHC. Figure 12 shows examples of sequences for the 2nd, 3rd, 4th and 5th major clusters. Because this method evaluates the indiscernibility degree of objects, each of the generated clusters contains strongly similar sets of sequences. Although populations in the clusters are not so large, one can clearly observe the representative of the in-

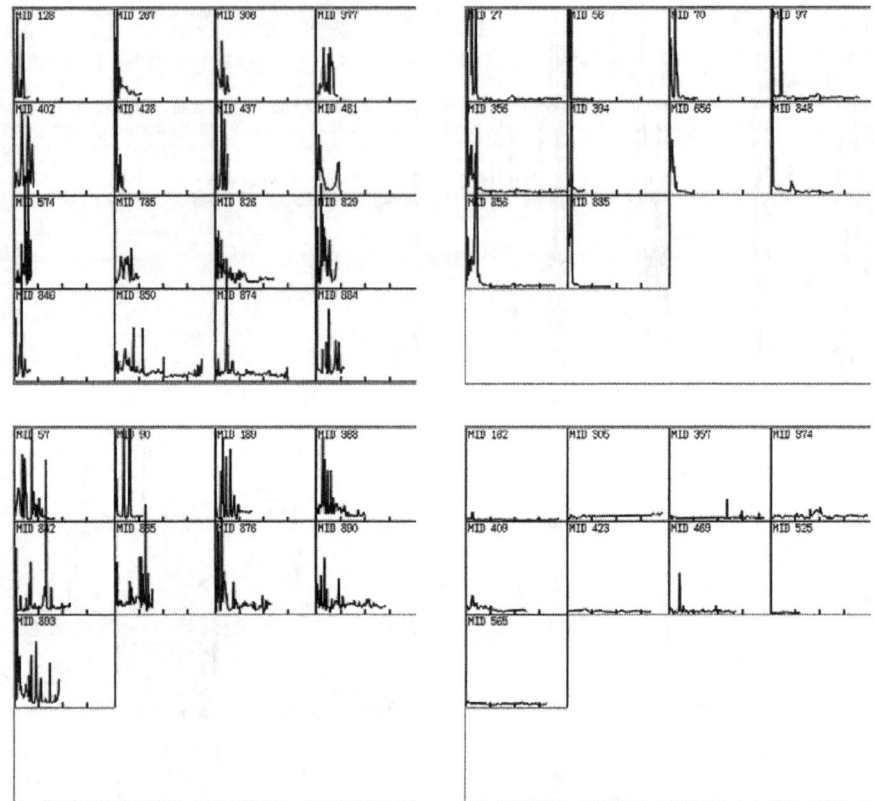

Fig. 12. Examples of the clustered GPT sequence for type B hepatitis patients. Comparison Method=DTW. Grouping method=RC. Top Left: 2nd cluster (16 cases), Top Right: 3rd cluster (10 cases), Bottom Left: 4th cluster (9 cases), Bottom Right; 5th cluster (9 cases)

teresting patterns described previously at CL-AHC. For example, the 2nd and 4th clusters contain cases with large vibration. Among them, the latter mostly contains cases followed by the vibration with the decreased level. The 3rd cluster contains clear cases of vibration followed by flattened patterns. Sequences in the 5th cluster represent obvious feature of flat patterns without large vibration.

Multiscale Matching and AHCs. Comparison of Multiscale Matching-AHC pairs with DTW-AHC pairs shows that Multiscale Matching's dissimilarities resulted in producing the larger number of clusters than DTW's dissimilarities.

One of the important issues in multiscale matching is treatment of 'no-match' sequences. Theoretically, any pairs of sequences can be matched because a sequence will become single segment at enough high scales. However, this is not a realistic approach because the use of many scales results in the unacceptable increase of computational time. If the upper bound of the scales is too low, the method may possibly fail to find the appropriate pairs of subsequences. For ex-

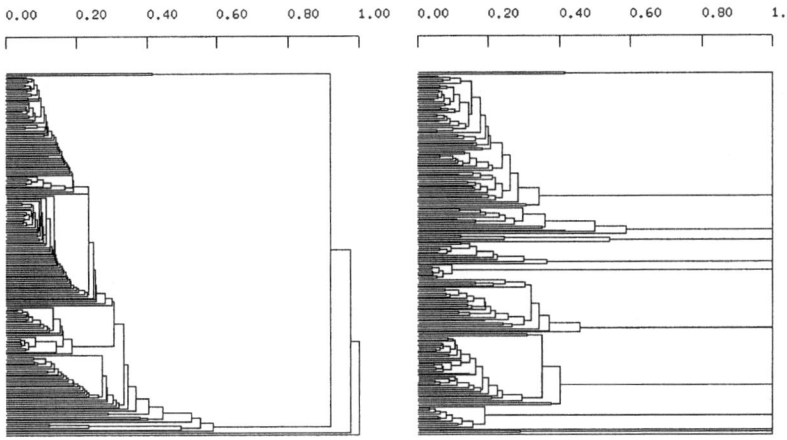

Fig. 13. Dendrograms for the GPT sequences of type C hepatitis patients with IFN therapy. Comparison Method=MSM. Grouping method = AL-AHC (left), CL-AHC (right)

ample, suppose we have two sequences, one is a short sequence containing only one segment and another is a long sequence containing hundreds of segments. The segments of the latter sequence will not be integrated into one segment until the scale becomes considerably high. If the range of scales we use does not cover such a high scale, the two sequences will never be matched. In this case, the method should return infinite dissimilarity, or a special number that identifies the failed matching.

This property prevents AHCs from working correctly. CL-AHC will never merge two clusters if any pair of 'no-match' sequences exist between them. AL-AHC fails to calculate average dissimilarity between two clusters. Figure 13 provides dendrograms for GPT sequences of Hepatitis C (with IFN) patients obtained by using multiscale matching and AHCs. In this experiment, we let the dissimilarity of 'no-match' pairs the same as the most dissimilar 'matched' pairs in order to elude computational problems. The dendrogram of AL-AHC is compressed to the small-dissimilarity side because there are several pairs that have excessively large dissimilarities. The dendrogram of CL-AHC demonstrates that the 'no-match' pairs will not be merged until the end of the merging process.

For AL-AHC, the method produced 8 clusters. However, similarly to the previous case, most of the sequences (182/196) were included in the same, largest cluster and no interesting information was found therein. For CL-AHC, the method produced 16 clusters containing 71, 39, 28, 12 ... sequences. Figure 14 provides examples of the sequences grouped into the four major clusters, respectively. Similar sequences were found in the clusters, however, obviously dissimilar sequences were also observed in their clusters.

Multiscale Matching and RC. Rough set-based clustering method produced 25 clusters containing 80, 60, 18, 6 ... sequences. Figures 15 represents examples

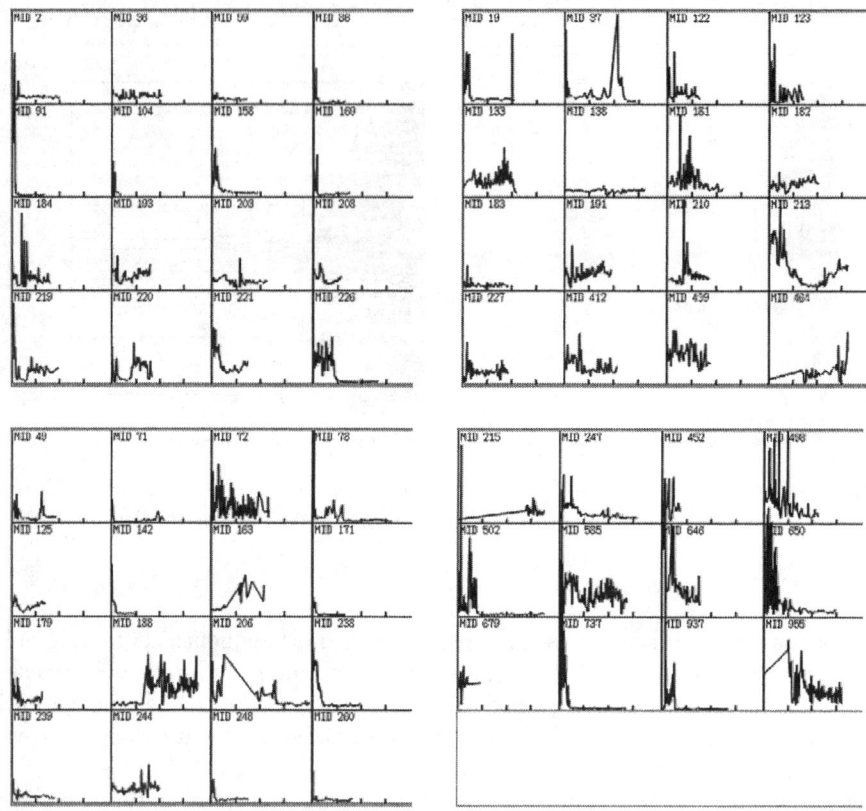

Fig. 14. Examples of the clustered GPT sequence for type C hepatitis patients with IFN therapy. Comparison Method=MSM. Grouping method=CL-AHC. Top Left: 1st cluster (71 cases), Top Right: 2nd cluster (39 cases), Bottom Left: 3rd cluster (28 cases), Bottom Right; 4th cluster (12 cases). Sequences are selected according to MID order

of the sequences grouped into the four major clusters. It can be observed that the sequences were properly clustered into the three major patterns: continuous, large vibration (1st cluster), flat after vibration (2nd cluster), and short (3rd cluster). Although the 4th cluster is likely to be intermediate of them and difficult to interpret, other results demonstrate the ability of the clustering method for handling relative proximity, which enables us to elude the problem of no-match cases occurring with MSM.

5   Conclusions

In this paper we have reported a comparative study about the characteristics of time-series comparison and clustering methods. First, we examined the basic characteristics of MSM and DTW using a simple sine wave and its variants.

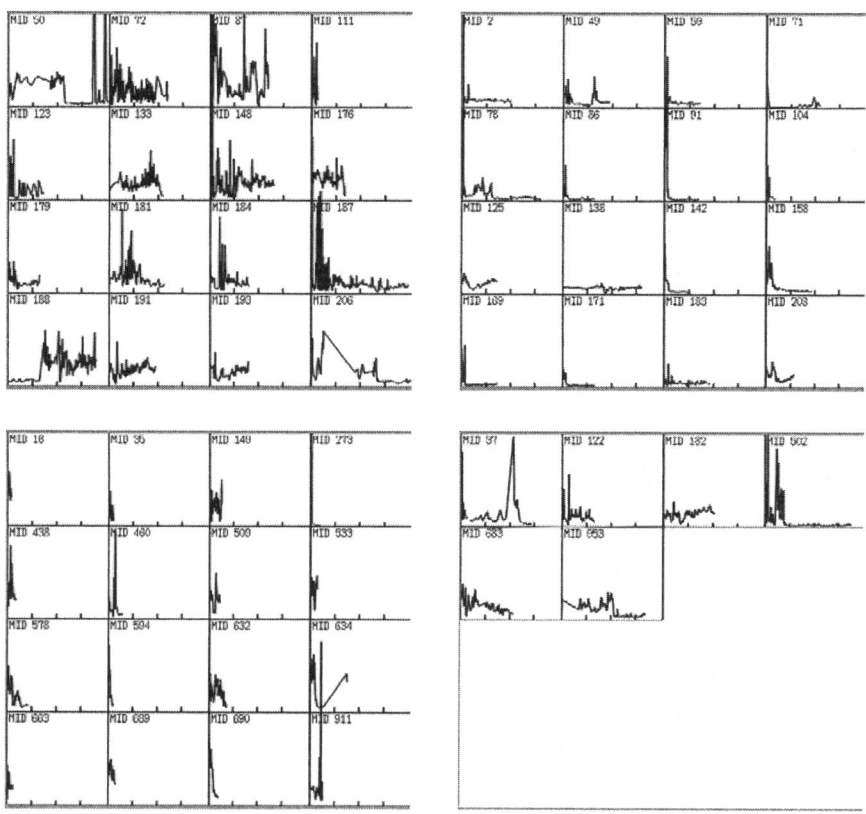

Fig. 15. Examples of the clustered GPT sequence for type C hepatitis patients with IFN therapy. Comparison Method=MSM. Grouping method=RC. Top Left: 1st cluster (80 cases), Top Right: 2nd cluster (60 cases), Bottom Left: 3rd cluster (18 cases), Bottom Right; 4th cluster (6 cases). Sequences are selected according to MID order

The result demonstrated that shape representation parameters in MSM could capture the structural feature of time series; for example, the difference of amplitude were successfully captured using rotation term, and that differences on phases and trends were also successfully reflected in the dissimilarity. However, it also revealed that the dissimilarity induced by MSM lacks linearity compared with DTW. Next, we examined the characteristics of combination of sequence comparison methods and clustering methods using time-series medical data. Although the subjects and conditions for comparison were limited, the results suggested that (1) complete-linkage criterion outperforms average-linkage criterion in terms of the interpret-ability of a dendrogram and clustering results, (2) combination of DTW and CL-AHC constantly produced interpretable results, (3) combination of DTW and RC would be used to find core sequences of the clusters. Multiscale matching may suffer from the problem of 'no-match' pairs, however, the problem may be eluded by using RC as a subsequent grouping method. In the future we extend this study to other types of databases and other types of clustering/comparison methods.

Acknowledgments

This work was supported in part by the Grant-in-Aid for Scientific Research on Priority Area (2) "Development of the Active Mining System in Medicine Based on Rough Sets" (No. 13131208) by the Ministry of Education, Culture, Science and Technology of Japan.

References

1. E. Keogh (2001): Mining and Indexing Time Series Data. Tutorial at the 2001 IEEE International Conference on Data Mining.
2. Chu, S., Keogh, E., Hart, D., Pazzani, M. (2002). Iterative Deepening Dynamic Time Warping for Time Series. In proceedings of the second SIAM International Conference on Data Mining.
3. D. Sankoff and J. Kruskal (1999): Time Warps, String Edits, and Macromolecules. CLSI Publications.
4. S. Hirano and S. Tsumoto (2002): Mining Similar Temporal Patterns in Long Time-series Data and Its Application to Medicine. Proceedings of the IEEE 2002 International Conference on Data Mining: pp. 219–226.
5. N. Ueda and S. Suzuki (1990): A Matching Algorithm of Deformed Planar Curves Using Multiscale Convex/Concave Structures. IEICE Transactions on Information and Systems, J73-D-II(7): 992–1000.
6. F. Mokhtarian and A. K. Mackworth (1986): Scale-based Description and Recognition of planar Curves and Two Dimensional Shapes. IEEE Transactions on Pattern Analysis and Machine Intelligence, PAMI-8(1): 24-43
7. URL: http://lisp.vse.cz/challenge/ecmlpkdd2003/
8. B. S. Everitt, S. Landau, and M. Leese (2001): Cluster Analysis Fourth Edition. Arnold Publishers.
9. S. Hirano and S. Tsumoto (2003): An Indiscernibility-based Clustering Method with Iterative Refinement of Equivalence Relations - Rough Clustering -. Journal of Advanced Computational Intelligence and Intelligent Informatics, 7(2):169–177
10. Lowe, D.G (1980): Organization of Smooth Image Curves at Multiple Scales. International Journal of Computer Vision, 3:119–130.
11. Z. Pawlak (1991): Rough Sets, Theoretical Aspects of Reasoning about Data. Kluwer Academic Publishers, Dordrecht.
12. A. P. Witkin (1983): Scale-space Filtering. Proceedings of the Eighth IJCAI, pp. 1019–1022.

Spiral Mining Using Attributes from 3D Molecular Structures

Takashi Okada, Masumi Yamakawa, and Hirotaka Niitsuma

Department of Informatics, Kwansei Gakuin University,
2-1 Gakuen, Sanda-shi, Hyogo 669-1337, Japan
okada-office@ksc.kwansei.ac.jp

Abstract. Active responses from analysts play an essential role in obtaining insights into structure activity relationships (SAR) from drug data. Experts often think of hypotheses, and they want to reflect these ideas in the attribute generation and selection process. We analyzed the SAR of dopamine agonists and antagonists using the cascade model. The presence or absence of linear fragments in molecules constitutes the core attribute in the mining. In this paper, we generated attributes indicating the presence of hydrogen bonds from 3D coordinates of molecules. Various improvements in the fragment expressions are also introduced following the suggestions of chemists. Attribute selection from the generated fragments is another key step in mining. Close interactions between chemists and system developers have enabled spiral mining, in which the analysis results are incorporated into the development of new functions in the mining system. All these factors are necessary for success in SAR mining.

1 Introduction

The importance of structure-activity relationship (SAR) studies relating chemical structures and biological activity is well recognized. Early studies used statistical techniques, and concentrated on establishing quantitative structure activity relationships involving compounds sharing a common skeleton. However, it is more natural to treat a variety of structures together, and to identify the characteristic substructures responsible for a given biological activity. Recent innovations in high-throughput screening technology have produced vast quantities of SAR data, and there is an increasing need for new data mining methods to facilitate drug development.

Several SARs [3, 4] have been analyzed using the cascade model that we developed [5]. More recently the importance of a "datascape survey" in the mining process was emphasized in order to obtain more valuable insights. We added several functions to the mining software of the cascade model to facilitate the datascape survey [6, 7].

This new method was recently used in a preliminary study of the SAR of the antagonist activity of dopamine receptors [8]. The resulting interpretations of the rules were highly regarded by experts in drug design, as they were able to identify some

S. Tsumoto et al. (Eds.): AM 2003, LNAI 3430, pp. 287–302, 2005.

characteristic substructures that had not been recognized previously. However, the interpretation process required the visual inspection of supporting chemical structures as an essential step. Therefore, the user had to be very careful not to miss characteristic substructures. The resulting information was insufficient for drug design, as the results often provided fragments so simple that they appear in multitudes of compounds. In order to overcome this difficulty, we incorporated further functions in the cascade model, and we tried to improve the expressions for linear fragments.

Fruitful mining results will never be obtained without a response from active users. This paper reports an attempt to reflect expert ideas in the process of attribute generation and selection. These processes really constitute spiral mining, in which chemists and system developers conduct analyses alternately. We briefly describe the aims of mining and introduce the mining method used. Fragment generation is described in Section 3, and attempts to select attributes from fragments are reported in Section 4. Typical rules and their interpretations for dopamine D1 agonists are given in Section 5.

2 Aims and Basic Methods

2.1 Aims and Data Source for the Dopamine Antagonists Analysis

Dopamine is a neurotransmitter in the brain. Neural signals are transmitted via the interaction between dopamine and proteins known as dopamine receptors. There are six different receptor proteins, D1 – D5, and the dopamine autoreceptor (D$auto$), each of which has a different biological function. Their amino acid sequences are known, but their 3D structures have not been established.

Certain chemicals act as agonists or antagonists for these receptors. An agonist binds to the receptor, and it in turn stimulates a neuron. Conversely, an antagonist binds to the receptor, but its function is to occupy the binding site and to block the neurotransmitter function of a dopamine molecule. Antagonists for these receptors might be used to treat schizophrenia or Parkinson's disease. The structural characterization of these agonists and antagonists is an important step in developing new drugs.

We used the MDDR database (version 2001.1) of MDL Inc. as the data source. It contains about 120,000 drug records, including 400 records that describe dopamine (D1, D2, and D$auto$) agonist activities and 1,349 records that describe dopamine (D1, D2, D3, and D4) antagonist activities. Some of the compounds affect multiple receptors. Some of the compounds contain salts, and these parts were omitted from the structural formulae. The problem is to discover the structural characteristics responsible for each type of activity.

2.2 The Cascade Model

The cascade model can be considered an extension of association rule mining [5]. The method creates an itemset lattice in which an [attribute: value] pair is used as an item to constitute itemsets. Links in the lattice are selected and interpreted as rules. That is, we observe the distribution of the RHS (right hand side) attribute values along all links, and if a distinct change in the distribution appears along some link, then we focus on the two terminal nodes of the link. Consider that the itemset at the upper end of a link is [A: y] and item [B: n] is added along the link. If a marked activity change occurs along this link, we can write the rule:

```
Cases: 200 ==> 50            BSS=12.5
IF [B: n] added on [A: y]
THEN [Activity]:     .80 .20 ==> .30 .70 (y n)
THEN [C]:            .50 .50 ==> .94 .06 (y n)
Ridge [A: n]:    .70 .30/100 ==> .70 .30/50 (y n)
```

where the added item [B: n] is the main condition of the rule, and the items at the upper end of the link ([A: y]) are considered preconditions. The main condition changes the ratio of the active compounds from 0.8 to 0.3, while the number of supporting instances decreases from 200 to 50. *BSS* means the between-groups sum of squares, which is derived from the decomposition of the sum of squares for a categorical variable. Its value can be used as a measure of the strength of a rule. The second "THEN" clause indicates that the distribution of the values of attribute [C] also changes sharply with the application of the main condition. This description is called the *collateral correlation*, which plays a very important role in the interpretation of the rules.

2.3 Functions for the Datascape Survey

Three new points were added to DISCAS, the mining software for the cascade model. The main subject of the first two points is decreasing the number of resulting rules [6]. A rule candidate link found in the lattice is first greedily optimized in order to give the rule with the local maximum *BSS* value, changing the main and pre-conditions. Let us consider two candidate links: (M added on P) and (M added on P'). Here, their main conditions, M, are the same. If the difference between preconditions P and P' is the presence/absence of one precondition clause, the rules starting from these links converge on the same rule expression, which is useful for decreasing the number of resulting rules.

The second point is the facility to organize rules into principal and relative rules. In the association rule system, a pair of rules, R and R', are always considered independent entities, even if their supporting instances overlap completely. We think that these rules show two different aspects of a single phenomenon. Therefore, a group of rules sharing a considerable number of supporting instances are expressed as a principal rule with the largest *BSS* value and its relative rules. This function is useful for decreasing the number of principal rules to be inspected, and to indicate the relationships among rules. Further, we omit rules, if most of their supporting instances are covered by the principal rule and if its distribution change in the activity is less than that of the principal rule.

The last point provides ridge information for a rule [7]. The last line in the aforementioned rule contains ridge information. This example describes [A: n], the ridge region detected, and the change in the distribution of "Activity" in this region. Compared with the large change in the activity distribution for the instances with [A: y], the distribution does not change on this ridge. This means that the *BSS* value decreases sharply if we expand the rule region to include this ridge region. This ridge information is expected to guide the survey of the datascape.

3   Scheme of Analysis and Linear Fragment Generation

3.1   Basic Scheme of Analysis

Figure 1 shows a brief scheme of the analysis. The structural formulae of all chemicals are stored in the SDF file format. We used two kinds of explanation attributes generated from the structural formulae of chemical compounds: physicochemical properties and the presence/absence of many linear fragments. We used four physicochemical estimates: the HOMO and LUMO energy levels, the dipole moment, and LogP. The first three values were estimated using molecular mechanics and molecular orbital calculations using the MM-AM1-Geo method provided in *Cache*. LogP values were calculated using the program ClogP in *Chemoffice*. The scheme used for fragment generation is discussed in the following section.

The number of fragments generated is huge, and some of them are selected to form the data table shown in the center of Fig. 1. The cascade model is applied to analyze data, and the resulting rules are interpreted. Often, chemists will browse the rules and try to make hypotheses, but they rarely reach a reasonable hypothesis from the rule

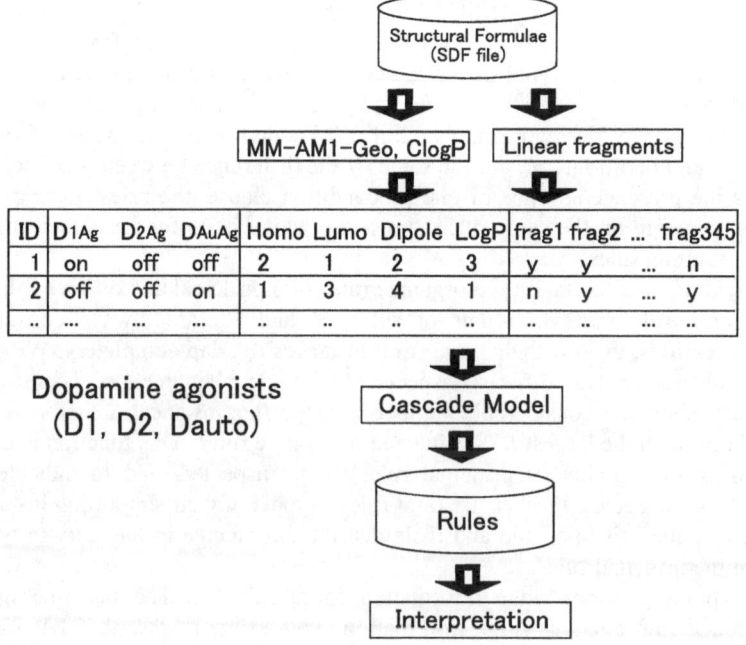

Fig. 1. Flow of the dopamine agonist analysis in the cascade model

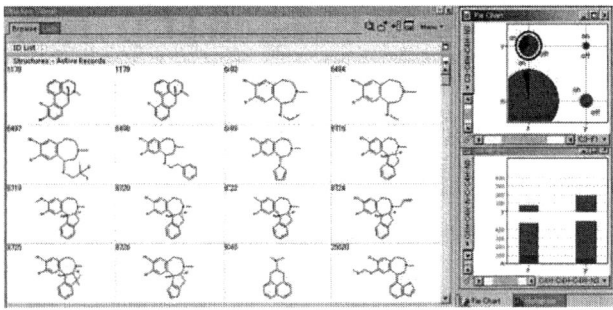

Fig. 2. Inspection of activity distributions and structural formulae

expression alone. *Spotfire* software can then be used, as it can visualize the structural formulae of the supporting compounds when the user specifies the rule conditions. Figure 2 shows a sample window from *Spotfire*. Here, the attributes appearing in a rule are used as the axes of pie and bar charts, and the structural formulae with the specified attribute values are depicted on the left side by clicking a chart. A chemist might then find meaningful substructures from a focused set of compound structures. This function was found to be essential in order to evoke active responses from a chemist.

3.2 Generation of Linear Fragments

The use of linear fragments as attributes has been described in a previous paper [3]. Klopman originally proposed this kind of scheme [1]. Kramer developed a similar kind of scheme independently from our work [2].

Figure 2 shows an example of a structural formula and a set of linear fragment patterns derived from it. Hydrogen atoms are regarded as attachments to heavy atoms. Here, every pattern consists of two terminal atoms and a connecting part along the shortest path. For example, the pattern at the bottom of the left column uses atoms <1> and <6> as terminals, and the connecting part is described by "=C–C–C–", which shows the sequence of bond types and element symbols along the path, <1>=<2>–<3>–<5>–<6>. An aromatic bond is denoted as "r". The description of a terminal atom includes the coordination number (number of adjacent atoms), as well as whether there are attached hydrogen atoms.

In this example, we require that at least one of the terminal atoms be a heteroatom or an unsaturated carbon atom. Therefore, in Fig. 3, no fragment appears between tetrahedral carbon atoms <3> and <5>. Fragments consisting of a single heavy atom like C3H and O2H have been added to the items, although they are not shown in the figure. The set of these fragments can be regarded as constituting a kind of fingerprint of the molecule.

The fragment patterns in Fig. 3 are just examples. The coordination number and hydrogen attachments in the terminal atom part may be omitted. The connecting part is also subject to change. For example, we can just use the number of intervening bonds as the connecting part. Conversely, we can add coordination numbers or the hydrogen attachment to the atom descriptions in the connecting part. There is no *a*

C3H=C3H	C3H-C4H	C4H-C-O2H
C3H=C-C4H	C3H-C-O2H	N3H-C-C-O2H
C3H=C-C-O2H	C3H-C-C4H	C4H-N3H
C3H=C-C-C4H	C3H-C-C-N3H	C4H-C-N3H
C3H=C-C-C-N3H	C4H-O2H	

Fig. 3. A sample structural formula and its linear fragments

priori criterion to judge the quality of various fragment expressions. Only after the discovery process can we judge which type of fragment expression is useful.

This fragment expression led to the discovery of new insights in the application to mutagenesis data. However, a preliminary examination of the rules resulting from dopamine antagonists was not as promising. For example, an aromatic ether substructure was found to be effective in D2 antagonist activity. This substructure appears in many compounds, and chemists concluded that the rules were not useful. Further, they suggested several points to improve the readability of the rules. Therefore, we decided to incorporate new features into the expression of fragments, as discussed in the following sections.

3.3 Extension of Terminal Parts and Omission of Element Symbols in the Connecting Part

Chemists have an image of a dopamine antagonist: the essential substructure is a combination of various components containing oxygen and nitrogen atoms as well as aromatic rings. Further, it often consists of multiple important components connected by a linker. The role of the linker is to locate the important components in the correct positions in 3D space, and its constituting elements have no meaning by themselves. For example, all the 6-membered rings with different constituent atoms in the following three structures will place components A and B in a similar stereochemical configuration, if we neglect the chirality of molecules.

When we describe all the element symbols in the fragment, the number of supporting compounds for a fragment decreases and none of the three fragments might be used as the attribute. If we express the connecting part using the number of intervening atoms, then all these structures contain the fragment "A-<4>-B". However, chemists rejected this expression, as it does not evoke structural formulae in their mind. Therefore, we tried to introduce a new mechanism that omits element and bond symbols from fragment expressions, while keeping the image of structural formula. The proposed fragment expression takes the following forms when applied to the above three structures.

A– – – – –B   if bond types are shown.

A^ ^ ^ ^ ^B   if an anonymous bond type is used.

Chemists rejected the latter notation, as the anonymous bond type hides the existence of an aromatic bond. When an aromatic bond appears in a fragment, it is not a linker, but is an essential component. Therefore, we used the former fragment expression depicting all bond types.

Another comment by chemists was directed to the expression of the terminal part of the fragment. That is, understanding the environment of the terminal components is very important, but the expression is too simple if they are denoted simply by an atom symbol along with its coordination numbers and the attachment of hydrogen atoms. Therefore, we extended the terminal part to include two atoms. The sample molecule in Fig. 2 is small, and the effect of this change in its fragments is limited to the longest one shown below. The element symbol C of the third atom from both ends is dropped in the new expression.

C3H=C-C-C-N3H   ➔   C3H=C--C-N3H

3.4 Hydrogen Bond Fragments

The hydrogen bond is a key concept in chemistry. A sample structure containing a hydrogen bond is illustrated in Fig. 4, where the hydrogen atom of the OH group has a weak bonding interaction with the nitrogen atom in the right ring.

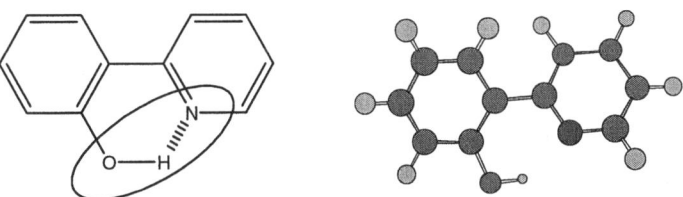

Fig. 4. An example of an intramolecular hydrogen bond

When we visualize chemical structures that satisfy rule conditions, we sometimes see a group of compounds that might be characterized by an intramolecular hydrogen bond, XH...Y, where X and Y are usually oxygen or nitrogen atoms. However, the above-mentioned fragment generation scheme uses only the graph topology of the molecular structure, and we cannot recognize the hydrogen bond.

The results of the MM-AM1-Geo calculation used to estimate the physicochemical properties provide 3D coordinates of atoms. Since their coordinates are obtained by energy minimization starting from the geometry of the structural formula drawing, some molecules converged on coordinates with a local minimum energy. However, we can detect the existence of a hydrogen bond using these 3D coordinates at the risk of missing some hydrogen bonds.

We judge the hydrogen bond XH…Y to exist when the following conditions are all satisfied.

1. Atom X is O, N, S or a 4-coordinated C with at least one hydrogen atom.
2. Atom Y is O, N, S, F, Cl or Br.
3. The distance between X and Y is less than 3.7 Å if Y is O, N or F; and it is less than 4.2 Å otherwise.
4. The structural formula does not contain fragments X-Y or X-Z-Y, including any bond type between atoms.

When these conditions are satisfied, we generate fragments: Xh.Y, V-Xh.Y, Xh.Y-W, and V-Xh.Y-W, where "h." denotes a hydrogen bond and neighboring atoms V and W are included. Other notations follow the basic scheme. The fragments derived from the sample structure in Fig. 4 are as follows.

O2Hh.n2 ,   c3-O2Hh.n2 ,   O2Hh.n2:c3 ,   O2Hh.n2:c3H ,
c3-O2Hh.n2:c3,   c3-O2Hh.n2:c3H

where we use the notation for the aromatic ring explained in the next section.

Application to the dopamine antagonist dataset resulted in 431 fragments, but the probability of the most frequent fragment was less than 0.1. Therefore, no hydrogen bond fragments were used in the standard attribute selection process.

3.5 Lowercase Letters for Atoms in an Aromatic Ring

So far, the element symbol of all carbon atoms has been expressed by the capital letter "C". Consider molecule I, shown below. Its fragments contain C3-C3-N3H and C3-C3=O1, and we cannot judge whether these C3 atoms are in an aromatic ring or are part of a double bond. It is important to know whether an atom is in an aromatic ring. Therefore, we introduced a mechanism to indicate aromatic rings; we describe aromatic atoms in lowercase letters. The above fragments are now written c3-C3-N3H and c3-C3=O1, so chemists can easily recognize the molecular environment of the fragment.

I

Further, we changed the bond notation for an aromatic ring from "r" to ":", as the latter is used in SMILES notation, a well-known chemical structure notation system.

3.6 United Atom Expression for a Carbonyl Group

A carbonyl group (>C=O) has a marked effect on the chemical properties of a molecule. It appears alone in a skeleton as a ketone (C-CO-C), or it appears as an amide (-CO-NH-) or ester (-CO-O-) group when combined with nitrogen and oxygen atoms, respectively. When a chemist looks at a carbonyl group in the fragment of a rule, he/she always asks whether it is a ketone, amide, or ester group. For example, structure I can generate three fragments: c3-C3-N3H, c3-C3=O1, and O1=C3-N3H.

If these fragments appear in a rule, chemists will wonder whether they constitute an amide group like I, or if they appear in separate positions in the molecule.

In order to overcome this difficulty, we introduced a united atom symbol "CO" for a carbonyl group with two neighboring atoms. Then, the above fragment can be written as c3-CO2-N3H. Chemists felt that this expression improves the readability of rules greatly. A similar notation was used in the *CASE* system adopted by Klopman [1].

4 Attribute Selection and Spiral Mining

The number of all possible fragments is obviously too large to be used in data mining. Therefore, we limited the length of linear fragments to be less than or equal to 10, and omitted those fragments with a single functional group: a heteroatom or an olefin. However, there are still several thousand fragments, which is too many for analysis using the current implementation of the cascade model. Therefore, we omitted a fragment from the attribute set, unless the probability of its appearance satisfies the condition: $edge < P(\text{fragment}) < 1.0 - edge$. This is reasonable, since a fragment appearing in only a few compounds will not help in discerning the activity relationship.

However, we were forced to set the *edge* value to $0.1 - 0.15$, and to use about $100 - 150$ fragments for the analysis, as the combinatorial explosion in the lattice size prohibits the analysis if we use more attributes. This selection of attributes has always been a weak point in the analysis scheme. In fact, chemists noticed that some fragments with lower support should appear in the rules, when browsing structural formulae of active compounds.

4.1 The First Attempt

We provided a mechanism to add specified fragments as the attribute used in mining, even if their support is lower than the specified *edge* value. Consequently, a user can repeat the following steps, in order to discover better characteristic substructures.

1. Prepare fragment attributes using the basic scheme.
2. Compute rules.
3. Read the resulting rules and make hypotheses in terms of chemistry.
4. Confirm the hypothesis by browsing the supporting structural formulae.
5. If one notices a characteristic fragment that does not appear in the rule, add the fragment as an attribute. Go to step 2.
6. Repeat until satisfactory results are obtained.

Since an expert can incorporate his/her ideas in the mining process, the addition of fragments and the reading of rules were expected to provide an interesting study.

4.1.1 D2 Antagonist Activity

The analysis of D2 antagonist activity was performed using the scheme described above. We selected 73 fragments using the *edge* value 0.15. We added 32 fragments after reading rules and inspecting chemical structures. They included 27 hydrogen bond fragments for which the probability of appearance was > 0.02, as well as five other fragments: N3-c3:c3-O2, N3H-c3:c3-O2, N3-c3:c3-O2H, N3H-c3:c3-O2H, O1=S4.

The strongest rule indicating active compounds takes the following form, unless we add 32 fragments as attributes.

```
IF [C4H-C4H-O2: y] added on    [ ]
THEN D2AN:                      0.32   ==>   0.62  (on)
THEN c3-O2:                     0.42   ==>   0.89  (y)
THEN c3H:c3-O2:                 0.33   ==>   0.70  (y)
Ridge [c3H:c3H::c3-N3: y] 0.49/246 -->  0.92/71  (on)
```

No preconditions appear, and the main condition shows that an oxygen atom bonded to an alkyl carbon is important. However, this finding is so different from the common sense of chemists, and it will never be accepted as a useful suggestion. In fact, the ratio of active compounds is only 62%. Collateral correlations suggest that the oxygen atom is representative of aromatic ethers, and the ridge information indicates the relevance of aromatic amines. Nevertheless, it is still difficult for an expert to make a reasonable hypothesis.

Chemists found a group of compounds sharing the skeleton shown below, on browsing the supporting structures. Therefore, they added fragments consisting of two aromatic carbons bonded to N3 and O2. This addition did not change the strongest rule, but the following new relative rule appeared.

```
IF [N3-c3:c3-O2: y]   added on    [ ]
THEN D2AN:                      0.31 ==>  0.83  (on)
THEN HOMO:                 .16.51.33 ==>  .00.19 .81 (low medium high)
THEN c3H:c3---C4H-N3:           0.24 -->  0.83  (y)
```

This rule has a greater accuracy and it explains about 20% of the active compounds. The tendency observed in the HOMO value also gives us a useful insight. However, the collateral correlation on the last line suggests that most compounds supporting this rule have the skeleton shown above. Therefore, we cannot exclude the possibility that other parts of this skeleton are responsible for the activity.

4.1.2 D3 Antagonist Activity
The analysis of this activity is also complex, because more than 10 principal rules appeared. We suggested five characteristic substructures in the previous study. The strongest rule leading to this activity had the following form.

```
IF [O1: y] added on [c3-N3: n] [CO2: n]
THEN D3AN:                      0.21 ==>  0.94  (on)
THEN c3:n2:                     0.33 ==>  0.01  (y)
```

```
THEN O2:                0.45 ==> 0.76 (y)
THEN n3Hh.O2:           0.09 ==> 0.54 (y)
```

The main condition of this principal rule is an oxygen atom, and the preconditions used are the absence of two short fragments. Therefore, its interpretation was very difficult. After including hydrogen-bond fragments, the last line in the collateral correlations appeared, where a steep increase in n3Hh.O2 is observed. The relevance of this fragment was confirmed by the appearance of the following relative rule.

```
IF [n3Hh.O2: y] added on   [c3-N3H: n]
THEN D3AN:              0.12 ==> 0.95 (on)
```

In fact, this rule accounts for about half of the active compounds supported by the principal rule. Visual inspection of the supporting structures showed that the following skeleton leads to this activity. We must note that a hydrogen bond itself is not responsible for the activity.

4.1.3 Difficulties in Adding Fragments

The attempt introduced above seemed to evoke active responses from chemists at first. In fact, we identified new characteristic structures using the added fragments. However, the chemists finally rejected this approach. The first reason was because the chemists actually found the new characteristics through visual inspection of the compound structures, and they obtained no new insight. Another reason was the difficulty in selecting interesting fragments from the visual inspection of structures. The more deeply a chemist inspects structures, the more fragments he/she can find. The spirals involving interpreting rules and selecting fragments generated unending work for the chemists.

In this scheme, chemists are responsible all the mining results through the selection of fragments. This process intrinsically forced chemists to hypothesize on the characteristic structures, which was the original aim of mining.

4.2 The Second Attempt

We changed the direction of the mining scheme so that it used more attributes in mining to remove the burden placed on chemists in the first attempt. A correlation-based approach for attribute selection was introduced. This new scheme enabled the use of several hundred fragments as attributes. The details of the attribute-selection scheme will be published separately [9].

When we applied the new scheme to agonist data, 4,626 fragments were generated. We omitted a fragment from the attribute set, unless the probability of its appearance satisfied the condition: $0.03 < P(\text{fragment}) < 0.97$. This gave 660 fragments as candidates of attributes. Then, we omitted a fragment in a correlated pair, if the correlation coefficient was greater than 0.9. The fragment with the longer string was selected, as it was thought to possess more information. The number of fragments decreased to 306 at this stage.

However, the resulting rules caused some difficulty in the rule interpretation process. That is, chemists found that some important fragments were omitted in the attribute selection process. Therefore, we developed a mechanism to replace and add user-designated fragments. Chemists specified some fragments to be included in the attribute set after consulting the output of the correlated fragment pairs. The final number of fragments in the dopamine agonist study was 345. We were able to obtain fruitful results from this attempt, which are presented in the next section.

5 Results and Discussion

We used 345 fragments and four physicochemical properties to construct the itemset lattice. The *thres* parameter value was set to 0.125, and this controls the details of the lattice search [5]. The resulting lattice contained 9,508 nodes, and we selected 1,762 links ($BSS > 2.583 = 0.007$*#compounds) as rule candidates in the D1 agonist analysis. Greedy Optimization of these links resulted in 407 rules ($BSS > 5.535 = 0.015$*#compounds). Organization of these rules gave us 14 principal rules and 53 relative rules. Many rules indicated characteristics leading to inactive compounds or had few supporting compounds, and we omitted those rules with an activity ratio < 0.8 and those with #compounds < 10 after applying the main condition. The final number of rules we inspected decreased to two principal and 14 relative rules.

We inspected all the rules in the final rule set, browsing the supporting chemical structures using *Spotfire*. Table 1 summarizes the important features of valuable rules that guided us to characteristic substructures for D1 agonist activity.

R1 was the strongest rule derived in the D1 agonist study. There are no preconditions, and the activity ratio increases from 17% in 369 compounds to 96% in 52 compounds by including the catechol structure (O2H-c3:c3-O2H). This main condition reduces D*auto* activity to 0%. Other collateral correlations suggest the existence of N3H-C4H-C4H-c3, and OH groups are thought to exist at the positions *meta* and *para* to this ethylamine substituent. However, this ethylamine group is not an indispensable substructure, as the appearance of the N3H-C4H-C4H-c3 fragment is limited to 81% of the supporting compounds.

This observation is also supported by the ridge information. That is, the selection of a region inside the rule by adding a condition [N3H-C4H--:::c3-O2H: y] results in 53 (35 active, 18 inactive) and 35 (34 active, 1 inactive) compounds before and after the application of the main condition, respectively. This means that there are 1 active and 17 inactive compounds when the catechol structure does not exist, and we can say that N3H-C4H--:::c3-O2H cannot show D1Ag activity without catechol. Therefore, we can hypothesize that for D1Ag activity catechol is the active site and it is supported by a primary or secondary ethylamine substituent at the *meta* and *para* positions as the binding site.

Table 1. Rules suggesting the characteristics of D1 agonist activity

Rule ID	Number of compounds and conditions of a rule		Distribution changes in D1Ag and collateral correlations		
			Descriptor	before	after
R1	#compounds	369 → 52	D1Ag:	17% →	96%
			DAuAg:	50% →	0%
	Main condition	[O2H-c3:c3-O2H: y]	C4H-C4H-:::c3-O2H	19% →	92%
			C4H-C4H-::c3-O2H:	18% →	98%
			N3H-C4H--:::c3-O2H:	14% →	67%
	Preconditions	none	N3H-C4H--::c3-O2H:	10% →	69%
			N3H-C4H-C4H-c3:	18% →	81%
			C4H-N3H--C4H-c3	15% →	62%
	Ridge 1: new inside		[N3H-C4H--:::c3-O2H: y]	66%/53 →	97%/35
R1-UL9	#compounds	288 → 16	D1Ag:	19% →	100%
			DAuAg	51% →	0%
	Main condition	[C4H-N3----:c3-O2H: y]	D2Ag:	36% →	100%
			C4H-N3---:::c3-O2H:	5% →	87%
	Preconditions	[N3H: y]	C4H-N3---C4H-c3:	11% →	100%
			O2H-c3:c3-O2H:	17% →	100%
R1-UL12	#compounds	170 → 12	D1Ag:	14% →	100%
			DAuAg	40% →	0%
	Main condition	[N3H-C4H---::c3-O2H: y]	D2Ag:	50% →	0%
			C4H-N3---:::c3-O2H:	8% →	100%
			C4H-N3---C4H-c3:	7% →	100%
	Preconditions	[N3H-C4H--:c3H:c3H: n]	C4H-N3H-C4H-c3:	8% →	100%
		[O2-c3:c3: n]	O2H-c3:c3-O2H	12% →	100%
			O2H-c3:::-C4H-c3:	7% →	100%
			O2H-c3::-C4H-c3:	7% →	100%
R14	#compounds	72 → 11			
	Main condition	[C4H-C4H-O2-c3: n]	D1Ag:	15% →	91%
			DAuAg:	72% →	0%
	Preconditions	[LUMO: 1-3]	CO2-O2-c3:c3H:	31% →	64%
		[C4H-N3---c3:c3: n]	O2-c3:c3:c3-O2:	32% →	64%
		[O2-c3:c3:c3H: y]	N3H-C4H---:c3H:c3H:	7% →	45%

A catechol supported by an ethylamine substituent is the structure of dopamine molecule D1-A, and this covers 50 compounds out of 63 D1 agonists. Therefore, this hypothesis can be evaluated as a rational one.

D1-A

Fourteen relative rules are associated with principal rule R1. Some of them use [N3H-C4H--::c3-O2H: y] and [O2H-c3:c3: y] as the main condition with a variety of preconditions. Another relative rule has the main condition [N3: n] and preconditions [C4H-O2-c3: n] and [C4H-C4H----:::c3-O2H: n]; characterization depending on the absence of substructures was difficult. Nevertheless, the supporting compounds for these relative rules overlap those of R1, and the inspection of their structures supported the hypothesis drawn from R1.

The third entry in Table 1, R1-UL12, seems to suggest a new substructure. Its collateral correlations indicate an N3H group at a position separated by 1, 2, and 3 atoms from an aromatic ring, as well as a diphenylmethane structure. The supporting structures are found to have skeleton D1-B, where the thiophene ring can also be benzene or a furan ring. Therefore, we do not need to change the hypothesis since it contains the dopamine structure D1-A.

D1-B

The only exceptional relative rule was R1-UL9, which is shown as the second entry in Table 1. The interesting points of this rule are the 100% co-appearance of the D2 agonist activity, as well as the *tert*-amine structure in the main condition. These points make a sharp contrast to those found in R1, where *prim*- and *sec*-amines aid the appearance of D1Ag activity and D2Ag activity was found in 38% of the 52 compounds. The importance of the *prim*- or *sec*-amines, ethylamine substituent, and catechol structure are also suggested by the precondition and collateral correlations.

Inspection of the supporting structures showed that this rule was derived from compounds with skeleton D1-C. We found a dopamine structure around the phenyl ring at the right in some compounds, but it could not explain the D1Ag activity for all the supporting compounds. Therefore, we proposed a new hypothesis that the active site is the catechol in the left ring, while the binding site is the *sec*-amine in the middle of the long chain. This *sec*-amine can locate itself close to the catechol ring by folding the $(CH4)_n$ (n=6, 8) chain and it will act as the ethylamine substituent in D1-A.

D1-C

R14 is the second and final principal rule leading to D1Ag activity. Contrary to the R1 group rules, no OHs substituted to an aromatic ring played an essential role in this rule. It was difficult to interpret this rule, because the main condition and second precondition are designated by the absence of ether and *tert*-amine substructures. However, we found that 6 out of 11 compounds share the skeleton D1-D, where the vicinal OHs in catechol are transformed into esters. These esters are thought to be hydrolyzed to OH in the absorption process, and these compounds act as pro-drugs to provide the D1-A skeleton.

D1-D

6   Conclusion

The development of the cascade model along with improvements in linear fragment expressions led to the successful discovery of the characteristic substructure of D1 agonists. The proposed hypothesis bears a close resemblance to the dopamine molecule, and is not a remarkable one. Nevertheless, the hypotheses are rational and they have not been published elsewhere. Other agonists and antagonists are now being analyzed.

Close collaboration between chemists and system developers has been the key to our final success. In this project, the chemist had expertise in using computers in SAR study, while the system developer had a previous career in chemistry. These backgrounds enabled efficient, effective communication between the members of the research group. The chemist would briefly suggest points to improve, and the developer could accept the meaning without rational, detailed explanations by the chemist. The developer often tried to analyze the data in the preliminary analysis, and sometimes he could judge the shortcomings of his system before consulting the chemist. Therefore, the number of spirals in the system development process cannot be estimated easily. Such collaboration is not always possible, but we should note that the communication and trust among the persons involved might be a key factor in the success in this sort of mining.

Acknowledgements

The authors thank Ms. Naomi Kamiguchi of Takeda Chemical Industries for her preliminary analysis on dopamine activity data. This research was partially supported by the Ministry of Education, Science, Sports and Culture, Grant-in-Aid for Scientific Research on Priority Areas, 13131210 and by Grant-in-Aid for Scientific Research (A) 14208032.

References

1   Klopman, G.: Artificial Intelligence Approach to Structure-Activity Studies. J. Amer. Chem. Soc. 106 (1985) 7315-7321
2   Kramer, S., De Raedt, L., Helma, C.: Molecular feature mining in HIV data. In: Proc. of the Seventh ACM SIGKDD International Conference on Knowledge Discovery and Data Mining (KDD-01) (2001) 136-143
3   Okada, T.: Discovery of Structure Activity Relationships using the Cascade Model: the Mutagenicity of Aromatic Nitro Compounds. J. Computer Aided Chemistry 2 (2001) 79-86

4   Okada, T.: Characteristic Substructures and Properties in Chemical Carcinogens Studied by the Cascade Model. Bioinformatics 19 (2003) 1208-1215

5   Okada, T.: Efficient Detection of Local Interactions in the Cascade Model. In: Terano, T. *et al.* (eds.) Knowledge Discovery and Data Mining PAKDD-2000. LNAI 1805, Springer-Verlag (2000) 193-203.

6   Okada, T.: Datascape Survey using the Cascade Model. In: Satoh, K. *et al.* (eds.) Discovery Science 2002. LNCS 2534, Springer-Verlag (2002) 233-246

7   Okada, T.: Topographical Expression of a Rule for Active Mining. In: Motoda, H. (ed.) Active Mining. IOS Press, (2002) 247-257

8   Okada, T., Yamakawa, M.: Mining Characteristics of Lead Compounds using the Cascade Model (in Japanese). Proc. 30th Symposium on Structure-Activity Relationships (2002) 49-52

9   Okada, T.: A Correlation-Based Approach to Attribute Selection in Chemical Graph Mining. in press, JSAI Workshops 2004, LNAI, Springer-Verlag (2005)

Classification of Pharmacological Activity of Drugs Using Support Vector Machine

Yoshimasa Takahashi, Katsumi Nishikoori, and Satoshi Fujishima

Department of Knowledge-based Information Engineering,
Toyohashi University of Technology,
1-1 Hibarigaoka Tempaku-cho, Toyohashi 441-8580, Japan
{taka, katsumi, fujisima}@mis.tutkie.tut.ac.jp

Abstract. In the present work, we investigated an applicability of Support Vector Machine (SVM) to classify of pharmacological activities of drugs. The numerical description of each drug's chemical structure was based on the Topological Fragment Spectra (TFS) proposed by the authors. 1,227 Dopamine antagonists that interact with different types of receptors (D1, D2, D3 and D4) were used for training SVM. For a prediction set of 137 drugs not included in the training set, the obtained SVM classified 123 (89.8 %) drugs into their own activity classes correctly. The comparison between using SVM and artificial neural network will also be discussed.

1 Introduction

For half a century, a lot of efforts have been made to develop new drugs. It is true that such new drugs allow us to have better life. However, serious side effects have often been reported and raise a social problem. The aim of this research project is to establish a basis of computer-aided risk report for chemicals based on pattern recognition techniques and chemical similarity analysis.

The authors [1] proposed Topological Fragment Spectral (TFS) method for a numerical vector representation of the topological structure profile of a molecule. The TFS provides us a useful tool to evaluate structural similarity among molecules [2]. In our preceding work [3], we reported that an artificial neural network approach combined with input signals of the TFS allowed us to successfully classify type of activities for dopamine receptor antagonists, and it could be applied to the prediction of active class of unknown compounds. And we also suggested that similar structure searching based on TFS representation of molecules could provide us a chance to discover new insight or knowledge from a huge amount of data [4].

On the other hand, in the past few years, support vector machines (SVM) have attracted great interest in machine learning due to its superior generalization ability in various learning problems [5-7]. Support vector machine is originated from perceptron theory, but seldom causes some classical problems such as multiple local minima, curse of dimensionality and over-fitting in artificial neural network. Here we investigate the utility of support vector machine combined with TFS representation of chemical structures in classifying pharmacological drug activities.

S. Tsumoto et al. (Eds.): AM 2003, LNAI 3430, pp. 303–311, 2005.

2 Methods

2.1 Numerical Representation of Chemical Structure

In the present work, to describe structural information of drugs, Topological Fragment Spectra (TFS) method [1] is employed. TFS is based on enumeration of all the possible substructures from a chemical structure and their numerical characterization. A chemical structure can be regarded as a graph in terms of graph theory. For graph representation of chemical structures, hydrogen suppressed graph is often used. A schematic flow of TFS creation is shown in Fig. 1.

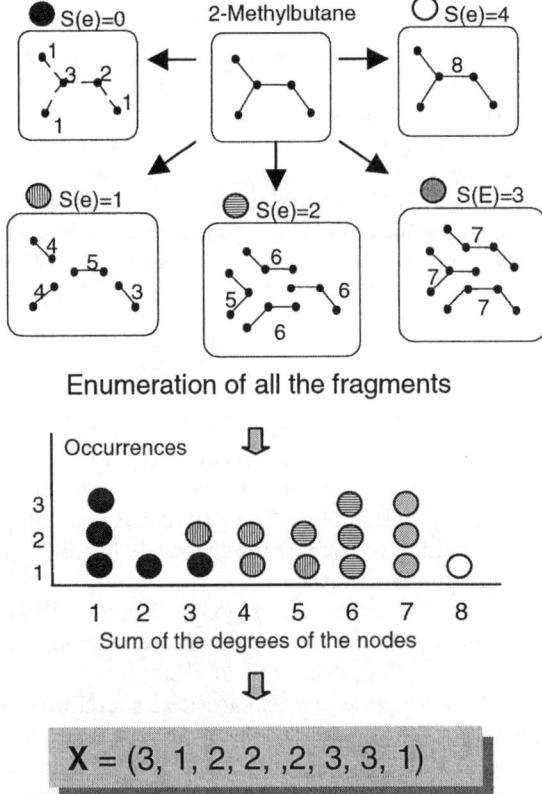

Fig. 1. A schematic flow of TFS generation. $S(e)$ is the number of edges (bonds) of generated fragments

To get TFS representation of a chemical structure, all the possible subgraphs with specified number of edges are enumerated. Subsequently, every subgraph is characterized with a numerical quantity defined in a characterization scheme in advance. In Fig.1 the sum of degree of vertex atoms is used as the characterization index of each subgraph. Alternative method can be also employed for the characterization such as the sum of mass numbers of the atoms (atomic groups) corresponding to the vertices of the subgraph. The histogram is defined as TFS obtained from frequency distribution of individually characterized subgraphs (i.e. substructures or structural fragments) according to their values of the characterization index. TFS of promazine characterized by the two different ways are shown in Fig. 2.

For the present work we used the latter characterization scheme to generate the TFS. In the characterization process, suppressed hydrogen atoms are considered as augmented atoms.

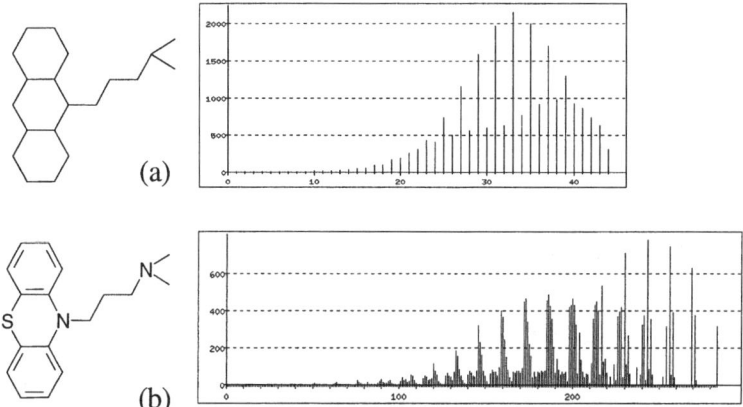

Fig. 2. TFS of promazine generated by the different characterization methods. (a) is obtained by the characterization with the sum of degrees of vertex atoms of the fragments. (b) is obtained by another characterization scheme with the sum of atomic mass numbers of the fragments

TFS generated by this way is a digital representation of topological structural profile of a drug molecule. This is very similar to that of mass spectra of chemicals. Thus the TFS can be regarded as a function of chemical structure, i.e. *TFS= f(chemical structure)*.

Computational time required for exhaustive enumeration of all possible substructures is often very large especially for the molecules that involve highly fused rings. To avoid such a problem, the use of subspectrum was employed for the present work, in which each spectrum could be described with structural fragments up to a specified size in the number of edges (bonds).

Obviously, the fragment spectrum obtained by these methods can be described as a kind of multidimensional pattern vector. However, the number of dimensions of the TFS pattern description vector depends on individual chemical structures. The different dimensionalities of the spectra to be compared are adjusted as follows,

$$\text{if } X_i = (x_{i1}, x_{i2}, ..., x_{iq}) \text{ and } X_j = (x_{j1}, x_{j2}, ..., x_{jq}, x_{j(q+1)}, ..., x_{jp}) \text{ (q<p)}, \quad (1)$$

$$\text{then } X_i \text{ is redefined as } X_i = (x_{i1}, x_{i2}, ..., x_{iq}, x_{i(q+1)}, ..., x_{ip})$$

306 Y. Takahashi, K. Nishikoori, and S. Fujishima

here, $x_{i(q+1)} = x_{i(q+2)} = ... = x_{ip} = 0$

Where, x_{ik} is the intensity value of peak k of TFS for i-th molecule, and x_{jk} is that of peak k of TFS for the j-th molecule that have the highest value of the characterization index (in this work, the highest fragment mass number). For the prediction, each TFS is adjusted by padding with 0 or by cutting the higher mass region off to have the same dimensionality as that of the training set when a prediction sample is submitted.

2.2 Support Vector Machine

Support vector machine has been focused as a powerful nonlinear classifier in the last decade because it introduces kernel function trick [7]. The SVM implements the following basic idea: it maps the input vectors $\mathbf{x}$ into a higher dimensional feature space $\mathbf{z}$ through some nonlinear mapping, chosen a priori. In this space, an optimal discriminant surface with maximum margin is constructed (Fig.2). Given a training dataset represented by $\mathbf{X}(\mathbf{x}_1,...,\mathbf{x}_i,...,\mathbf{x}_n)$, $\mathbf{x}_i$ that are linearly separable with class labels $y_i \in \{-1,1\}, i=1,...,n$, the discriminant function can be described in the following equation.

$$f(\mathbf{x}_i) = (\mathbf{w} \cdot \mathbf{x}_i) + b \qquad (2)$$

Where $\mathbf{w}$ is a weight vector, b is a bias. The discriminant surface can be represented as $f(\mathbf{x}_i) = 0$. The maximum margin can be obtained by minimizing square of the norm of weight vector $\mathbf{w}$,

$$\|\mathbf{w}\|^2 = \mathbf{w} \cdot \mathbf{w} = \sum_{l=1}^{d} w_l^2 \qquad (3)$$

with the constraints $y_i(\mathbf{w} \cdot \mathbf{x}_i + b) \geq 1 \quad (i=1,...,n)$

The decision function is described as $S(\mathbf{x}) = sign(\mathbf{w} \cdot \mathbf{x} + b)$ for classification, where $sign$ is a sign function that returns 1 for positive value and -1 for negative value. This basic idea can be extended to a linearly inseparable case by introducing slack variables ξ and minimizing the following quantity,

$$\frac{1}{2}\mathbf{w} \cdot \mathbf{w} + C\sum_{i=1}^{n} \xi_i \qquad (4)$$

with the constraints $y_i = (\mathbf{w} \cdot \mathbf{x}_i + b) \geq 1 - \xi_i$ and $\xi_i \geq 0$.

This optimization problem reduces to the previous one for separable data when constant C is large enough. This quadratic optimization problem with constraints can be reformulated by introducing Lagrangian multipliers α.

$$W(\alpha) = \frac{1}{2}\sum_{i,j=1}^{n} \alpha_i \alpha_j y_i y_j \mathbf{x}_i \cdot \mathbf{x}_j - \sum_{i=1}^{n} \alpha_i \qquad (5)$$

with the constraints $0 \leq \alpha_i \leq C$ and $\sum_{i=1}^{n} \alpha_i y_i = 0$.

Since the training points $\mathbf{x}_i$ do appear in the final solution only via dot products, this formulation can be extended to general nonlinear functions by using the concepts of nonlinear mappings and kernels [6]. Given a mapping, $\mathbf{x} \rightarrow \phi(\mathbf{x})$, the dot product in the final space can be replaced by a kernel function.

$$f(\mathbf{x}) = g(\phi(\mathbf{x})) = \sum_{i=1}^{n} \alpha_i y_i K(\mathbf{x}, \mathbf{x}_i) + b \tag{6}$$

Here we used radial basis function as the kernel function for mapping the data into a higher dimensional space.

$$K(\mathbf{x}, \mathbf{x}') = \exp\left(-\frac{\|\mathbf{x} - \mathbf{x}'\|^2}{\sigma^2}\right) \tag{7}$$

An illustrative scheme of nonlinear separation of data space by SVM is shown in Fig.3.

Basically, SVM is a binary classifier. For classification problem of three or more categorical data, plural discrimination functions are required for the current multi categorical classification. In this work, one-against-the-rest approach was used for the case. The TFS were used as input feature vectors to the SVM. All the SVM analyses were carried out using a computer program developed by the authors according to Platt's algorithm [8].

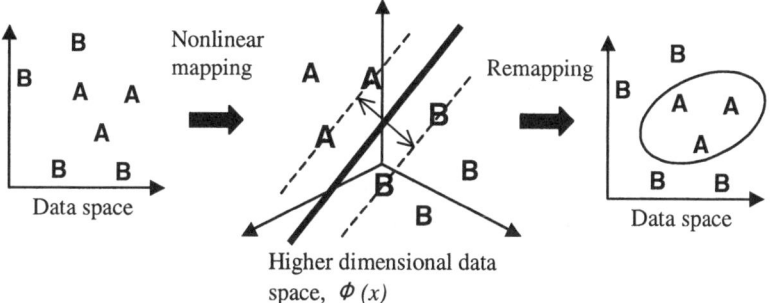

Fig. 3. Illustrative scheme of nonlinear separation of two classes by SVM with a kernel trick

2.3 Neural Network

Discrimination of pharmacological activity classes of chemicals was investigated using artificial neural network (ANN). Three-layer learning network with a complete connection among layers was used. The TFS was submitted to the ANN as input signals for the input neurons. The number of neurons in the input layer was 165, that is the same as the value of dimensionality of the TFS. The number of neurons in the single hidden layer was determined by trial and error. Training of the ANN was carried out by error back propagation method. All the neural network analyses in this work were carried out using a computer program, NNQSAR, developed by the authors [9].

2.4 Data Set

In this work we employed 1364 dopamine antagonists that interact with four different types of receptors (D1, D2, D3 and D4 receptors of dopamine). Dopamine is one of representative neurotransmitters. Decreasing of dopamine causes to various neuropathy. It's closely related to Parkinson's disease. Several G protein-coupled receptors, GPCR(s) are known. On the contrary, Dopamine antagonists interact to dopamine receptors and then inhibit the role of dopamine. The data are taken from MDDR [10] database that is a structure database of investigative new drugs, and they are all the data of dopamine receptor antagonists that are available on it. The data set was divided into two groups; training set and prediction set. The training set consists of 1227 compounds (90% of the total data), and the prediction set consists of 137 compounds (10% of the total data) remained. They were randomly chosen.

3   Results and Discussion

3.1 Classification and Prediction of Pharmacological Activity of Dopamine Receptor Antagonists by SVM

Applicability of SVM combined with TFS representation of chemical structures was validated in discriminating active classes of pharmaceutical drugs. Here, 1,227

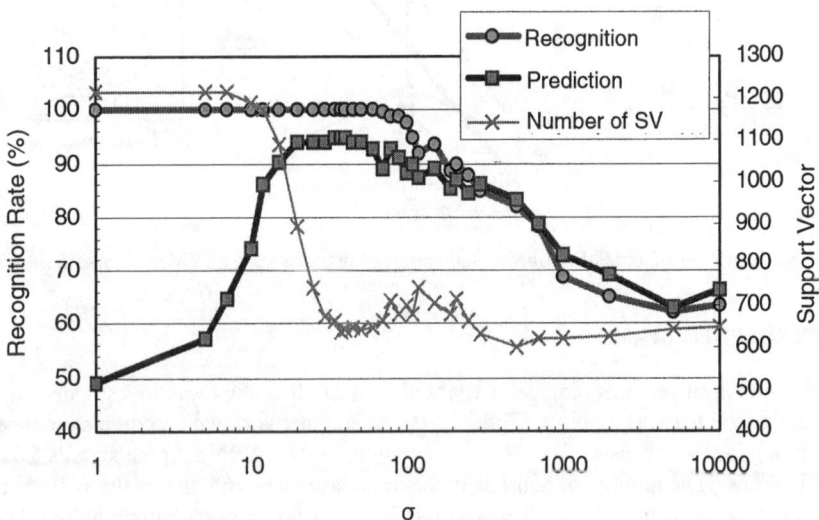

Fig. 4. Variation of the recognition rate, prediction rate and support vectors

Dopamine antagonists that interact with different type of receptors (D1, D2, D3 and D4) were used for training SVM with their TFS to classify the type of activity. SVM model was able to learn to classify all the compounds into own active classes correctly. However, the prediction ability is sensitive to the value of σ in the kernel function used. For the reason, we investigated the optimum value of σ parameter in preliminary computational experiments. Figure 4 shows plots of the performances with different values of the σ parameter. The plots show that the small values of σ gave us better training results but they gave us poor results for the predictions. It is clear that there is an optimum for the value. For the present case, it was concluded the optimum value 40.

Then, the trained SVM model was used to predict activity for unknown compounds. For 137 separately prepared compounds in advance, the activity classes of 123 compounds (89.8%) were correctly predicted. The results are summarized in Table 1. Out of the four classes, the prediction result for D4 receptor antagonists is better than the others in both of the training and the prediction. Supposedly it obtains well defined support vectors from the training set with a lot more samples than the rest. These results show that SVM provides us a very powerful tool for classification and prediction of pharmaceutical drug activities, and that TFS representation is suitable as input signal to SVM in the case.

Table 1. Results of SVM analyses for 1364 dopamine antagonists

Class	Training		Prediction	
	Data	%Correct	Data	%Correct
All	**1227**	**100**	**123/137**	**89.8**
D1	155	100	15/18	83.3
D2	356	100	31/39	79.5
D3	216	100	22/24	91.7
D4	500	100	55/56	98.2

3.2 Cross Validation Test

In the previous section, the TFS-based support vector machine (TFS/SVM) successfully classified and predicted most of the dopamine antagonists into their own active classes. We also tested the validity of the results using a cross-validation technique. For the same data set of 1364 compounds that contain both the training set and prediction set, ten different trial datasets were generated. For making these trial datasets the whole data was randomly divided into 10 subsets that had almost same number of samples for (136 or 137 compounds for each). Each trial dataset was used as the test set for the prediction and the remaining of the datasets were employed for the training of the TFS/SVM. The results of these computational trials were summarized in Table 2.

Table 2. Results of ten-fold cross validation test for TFS/SVM

Class	Prediction results (%)				
	D1	**D2**	**D3**	**D4**	**All**
Max	100	94.8	91.7	100	93.4
Min	76.5	79.5	83.3	90.9	87.6
Average	87.5	86.1	88.3	95.5	90.6

In the cross validation test, the total prediction rates for ten trials of the training were 87.6 % to 93.4 %. The total average of prediction rates was 90.6 %. These values are quite similar to them described in the previous section. It is considered that the present results strongly validate the utility of the TFS-based support vector machine approach to the problems for classification and prediction of pharmacologically active compounds.

3.3 Comparison Between SVM and ANN

In the preceding work [2], the authors reported that an artificial neural network based on TFS gives us a successful tool to discriminate active drug classes. To evaluate better performance of SVM approach for the current problem, here, we tried to compare the results by SVM with those by artificial neural network (ANN). The data set of 1364 drugs used in the above section was employed for the analysis as well. Ten-fold cross validation technique was used for the computational trial. The results were summarized in Table 2.

Table 3. Comparison between SVM and ANN by ten-fold cross validation test

Active Class	SVM		ANN	
	Training %Correct	Prediction %Correct	Training %Correct	Prediction %Correct
All	**100**	**90.6**	**87.5**	**81.1**
D1	100	87.5	76.0	70.7
D2	100	86.1	80.7	69.9
D3	100	88.3	90.9	85.8
D4	100	95.5	94.5	90.5

The table shows that the results obtained by SVM were better than those obtained by ANN for every case in these trials. These results show that TFS-based support vector machine was more successful results than TFS-based artificial neural network for the current problem.

4 Conclusions and Future Work

In this work, we investigated the usage of support vector machine to classify pharmacological drug activities. Topological Fragment Spectra (TFS) method was used for the numerical description of chemical structure information of each drug. It is concluded that TFS-based support vector machine can be successfully applied to predict drug molecule activity types. However, because many instances are required to establish predictive risk assessment and risk report of drugs and chemicals, further works would still be required to test the usage of TFS-based support vector machine with more drugs. In addition, it would also be interesting to identify support vectors chosen in training phase and to analyze structural features from the viewpoint of drug molecule structure-activity relationships.

This work was supported by Grant-In-Aid for Scientific Research on Priority Areas (B) 13131210.

References

1. Y. Takahashi, H. Ohoka, and Y. Ishiyama, Structural Similarity Analysis Based on Topological Fragment Spectra, *In "Advances in Molecular Similarity"*, **2**, (Eds. R. Carbo & P. Mezey), JAI Press, Greenwich, CT, (1998) 93-104
2. Y. Takahashi, M. Konji, S. Fujishima, MolSpace: A Computer Desktop Tool for Visualization of Massive Molecular Data, *J. Mol. Graph. Model.*, **21** (2003) 333-339
3. Y. Takahashi, S. Fujishima and K. Yokoe: Chemical Data Mining Based on Structural Similarity, International Workshop on Active Mining, The 2002 IEEE International Conference on Data Mining, Maebashi (2002) 132-135
4. Y. Takahashi, S. Fujishima, H. Kato, Chemical Data Mining Based on Structural Similarity, *J. Comput. Chem. Jpn.*, **2** (2003) 119-126
5. V.N. Vapnik : The Nature of Statistical Learning Theory, Springer, (1995)
6. C. J. Burges,. A Tutorial on Support Vector Machines for Pattern Recognition, Data Mining and Knowledge Discovery **2**, (1998) 121-167
7. S. W. Lee and A. Verri, Eds, Support Vector Machines 2002, LNCS 2388, (2002)
8. J. C. Platt : Sequential Minimal Optimization: A Fast Algorithm for Training Support Vector Machines, Microsoft Research Tech. Report MSR-TR-98-14, Microsoft Research, 1998.
9. H. Ando and Y. Takahashi, Artificial Neural Network Tool (NNQSAR) for Structure-Activity Studies, *Proceedings of the 24th Symposium on Chemical Information Sciences* (2000) 117-118
10. MDL Drug Data Report, MDL, ver. 2001.1, (2001)

Cooperative Scenario Mining from Blood Test Data of Hepatitis B and C

Yukio Ohsawa[1,4], Hajime Fujie[2], Akio Saiura[3], Naoaki Okazaki[4], and Naohiro Matsumura[5]

[1] Graduate School of Business Sciences, University of Tsukuba
osawa@gssm.otsuka.tsukuba.ac.jp
[2] Department of Gastroenterology, The University of Tokyo Hospital
[3] Department of Digestive Surgery, Cancer Institute Hospital, Tokyo
[4] Graduate School of Information Science and Technology, The University of Tokyo
[5] Faculty of Economics, Osaka University

Abstract. Chance discovery, to discover events significant for making a decision, can be regarded as the emergence of a scenario with extracting events at the turning points of valuable scenarios, by means of communications exchanging scenarios in the mind of participants. In this paper, we apply a method of chance discovery to the data of diagnosis of hepatitis patients, for obtaining scenarios of how the most essential symptoms appear in the patients of hepatitis of type B and C. In the process of discovery, the results are evaluated to be novel and potentially useful for treatment, under the mixture of objective facts and the subjective focus of the hepatologists' concerns. Hints of the relation between f iron metabolism and hepatitis cure, the effective condition for using interferon, etc. has got visualized.

1 Introduction: Scenarios in the Basis of Critical Decisions

A scenario is a sequence of events sharing a context. For example, suppose a customer of a drug store buys a number of items in series, a few items per month. He should do this because he has a certain persistent disease. In this case, a remedy of the disease suggested from his doctor is the context shared over the event-sequence, where an event is this patient's purchase of a set of drugs. This event-sequence is a scenario under the context proposed by the doctor. However, the patient may hear about a new drug, and begin to buy it to change the context, from the remedy he followed so far to a new remedy to seep up his cure. In other words, the patient introduces a new scenario. After a month, his doctor gets upset hearing this change due to the patient's ignorance about the risk of the new drug. The doctor urgently introduces a powerful method to overcome all the by-effects of the risky new drug – changing to the third scenario.

In this example, we find two "chances" in the three scenarios. The first chance is the information about the new drug which changed from the first remedy scenario to the second, risky one. Then the doctor's surprise came to be the second chance to turn to the third scenario. Under the definition of "chance" in [Ohsawa and McBurney

S. Tsumoto et al. (Eds.): AM 2003, LNAI 3430, pp. 312–335, 2005.

2003], i.e., an event or a situation significant for decision making, a chance occurs at the cross point of multiple scenarios as in the example above because a decision is to select one scenario in the future. Generally speaking, a set of scenarios form a basis of decision making, in domains where the choice of a sequence of events affects the future significantly. Based on this concept, the methods of chance discovery have been making successful contributions to science and business domains [Chance Discovery Consortium 2004].

Now let us stand on the position of a surgeon looking at the time series of symptoms during the progress of an individual patient's disease. The surgeon should make appropriate actions for curing this patient, at appropriate times. If he does so, the patient's disease may be cured. However, otherwise the patient's health condition might be worsened radically. The problem here can be described as choosing one from multiple scenarios. For example, suppose states 4 and 5 in Eq. (1) mean two opposite situations.

Scenario 1 = {state0 -> state 1 -> state2 -> state3 -> state4 (a normal condition)}.

Scenario 2 = {state 4 -> state5 -> state6 (a fatal condition)}.   (1)

Each event-sequence in Eq.(1) is called a *scenario* if the events in it share some common context. For example, Scenario 1 is a scenario in the context of cure, and Scenario 2 is a scenario in the context of disease progress. Here, suppose there is a hidden state 11, which may come shortly after or before state 2 and state 5. The surgeon should choose an effective action at the time of state 2, in order to turn this patient to state 3 and state 4 rather than to state 5, if possible. Such a state as state 2, essential for making a decision, is a *chance* in this case.

Detecting an event at a crossover point among multiple scenarios, as state 2 above, and selecting the scenario going through such a cross point means a chance discovery. In general, the meaning of a scenario with an explanatory context is easier to understand than an event shown alone. In the example of the two scenarios above, the scenario leading to cure is apparently better than the other scenario leading to a fatal condition. However, the meaning of chance events, which occurs on the bridge from a normal scenario to a fatal scenario, i.e., state 2, state 11, and state 5 in Fig.1, are hard to understand if they are shown independently of more familiar events. For example, if you are a doctor and find polyp is in a patient's stomach, it would be hard to decide to cut it away or to do nothing else than leaving it at the current position. On the other hand, suppose the you find the patient is at the turning point of two scenarios – in one, the polyp will turn larger and gets worsened. In the other, the polyp will be cut away and the patient will be cured. Having such understanding of possible scenarios, you can easily choose the latter choice.

Consequently, an event should be regarded as a valuable chance if the difference of the merits of scenarios including the event is large, and this difference is an easy measure of the utility of the chance. Discovering a chance and taking it into consideration is required for making useful scenarios, and proposing a number of scenarios even if some are useless is desired in advance for realizing chance discovery. For realizing these understandings, visualizing the scenario map showing the relations between states as in Fig.1 is expected to be useful. Here, let us each familiar scenario, such as Scenario 1 or Scenario 2 , an *island*. And, let us call the link between islands a *bridge*. In chance discovery, the problem is to have the user obtain bridges between islands, in order to explain the meaning of the connections among islands via bridges, as a scenario expressed in understandable language for the user him/herself.

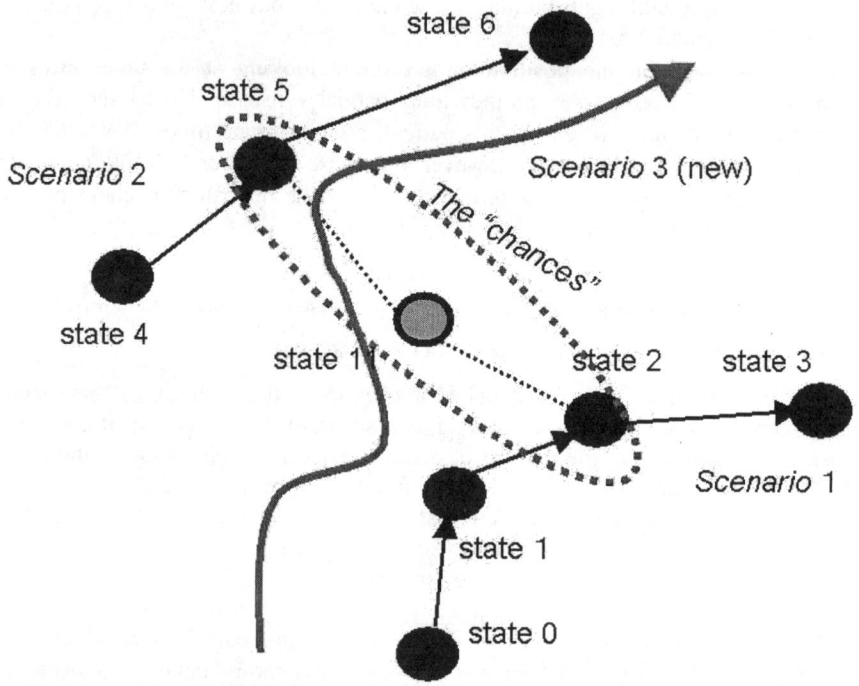

Fig. 1. A chance existing at the cross point of scenarios. The scenario in the thick arrows emerged from Scenario 1 and Scenario 2

2 Scenario "Emergence" in the Mind of Experts

In the term "scenario development", a scenario may sound like something to be "developed" by human(s) who consciously rules the process of making a scenario. However, valuable scenarios really "emerge" by unconscious interaction of humans and their environment. For example, a *scenario workshop* developed by the Danish Board of Technology (2003) starts from scenarios preset by writers, then experts in the domain corresponding to the preset scenarios discuss to improve the scenarios. The discussants write down their opinions during the workshop, but it is rare they notice all the reasons why those opinions came out and why the scenarios have got obtained finally.

This process of scenario workshop can be compared with the KJ (Kawakita Jiro) method, the method in the origin of creation aid, where participants write down their initial ideas on KJ cards and arrange the cards in a 2D-space in co-working for finding good plans. Here, the idea on each card reflects the future scenario in a participants' mind. The new combination of proposed scenarios, made during the arrangement and the rearrangements of KJ cards, helps the emergence of new valuable scenarios, putting in our terminology. In some design processes, on the other hand, it has been pointed out that ambiguous information can trigger creations [Gaver et al 2003]. The common points among the scenario "workshop", the "combination" of ideas in KJ method, and the "ambiguity" of the information to a designer is that scenarios presented from the viewpoint of each participant's environment, are bridged via ambiguous pieces of information about different mental worlds they attend. From these bridges, each participant recognizes situations or events which may work as "chances" to import others' scenarios to get combined with one's own. This can be extended to other domains than designing. In the example of Eq.(1), a surgeon who almost gave up because he guessed his patient is in Scenario 2, may obtain a new hope in Scenario 1 proposed by his colleague who noticed that state 2 is common to both scenarios – only if it is still before or at the time of state 2. Here, state 2 is uncertain in that its future can potentially go in two directions, and this uncertainty can make a chance, an opportunity not only a risk.

In this paper we apply a method for aiding scenario emergence, by means of interaction with real data using two tools of chance discovery, KeyGraph in [Ohsawa 2003b] and TextDrop [Okazaki 2003]. Here, KeyGraph with additional causal directions in the co-occurrence relations between values of variables in blood-test data of hepatitis patients (let us call this a *scenario map*), and TextDrop helps in extracting the part of data corresponding to the concern of an expert, a surgeon and a physician here.

These tools aid in obtaining useful scenarios of the hepatitis progress and cure, reasonably restricted to an understandable type of patience, from the complex real data taken from the mixture of various scenarios. The scenarios obtained for hepatitis were evaluated by two hepatologists, a hepatic surgeon and a hepatic physician, to be useful in finding a good timing to make actions in treating hepatitis patients. This evaluation is subjective in the sense that too small part of the large number of patients in the data were observed to follow the entire scenarios obtained. That is, a scenario corresponding to fewer patients may seem less trustworthy. However, we can say our discovery process was made quite well under the hard condition that it is very rare that the full scenarios of really critical worsening or exceptionally successful treatment occur. We can say a new and useful scenario can be created merging the subjective interests of experts reflecting their real-world experiences and the objective tendencies in the data. Rather than discussing about data-based discovery, our point is the humans' role in discoveries.

3 The Double Helix Process of Chance Discovery

In the studies of chance discovery, the discovery process has been supposed to follow the Double Helix (DH) model [Ohsawa 2003a] as in Fig. 2. The DH process starts from a state of user's mind concerned with catching a new chance, and this *concern* is reflected to acquiring *object data* to be analyzed by data-mining tools specifically designed for chance discovery. Looking at the visualized result of this analysis, possible scenarios and their meanings rise in each user's mind. Then users get to be participants of a co-working group for chance discovery, sharing the same visual result. Then, words corresponding to bridges among the various daily contexts of participants are visualized in the next step of visual data mining applied to the *subject data*, i.e., the text data recording the thoughts and opinions in the discussion. Via the participants' understanding of these bridges, the islands get connected and form novel scenarios.

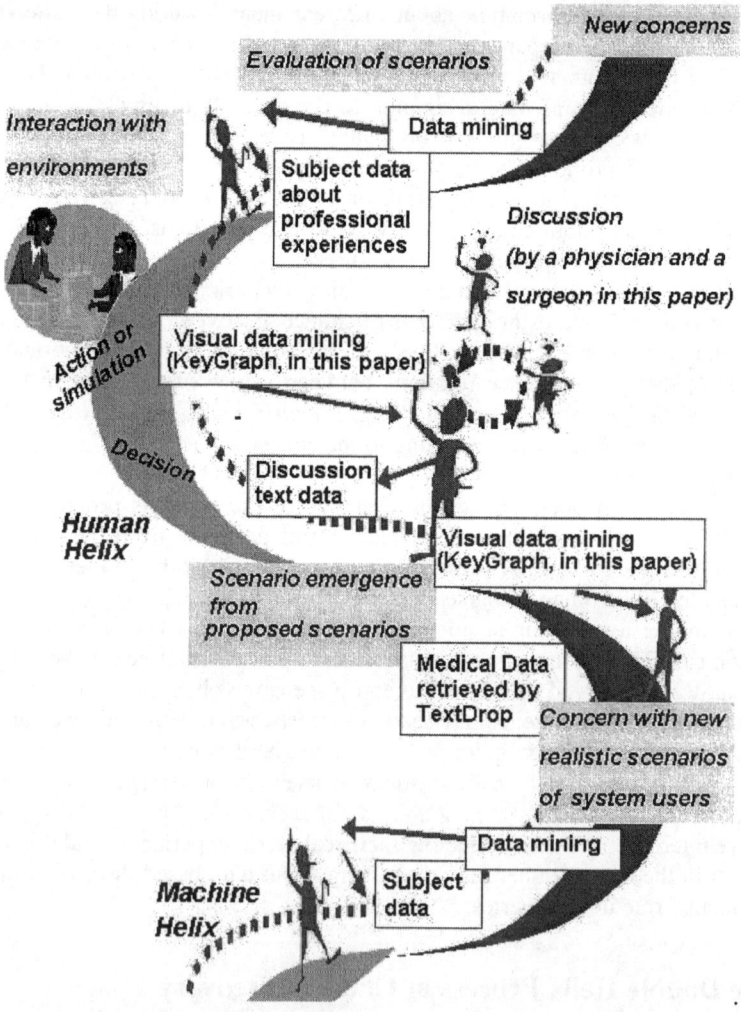

Fig. 2. The DH Model: A process model of chance discovery

By this time, the participants may have discovered chances on the bridges, because each visualized island corresponds to a certain scenario familiar to some of the participants and a bridge means a cross-point of those familiar scenarios. Based on these chances, the user(s) make actions, or simulate actions in a virtual environment, and obtain concerns with new chances – the helical process returns to the initial step of the next cycle. DH is embodied in this paper, in the application to obtaining hepatitis scenarios. Users watch and discuss on KeyGraph [Ohsawa 2003b] applied to the subject data and the object data in the process, thinking and talking about scenarios the diagram may imply.

4 Tools for Accelerating DH

4.1 KeyGraph for Visualizing Scenario Map

KeyGraph is a computer-aided tool for visualizing the map of event relations in the environment, in order to aid in the process of chance discovery. If the environment represents a place of discussion, an event may represent a word in by a participant. By visualizing the map where the words appear connected in a graph, one can see the overview of participants' interest. Suppose text-like data (string-sequence) D is given, describing an event-sequence sorted by time, with periods (``.'') inserted at the parts corresponding to the moments of major changes. For example, let text D be:

$$
\begin{aligned}
D \quad = \quad & a1, a2, a4, a5 \dots . \\
& a4, a5, a3, \dots . \\
& a1, a2, a6, \dots . \\
& \qquad \dots a4, a5 . \\
& a1, a2, , a5, \dots , a10. \\
& a1, a2, a4, , \dots , , \dots a10. \\
& \dots .
\end{aligned}
$$

$$(2)$$

On data D, KeyGraph runs in the following procudure.

KeyGraph-Step 1: Clusters of co-occurring frequent items (words in a document, or events in a sequence) are obtained as basic clusters, called *islands*. That is, items appearing many times in the data (e.g., the word "market" in Eq.(2)) are depicted with black nodes, and each pair of these items occurring often in the same sequence unit is linked to each other with a solid line. Each connected graph obtained here forms one island, implying the existence of a common context underlying the belonging items. As in (1) and (2) of Fig.3, this step is realized by two sub-steps.

KeyGraph-Step 2: Items which may not be so frequent as the black nodes in islands, but co-occurring with items in more than one islands, e.g., ``restructuring" in Eq.(2), are obtained as *hubs*. A path of links connecting islands via hubs is called a *bridge*. If a hub is rarer than black nodes, it is colored in a different color (e.g. red). We can regard such a new hub as a candidate of *chance*, i.e., items significant (assertions in a document, or latent demand in a POS data) with respect to the structure of item-relations. This step corresponds to (3) in Fig.3.

As a result, the output of KeyGraph as shown in (3) of Fig.3 includes islands and bridges, and this is expected to work as a scenario map introduced in Section 1. In the example of Fig.4, on the text data of Eq.(3), Island (1) means the context that the

(1) Obtain the co-occurrence network

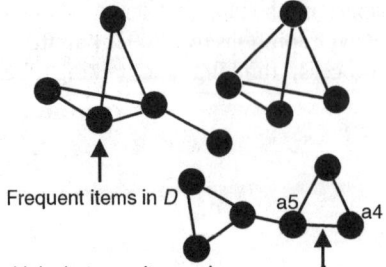

Frequent items in *D*

a5   a4

Links between item pairs, co-occurring
frequently in *D*.

Target data *D*:   a1, a2, a4, a5 ... .
                    a4, a5, a3, ...
                    a1, a2, a6, ...
                    ... a4, a5 .
                    ... .

(2) Obtain islands

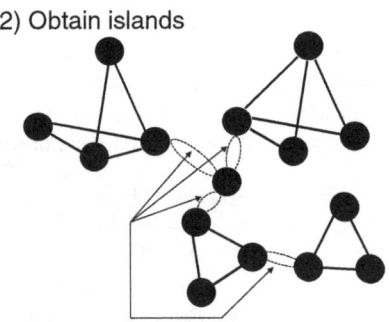

Separate into fundamental clusters,
i.e., islands.

**(3) Obtain bridges, on which chances
may exist**

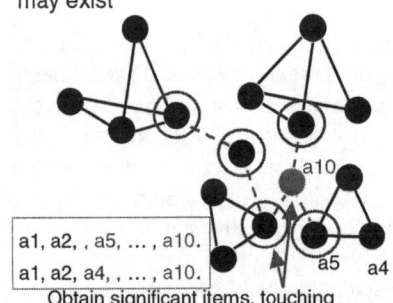

a10

a1, a2, , a5, ... , a10.
a1, a2, a4, , ... , a10.

a5   a4

Obtain significant items, touching
many node-cluster (green nodes)
bridges of frequent co-occurrence. If
the node is rarer than black nodes, it is
a new node put as a red one.

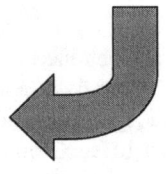

Fig. 3. The procedure of KeyGraph

market is losing customers, and Island (2) shows the context of a target company's
current state.   The bridge "restructuring" shows the company may introduce
restructuring, e.g. firing employees, for surviving in the bad state of the market.

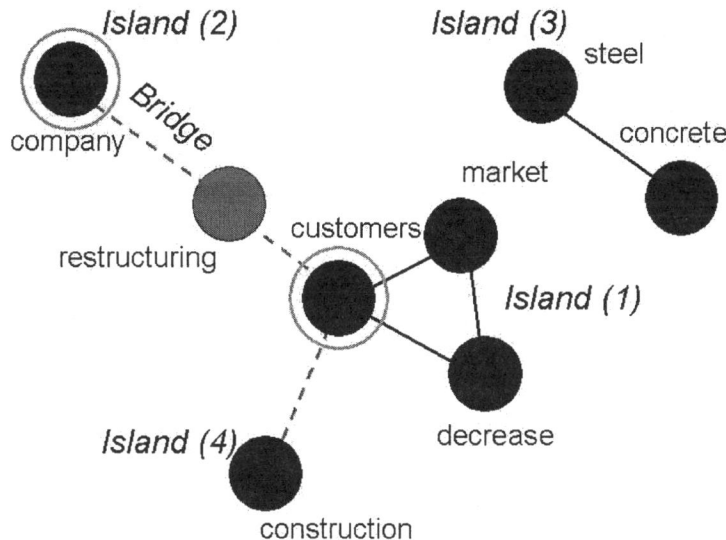

Fig. 4. KeyGraph for *D* in Eq.(2). Each island includs event-set {customers, decrease, market}, {steel, concrete}, {company}, etc. The double-circled node and the red ("restructuring") node show a frequent word and a rare word respectively, which forms hubs of bridges

"Restructuring" might be rare in the communication of the company staffs, but this expresses the concern of the employees about restructuring in the near future.

$D = $ "
    Speaker A : In the market of general construction, the customers decreased.
    Speaker B: Yes... My company build from concrete and steel, is in this bad trend.
    Speaker C: This state of the market induces a further decrease of customers. We may have to introduce restructuring, for satisfying customers.
    Speaker B: I agree. Then the company can reduce the production cost of concrete and steel. And, the price for the customers of construction...
    Speaker D: But, that may reduces power of the company. "   (3)

In the case of a document as in Eq.(3), periods are put at the end of each sentence, and the result shows the overview of the content. In the case of a sales (Position Of Sales: POS) data, periods are put in the end of each basket. *KeyGraph*, of the following steps, is applied to *D* ([Ohsawa 2003b] for details).

4.2 What Marketers Using KeyGraph Have Been Waiting for

In the case of marketing, users of KeyGraph sold out new products, and made real business profits [Usui and Ohsawa 2003]. The market researchers visualized the map of their market using KeyGraph, where nodes correspond to products and links corresponding to co-occurrences between products in the basket data of customers. In this map, market researchers found a valuable new scenario of the life-style of customers who may buy the product across a wide range in the market, whereas previous methods of data-based marketing helped in identifying focused segments of customers and the scenarios to be obtained have been restricted to ones of customers in each local segment. As a result, users successfully found promising new products, in a new desirable and realistic (i.e. possible to realize) scenario emerging from marketing discussions where scenarios of customers in various segments were exchanged. This realized hits of new products appearing in KeyGraph at bridges between islands, i.e. established customers.

However, a problem was that it is not efficient to follow the process of DH using KeyGraph solely, because the user cannot extract an interesting part of the data easily, when s/he has got a new concern with chances. For example, they may become concerned with a customer who buys product A or product B and also buys product C, but does not buy product D. Users has been waiting a tool to look into such customers matching with concern.

4.3 The Process Using TextDrop for Retrieving Data Relevant to User's Concern

TextDrop is a simple tool for Boolean-selection of the part of data corresponding to users' concern described in a Boolean formula, e.g,

$$concern = \text{``(product A | product B) \& product C \& !product D''}. \tag{3}$$

For this Boolean expression of user's concern, TextDrop obtains a focused data made of baskets including product A or product B, and product C, but not including product D. This becomes a revised input to KeyGraph, at the step where user acquires a new concern and seeks a corresponding data, in the DH process. TextDrop is convenient if the user can express his/her own concern in Boolean formula as in (3). The concern of user might be more ambiguous, especially in the beginning of the DH process. In such a case, the user is supposed to enter the formula "as much as" specifically representing one's own concern. Having KeyGraph, Text Drop, and the freedom to use these on necessity, the user can follow the procedure below to realize a speeding up of DH process.

[The DH process supported by KeyGraph and Text Drop]

Step 1) Extract a part of the object data with TextDrop, corresponding to user's concern with events or with the combination of events expressed in a Boolean formula.

Step 2) Apply KeyGraph to the data in Step 1) to visualize the map representing the relations between events, and attach causal arrows as much as possible with the help of expert of the domain.

Step 3) Co-manipulate KeyGraph with domain expert of the as follows:

    3-1) Move nodes and links to the positions in the 2D output of KeyGraph, or remove nodes and links obviously meaningless in the target domain.

    3-2) Write down comments about scenarios, proposed on KeyGraph.

Step 4) Read or visualize (with KeyGraph) the subject data, i.e., the participants' comments obtained in 3-2), and choose noteworthy and realistic scenarios.

Step 5) Execute or simulate (draw concrete images of the future) the scenarios obtained in Step 4), and, based on this experience, refine the statement of the new concern in concrete words. Go to Step 1).

5 Results for the Diagnosis Data of Hepatitis

5.1 The Hepatitis Data

The following shows the style of data obtained from blood-tests of hepatitis cases. Each event represents a pair, of a variable and its observed value. That is, an event put as "a_b" means a piece of information that the value of variable a was b. For example, T-CHO_high (T-CHO_low) means T-CHO (total cholesterol) was higher (lower) than a predetermined upper (lower) bound of normal range. lower than the lower threshold, if the liver is in a normal state. Note that the lower (higher) bound of each variable was set higher (lower) than values defined in hospitals, in order to be sensitive to moments the variables take unusual values. Each sentence in the data, i.e., a part delimited by '.' represents the sequence of blood-test results for the case of one patient. See Eq. (3).

Case1 = {event1, event2, ..., event m1}.

Case2 = {event 2, event 3, ..., event m2}.

Case3 = {event 1, event 5, ..., event m3}.   (3)

As in Eq.(3), we can regard one patient as a unit of co-occurrence of events. That is, there are various cases of patients and the sequence of one patient's events means his/her scenario of wandering in the map of symptoms.

For example, suppose we have the data as follows, where each event means a value of a certain attribute of blood, e.g. GPT_high means the state of a patient whose value of GPT exceeded its upper bound of normal range. Values of the upper and the lower bounds for each attribute are pre-set according to the standard values shared socially. Each period ('.') represents the end of one patient's case. If the doctor becomes interested in patients having experiences of both GPT_high and TP_low, then s/he eanters "GPT_high & TP_low" to TextDrop in Step 1), corresponding to the underlined items below. As a result, the italic sentences are extracted and given to KeyGraph in Step 2).

[An Example of Blood Test Data for KeyGraph]

GPT_high TP_low   TP_low   GPT_high TP_low   GPT_high   TP_low . (**input to KeyGraph**)

ALP_low F-ALB_low GOT_high GPT_high HBD_low LAP_high LDH_low TTT_high ZTT_high ALP_low CHE_high D-BIL_high F-ALB_low F-B_GL_low.

GOT_high GPT_high LAP_high LDH_low TTT_high ZTT_high F-ALB_low F-B_GL_low G_GL_high GOT_high GPT_high I-BIL_high LAP_high LDH_low

TTT_high ZTT_high GOT_high GPT_high LAP_high LDH_low TP_low TTT_high ZTT_high B-type CAH2A .

D-BIL_high   F-CHO_high   GOT_high   GPT_high   K_high   LAP_high   LDH_low TP_low. (**input to KeyGraph**)

UN_high T-BIL_high ALP_high D-BIL_high GPT_high I-BIL_high LDH_high T-BIL_high B-type CAH2B.

By applying KeyGraph to data as in Eq.(3), the following components are obtained:
- *Islands of events*: A group of events co-occurring frequently, i.e. occurring to many same patients. The doctor is expected to know what kind of patient each island corresponds to, in KeyGraph, corresponding to his/her experiences.
- *Bridges across islands*: A patient may switch from one island to another, in the progress of the disease or cure.

The data dealt with here was 771 cases, taken from 1981 through 2001. Fig. 5 is the KeyGraph obtained first, for all cases of hepatitis B in the data. The causal arrows in Step 2) of DH Process, which does not appear in the original KeyGraph of Ohsawa (2003), depict approximate causations. That is, "X -> Y" means event X precedes Y, in the scenario telling the causal explanation of event occurrences. Even if there are relations where the order of causality and time are opposite (i.e. if X is the cause of Y but was observed after Y due to the delay of appearance of symptom, or due to a high upper bound or a low lower bound of the variable in the blood test which makes it hard to detect symptom X), we should express a scenario including "X->Y."

If the direction from X to Y is apparent for an expert, we put the arrow in the graph. If this direction is not apparent, we compared the two results of KeyGraph, one for data retrieved for entry "X" with TextDrop, and the other for data retrieved for entry "Y." If the expert judges the former includes more causal events than the latter and if the latter includes more consequent events than the former, X is regarded as a preceding event of Y in a scenario. If the order of causality and the order of occurrence time are opposite.

For example, the upper threshold of ZTT may be set low and easy to exceed than that of G_GL, which makes ZTT_high appear before G_GL_high even though ZTT_high is a result of G_GL_high. In such a case, we compare the results of KeyGraph, one for data including G_GL_high and the other for data including ZTT_high. Then, if the latter includes F1, an early stage of fibrosis, and the former includes F2, a later stage, we can understand G_GL_high was really preceding ZTT_high. Let us call a KeyGraph with the arrows made in the way mentioned here, a *scenario map*.

5.2 The Results for Hepatitis B

The scenario map in Fig.5, for all data of hepatitis B extracted by TextDrop entering query "type-B," was shown to a hepatic surgeon and a hepatic physician at Step 2) above, in the first cycle. This scenario map was co-manipulated by a technical expert of KeyGraph and these hepatologists at Step 3), with talking about scenarios of hepatitis cases. Each cycle was executed similarly, presenting a scenario map for the data extracted according to the newest concern of the hepatologists. For example, in Fig.5, the dotted links show the bridges between events co-occurring more often than a given threshold of frequency. If there is a group of three or more events co-occurring often, they become visualized as an island in KeyGraph.

At Step 3-1), participants grouped the nodes in the circles as in Fig.5, after getting rid of unessential nodes from the figure and resolving redundancies by unifying such items as "jaundice" and "T-BIL_high" (high total bilirubin) meaning the same into one of the those items. We wrote down the comments of hepatologists at Step 3-2), about scenarios of hepatitis progress/cure, looking at the KeyGraph. Each '?' in Fig. 5 is the part about which the hepatologists could not understand clearly enough to express in a scenario, but said interesting. In figures hereafter, the dotted frames and their interpretations were drawn manually reflecting the hepatologists' comments. Yet, all obtained by this step were short parts of common-sense scenarios about hepatitis B, as follows:

(Scenario B1) Transition from/to types of hepatitis exist, e.g. CPH (chronic persistent hepatitis) to CAH (chronic aggressive hepatitis), CAH2A (non-severe CAH) to CAH2B (severe CAH), and so on.

(Scenario B2) Biliary blocks due to ALP_high , LAP_high, and G-GTP_high can lead to jaundice i.e., increase in the T-BIL. Considering D-BIL increases more keenly than I-BIL, this may be from the activation of lien, due to the critical illness of liver.

(Scenario B3) The increase in immunoglobulin (G_GL) leads to the increase in ZTT.

Then, at Step 4), we applied KeyGraph to the memo of comments obtained in Step 3-2). The comments lasted for two hours, so we can not put all the content here. The short part of is below, for example.

[Comments of a surgeon looking at Fig.5]

> *Hepatitis B is from virus, you know. This figure is a mixture of scenarios in various cases. For example, AFP/E is a marker of tumor. CHE increases faster than T-BIL and then decreases, as far as I have been finding. If cancer is found and grows, the value of CHE tents to decrease. However, it is rare that the cancer produces CHE.*
>
> *...*
>
> *Jaundice i.e., the increase in T-BIL, is a step after the hepatitis is critically progressed. Amylase from sialo and pancreas increase after operation of tumors and cancer, or in the complete fibrosis of liver.*
>
> *...*
>
> *PL is low in case liver is bad. In the complete fibrosis CRE decrease.*
>
> *...*
>
> *LDH increases and decreases quickly for fulminate hepatitis B..*
>
> *...*

From the KeyGraph applied to the comments above, we obtained Fig.6. According to Fig.6, their comments can be summarized as :

For treatment, diagnosis based on bad scenarios in which hepatitis grows is essential. However, this figure shows a complicated mixture of scenarios of various contexts, i.e. acute, fulminant, and other types of hepatitis. We can learn from this figure that a biliary trouble triggers the worsening of liver, to be observed with jaundice represented by high T-BIL (total bilirubin).

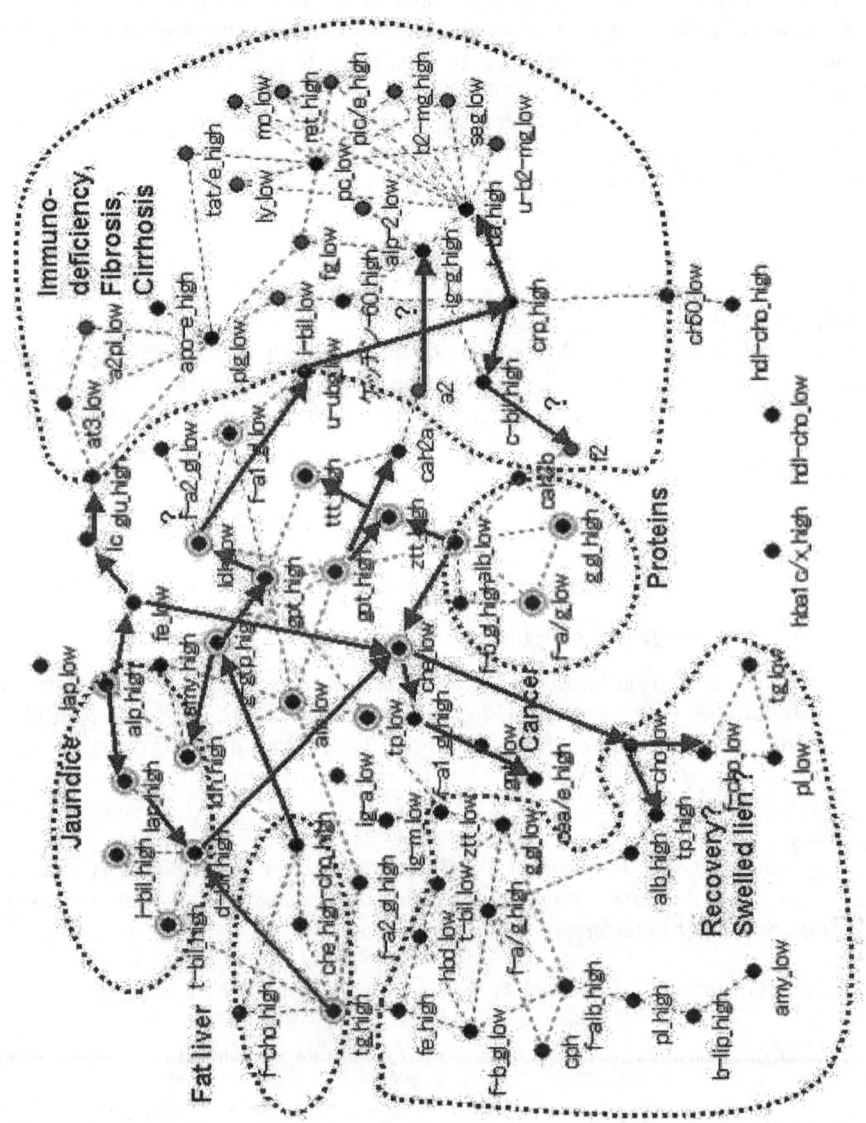

Fig. 5. The scenario map, at an intermediate step of manipulations for hepatitis B. In this case, all links are dotted lines because islands with multiple items were not obtained

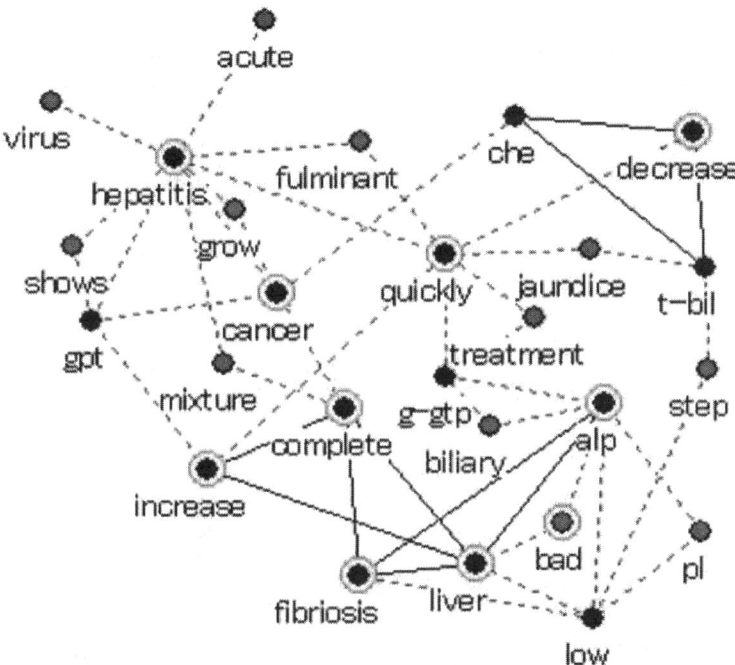

Fig. 6. KeyGraph to the memo of comments by hepatologists looking at Fig.4

An important new concern obtained here is that a scenario map illustrates a mixture of various scenarios, so it should be unfolded into scenarios of different contexts, say AH (acute hepatitis), CAH2B, CAH2A etc., by spotlighting events typical to each kind of scenario. For extracting acute hepatitis, we entered "AH" to Text Drop and obtained a scenario map for the extracted data as in Fig.7. This simple output corresponded precisely to the physician's and surgeon's experience plus knowledge. The increase in gamma globulin (IG_GL) is not found here, and this absence is a typical pattern for cases of acute hepatitis. Multiple areas of the cure of disease are found in this figure, and in fact AH is easier to be cured than other kinds of hepatitis.

Then we entered "CAH2B" to Tex Drop, and now obtained Fig.8. The early steps here are found to progress from symptoms common to most cases of hepatitis, e.g. GOT_high and GPT_high (corresponding to AST_high and ALT_high, in the current European and US terminologies), to heavier symptoms such as jaundice represented by I-BIL, D-BIL, and T-BIL. Items corresponding to the later steps in hepatitis, appearing in the lower left of the figure, is a complex mixture of cure and progress of hepatitis, difficult to understand even for hepatologists.

However, we acquired a new concern of hepatologists from the partial feature of Fig.8. That is, we could see that a quick sub-process from LDH_high to LDH_low (LDH: lactate dehydrogenase) can be a significant bridge from a light state of hepatitis to a critical state shown by the high value of T-BIL and the low value of CHE (choline esterase). A sudden increase in the value of LDH is sometimes observed in the introductory steps of fulminant hepatitis B, yet is ambiguous information for treatment because the high value of LDH is common to diseases of internal organs. However, according to the surgeon, the lower LDH is a rare event to appear in the two cases below:

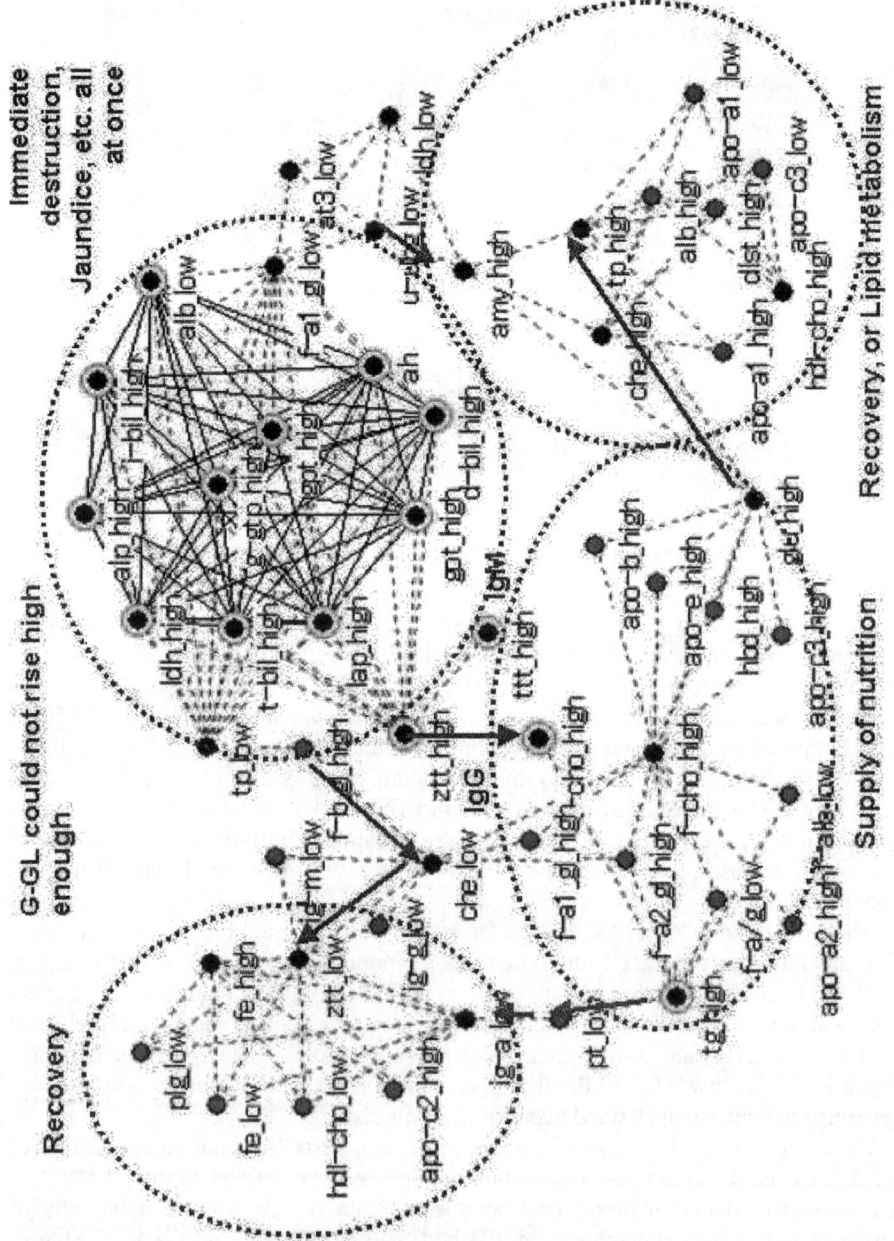

Fig. 7. The scenario map for acute hepatitis B

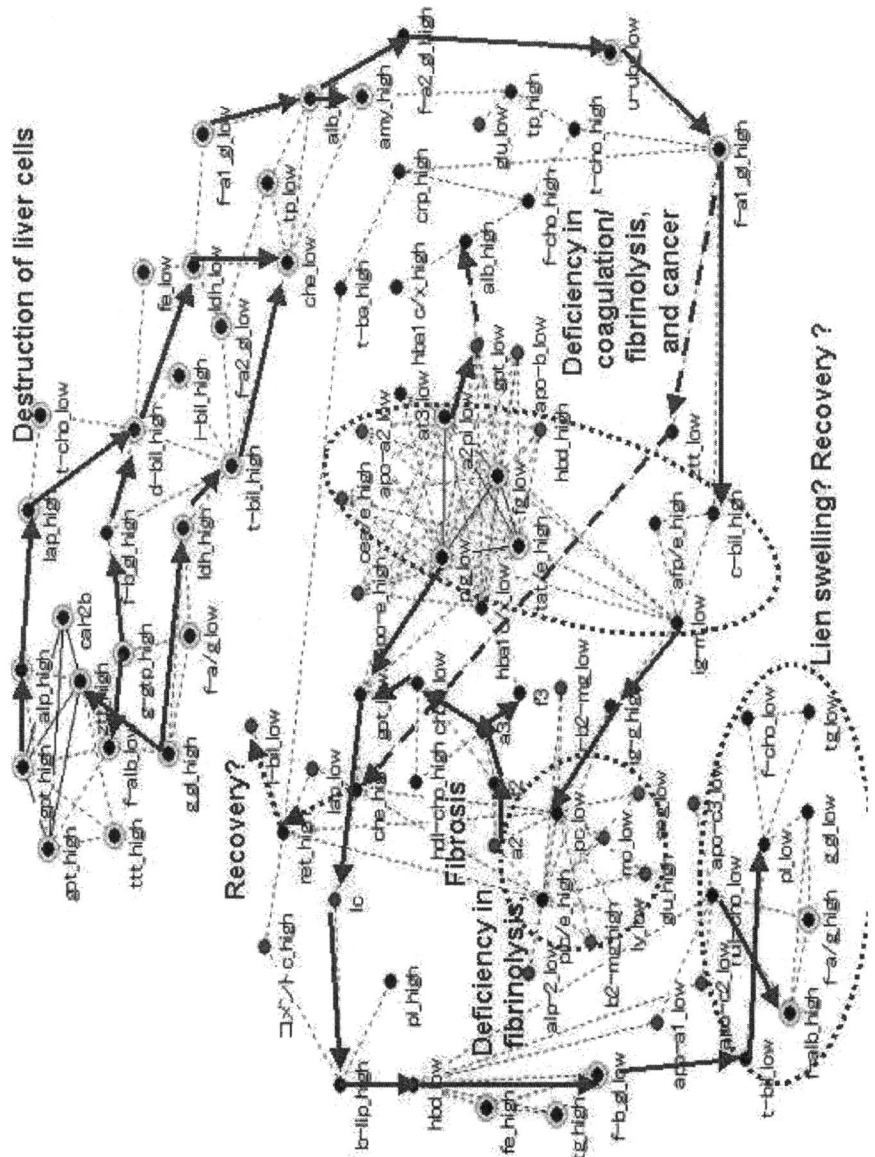

Fig. 8. The scenario map for severe chronic aggressive hepatitis, i.e. CAH2B

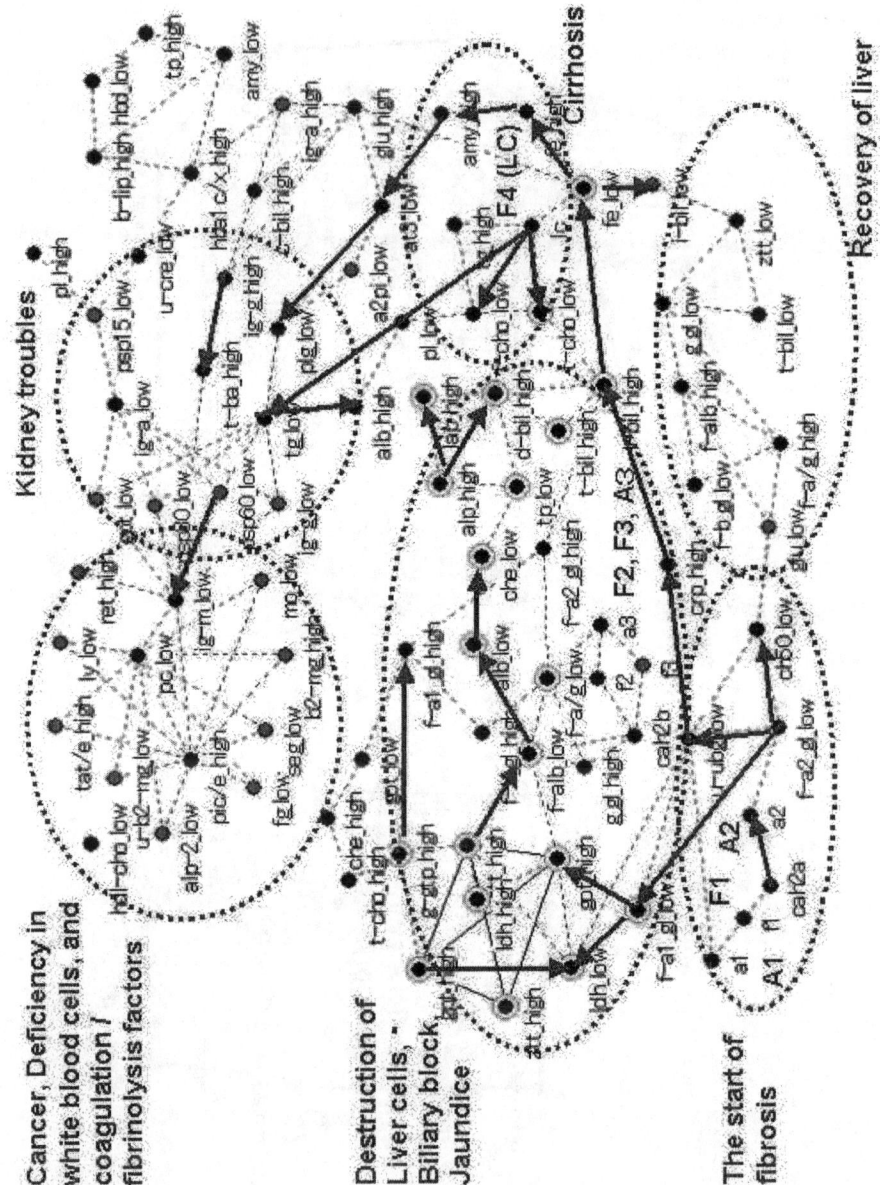

Fig. 9. The scenario map for hepatitis B, in the spotlight of F1, F2, F3, and F4 (LC)

1) A short time in the recovery from CAH and AH
2) The sudden progress (worsening) of fibrosis in fulminant hepatitis.

Especially, the surgeon's feeling in event 2) was his tacit experience reminded by KeyGraph obtained here, but has been published nowhere yet. These implications of Fig.8 drove us to separate the data to ones including progressive scenarios and others, so we extracted the stepwise progress of fibrosis denoted by F1, F2, F3, and F4 (or LC: liver cirrhosis). Fig. 9 is the scenario map for hepatitis B, corresponding to the spotlights of F1, F2, F3, and F4 (LC), i.e., for data extracted by TextDrop with entry "type-B & (F1 | F2 | F3 | F4 | LC)".

Fig.9 matched with hepatic experiences in the overall flow, as itemized below. These results are useful for understanding the state of a patient at a given time of observation in the transition process of symptoms, and for finding a suitable time and action to do in the treatment of hepatitis B.

- A chronic active hepatitis sometimes changes into a severe progressive hepatitis and then to cirrhosis or cancer, in the case of hepatitis B.
- The final states of critical cirrhosis co-occurs with kidney troubles, and get malignant tumors (cancer) with deficiencies of white blood cells.
- Recovery is possible from the earlier steps of fibrosis.
- The low LDH after the appearance of high LDH can be an early sign of fulminant hepatitis (see item 2) above).
- The low Fe level with cirrhosis can be a turning point to a better state of liver. In [Rubin et al 1995], it has been suggested here that iron reduction improves the response of chronic hepatitis B or C to interferon. Fig.9 does not show anything about the effect of interferon, but the appearance of FE_low, on the *only* bridge from cirrhosis to recovery, is very useful for finding the optimal timing to treat a patient of hepatitis B, and is relevant to Rubin's result in this sense.

5.3   The Results for Hepatitis C

For the cases of hepatitis C, as in Fig.10, we also found a mixture of scenarios, e.g.,
(Scenario C1) Transition from CPH to CAH
(Scenario C2) Transition to critical stages like cancer, jaundice, etc
These common-sense scenarios are similar to the scenarios in the cases of hepatitis B, but we also find "interferon" and a region of cure at the top (in the dotted ellipse) in Fig.10. GOT and GPT (i.e. AST and ALT, respectively) can be low both after the fatal progress of heavy hepatitis and when the disease is cured. The latter case is rare because GOT and GPT are expected to take "normal" value, i.e., between the lower and the upper threshold, rather than being "low" i.e. lower than the lower threshold of normal state.

However, due to the setting of lower bound of variables such as GOT and GPT to a high value, here we can find moments these variables take "low" values when the case changed to a normal states. As well, given the low value of ZTT in this region, we can judge the case is in the process to cure.

This suggested a new concern that the data with "interferon & ZTT_low" (i.e. interferon has been used, and the value of ZTT recovered) may clarify the role of interferon, i.e., how the process of curing hepatitis goes with giving interferon to the patient. Fig. 11 was obtained, for the data corresponding to this concern and extracted using TextDrop. In Fig.11, we find features as follows:

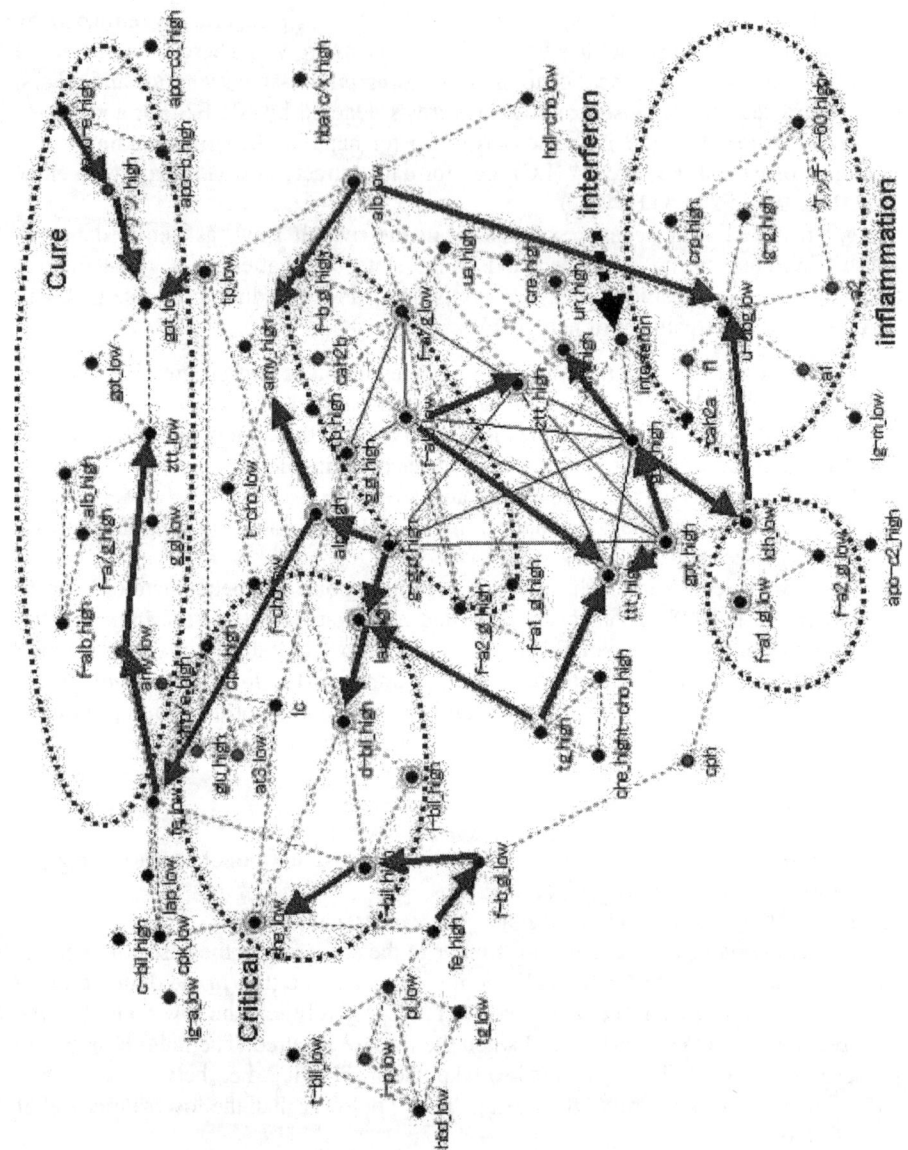

Fig. 10. The scenario map for all the cases of hepatitis C

- The values of GPT and GOT are lessened with the treatment using interferon, and then ZTT decreased.
- Both scenarios of cure and worsening progress are found, following the decrease in ZTT. In the worse scenarios, typical bad symptoms such as jaundice and low values of CHE and ALB (albumin) appear as a set. In the better, the recovery of various factors such as blood platelets (PL_high) are obvious.
- In the worse (former) scenario, blood components such as PL are lessened.

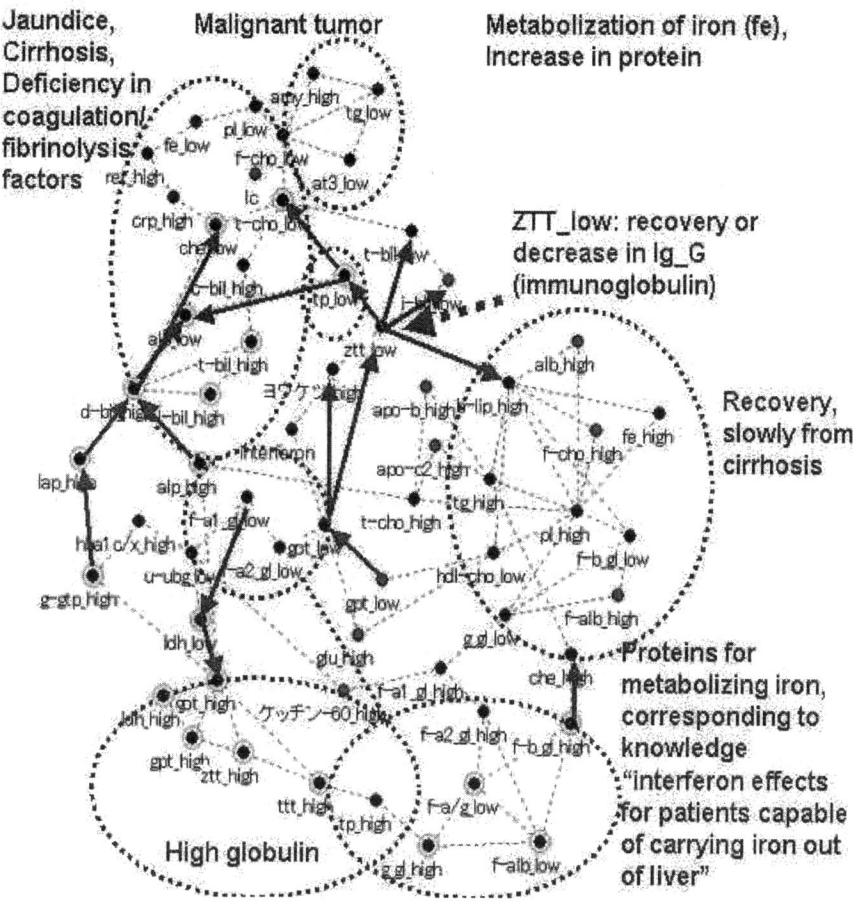

Fig. 11. Scenario map for cases with interferon and low values of ZTT

In the better (latter) scenario, changes in the quantity of proteins are remarkable. Among these, F-A2_GL (a2 globulin, mostly composed of haptoglobin, which prevents the critical decrease in iron by being coupled with hemoglobin before hemoglobin gets destroyed to make isolated iron) and F-B_GL (beta globulin, composed mostly of transferrin which carries iron for reusing it to make new hemoglobin) are relevant to the metabolism of iron (FE).

The realities and the significance of these scenarios were supported by the physician and the surgeon. To summarize those scenarios briefly, the effect of interferon works for cure only if the recycling mechanism of iron is active. In fact, the relevance of hepatitis and iron has been a rising concern of hepatologists working on hepatitis C, since Hayashi et al (1994) verified the effect of iron reduction in curing hepatitis C.

Supposing that the change in F-A2_GL is relevant to the role of interferon in curing hepatitis C, we finally obtained the scenario map as in Fig.12 showing that cases treated with interferon and changed in the value of F-A2_GL (i.e., taken by Text Drop for the entry "F-A2_GL_low & F-A2_GL_high & interferon & type-C") had a significant turning point to recovery, with the increase in the value of TP (total protein). Further more, the event TP_high is linked with F-B_GL_high, the iron-carrier protein called transferring mentioned above. In the dot-framed region of Fig.12, the decrease in GOT and GPT followed by low ZTT matches with the result in Tsumoto et al (2003). Also the antibody HCV-AB of HCV (virus of hepatitis C) decreased in the process to cure.

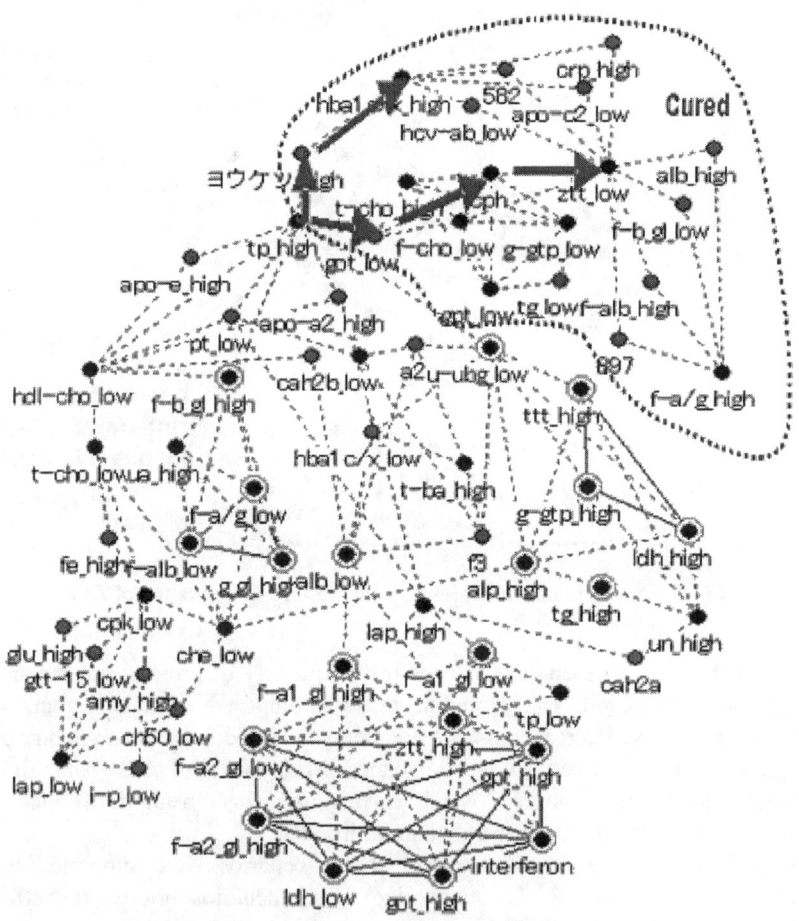

Fig. 12. Scenario map for cases with F-A2_GL_high & F_A2_GL_low, and interferon. The effect of interferon is clarified at the top of the map

6 Discussion: Subjective but Trustworthy

We obtained some qualitative new findings. For example, the low value as well as the high value of LDH is relevant to the turning point of fulminant hepatitis B, in shifting to critical stages. This means a doctor must not be relieved with finding that the value of LDH decreased, only because the opposite symptom i.e. the increase in LDH means a sign of hepatitis progress.

And, the effect of interferon is relevant to the change in the quantity of protein, especially ones relevant to iron metabolism (e.g. F-A2_GL and F-B_GL). The effect of interferon, as a result, appears to begin with the recovery of TP. These tendencies are apparent from both Fig.11 and Fig.12, but it is still an open problem if interferon is affected from such proteins as globulins or iron metabolism and interferon are two co-operating factors of cure. All in all, "reasonable, and sometimes novel and useful" scenarios of the hepatitis were obtained according to the surgeon and the physician.

Although not covered here, we also found other scenarios to approach significant situations. For example, the increase in AMY (amylase) in Fig.5, Fig.8, Fig.9, and Fig.10, can be relevant to surgical operations or liver cancers. The relevance of amylase corresponds to Miyagawa et al (1996), and its relevance to cancer has been pointed out in a number of references such as Chougle (1992) and also in commercial web sources such as Ruben (2003).

These are the effects of double helix (DH), the concern-focusing process of user in the interaction with the target data. Apparently, the subjective bias of hepatologists' concern influenced the results to be obtained in this manner, and this subjectivity sometimes becomes the reason why scientists discount the value of results obtained by DH. However, the results are trustworthy because they just show the summary of objective facts selected on the subjective focus of hepatologists' concerns.

As a positive face of this combination of subjectivity and objectivity, we discovered a broad range of knowledge useful in real-decisions, expressed in the form of scenarios. We say this, because subjectivity has the effect of choosing interesting part of the wide objective environment, and this subjective feeling of interestingness comes from the desire for useful knowledge.

7 Conclusions

Scenario emergence, a new side of chance discovery, is useful for decisions in the real world where events occur dynamically and one is required to make a decision promptly at the time a chance, i.e. a significant event occurring. In this paper we showed an application of scenario emergence with discovering triggering events of essential scenarios, in the domain of hepatitis progress and treatment. Realistic and novel scenarios were obtained according to experts of the target domain.

In the method presented here, the widening of user's view was aided by the projection of users' personal experiences to the objective scenario map representing a mixture of contexts in the wide real-world. The narrowing, i.e. data-choosing, was aided by user's focused concern and TextDrop. Like a human wandering in an unknown island, a doctor wondering which way the current patient can go will be helped by watching the overall scenario map corresponding to the objective facts in the environment and a focused range of the map corresponding to his temporary concern with the patient. This effect is the stronger, the newer the symptom is and the more ambiguous the future scenario is. We are currently developing tools to aid the process of double helix more efficiently by combining the functions of KeyGraph and TextDrop, and further integrating with visual interfaces enabling to feedback user's new concerns to news cycles of the spiral process.

Acknowledgment

The study has been conducted in the Scientific Research on Priority Area "Active Mining." We appreciate Chiba University Hospital for serving us with the priceless data, under the convenient contract of its use for research.

References

Chance Discovery Consortium 2004, http://www.chancediscovery.com

Chougle A; Hussain S; Singh PP; Shrimali R., 1992, Estimation of serum amylase levels in patients of cancer head and neck and cervix treated by radiotherapy, Journal of Clinical Radiotherapy and Oncology. 1992 Sept; 7(2): 24-26

Gaver W.W., Beaver J., and Benford S., 2003, Ambiguity as a Resource for Design, in Proceedings of Computer Human Interactions

Hayashi, H., T. Takikawa, N. Nishimura, M. Yano, T. Isomura, and N. Sakamoto. 1994. Improvement of serum aminotransferase levels after phlebotomy in patients with chronic active hepatitis C and excess hepatic iron, American Journal of Gastroenterol. 89: 986-988

Miyagawa S, Makuuchi M, Kawasaki S, Kakazu T, Hayashi K, and Kasai H., 1996, Serum Amylase elevation following hepatic resection in patients with chronic liver disease., Am. J. Surg. 1996 Feb;171(2):235-238

Miyagawa S, Makuuchi M, Kawasaki S, and Kakazu T., 1994, Changes in serum amylase level following hepatic resection in chronic liver disease, Arch Surg. 1994 Jun;129(6):634-638

Ohsawa Y and McBurney P. eds, 2003, Chance Discovery, Springer Verlag

Ohsawa Y., 2003a, Modeling the Process of Chance Discovery, Ohsawa, Y. and McBurney eds, Chance Discovery, Springer Verlag pp.2—15

Ohsawa Y, 2003b, KeyGraph: Visualized Structure Among Event Clusters, in Ohsawa Y and McBurney P. eds, 2003, Chance Discovery, Springer Verlag: 262-275

Okazaki N, 2003, Naoaki Okazaki and Yukio Ohsawa, "Polaris: An Integrated Data Miner for Chance Discovery" In Proceedings of The Third International Workshop on Chance Discovery and Its Management, Crete, Greece.

Rubin RB, Barton AL, Banner BF, Bonkovsky HL., 1995, Iron and chronic viral hepatitis: emerging evidence for an important interaction. in Digestive Diseases

Ruben D., 2003, Understanding Blood Work: The Biochemical Profile, http://petplace.netscape.com/articles/artShow.asp?artID=3436

The Danish Board of Technology, 2003, European Participatory Technology Assessment: Participatory Methods in Technology Assessment and Technology Decision-Making,. http://www.tekno.dk/europta

Tsumoto S., Takabayashi K., Nagira N., adn Hirano S., 2003, Trend-evaluating Multiscale Analysis of the Hepatitis Dataset, Annual Report of Active Mining, Scientific Research on Priority Areas, 191-198

Usui M., and Ohsawa Y., 2003, Chance Discovery in Textile Market by Group Meeting with Touchable Key Graph, On-line Proceedings of Social Intelligence Design International Concerence,. Published at:
http://www.rhul.ac.uk/Management/News-and-Events/conferences/SID2003/tracks.html

Integrated Mining for Cancer Incidence Factors from Healthcare Data

Xiaolong Zhang[1] and Tetsuo Narita[2]

[1]School of Computer Science and Technology,
Wuhan University of Science and Technology, Wuhan 430081, China
xiaolong.zhang@mail.wust.edu.cn
[2] ISV Solutions, IBM-Japan Application Solution Co., Ltd.
1-14 Nissin-cho, Kawasaki-ku, Kanagawa 210-8550, Japan
narita4@jp.ibm.com

Abstract. This paper describes how data mining is being used to identify primary factors of cancer incidences and living habits of cancer patients from a set of health and living habit questionnaires. Decision tree,
radial basis function and back propagation neural network have been
employed in this case study. Decision tree classification uncovers the primary factors of cancer patients from rules. Radial basis function method
has advantages in comparing the living habits between a group of cancer
patients and a group of healthy people. Back propagation neural network
contributes to elicit the important factors of cancer incidences. This case
study provides a useful data mining template for characteristics identification in healthcare and other areas.

Keywords: Knowledge acquisition, Data mining, Model sensitivity analysis, Healthcare, Cancer control and prevention.

1 Introduction

With the development of data mining approaches and techniques, the applications of data mining can be found in many organizations, such as banking,
insurance, industries, and government. Large volumes of data are produced in
every social organization, which can be from scientific research or business. For
example, the human genome data is being created and collected at a tremendous
rate, so the maximization of the value from this complex data is very necessary.
Since the ever increasing data becomes more and more difficult to be analyzed
with traditional data analysis methods, data mining has earned an impressive
reputation in data analysis and knowledge acquisition. Recently data mining
methods have been applied to many areas including banking, finance, insurance,
retail, healthcare and pharmaceutical industries as well as gene analysis[1, 2].

Data mining methods [3, 4, 5] are used to extract valid, previously unknown,
and ultimately comprehensible information from large data sources. The extracted information can be used to form a prediction or classification model,

S. Tsumoto et al. (Eds.): AM 2003, LNAI 3430, pp. 336–347, 2005.

identifying relations within database records. Data mining consists of a number of operations each of which is supported by a variety of techniques such as rule induction, neural networks, conceptual clustering, association discovery, etc. Usually, it is necessary to apply several mining methods to a data set to identify discovered rules and patterns with each other. Data mining methods allow us to apply multi-methods to broadly and deeply discover knowledge from data sets. For example, there is a special issue about the comparison and evaluation of KDD methods with common medical databases [6], where researchers employed several mining algorithms to discover rules from common medical databases.

This paper presents a mining process with a set of health and living habit questionnaire data. The task is to discover the primary factors and living habits of cancer patients via questionnaires. Discovered knowledge is helpful for cancer control and cancer incidence prevention. Several mining methods have been used in the mining process. Decision tree, radial basis function (RBF) and back propagation neural network (BPN) are included. Decision tree method helps to generate important rules hidden behind the data, and facilitates useful rule interpretation. However, when the severity distribution of the objective variable (with its class values) exists, decision tree method is not effective, being highly skewed with generating a long thick tail tree (also pointed out by Epte et al. [7]). Moreover, decision tree rules do not give the information that can be used to compare living habits between a group of healthy people and a group of cancer patients. RBF, with its "divide and conquer" ability, performs well in predictions even though it is in presence of severity distribution and noisy data. With RBF, we can obtain patterns of cancer patients and non-cancer people as well, which is useful for the living habit comparison. On the other hand, back propagation neural network can be used for both prediction and classification. In this study, BPN is used as neural classification and sensitivity analysis [8]. Both predication (for a numerical variable) and classification (for a categorical variable) of BPN have been applied in many areas (e.g., in genome analysis [9, 10]).

This paper describes a multi-strategy data mining application. For example, with BPN's sensitivity analysis, irrelevant and redundant variables are removed, which leads to generate a decision tree in a more understandable way. By means of the combined mining methods, rules, patterns and critical factors can be effectively discovered. Of course, mining with the questionnaire data should carefully investigate the data contents in the data processing, since such a data set contains not only noise but also missing values.

In the rest of this paper, there is description of decision tree classification, RBF and BPN algorithms. There is description about how to build data marts, how to use the algorithms to perform a serial of effective mining processes. Finally, there is the related work and conclusion.

2   Data Mining Approach

Generally, there may be several methods available to a mining problem. Considering the number of variables and records, as well as the quality of training data, applying several mining methods on the given mining data is recommended. Since one mining algorithm may outperform another, more useful rules and patterns can be further revealed.

2.1   Classification Method

Classification method is very important for data mining, which has been extensively used in many data mining applications. It analyzes the input data and generate models to describe the *class* using the attributes in the input data. The input data for classification consists of multiple attributes. Among these attributes, there should be a label tagged with *class*. Classification is usually performed through decision tree classifiers. A decision-tree classifier creates a decision-tree model with tree-building phase and tree-pruning phase (e.g., CART [11], C4.5 [12] and SPRINT [13]).

In the tree-building phase, a decision tree is grown by repeatedly partitioning the training data based on values of a selected attribute. Therefore the training set is split into two or more partitions according to the selected attribute. The tree-building process is repeated recursively until a stop criterion is met. Such a stop criterion may be all the examples in each partition has its class label or the depth of tree reaches a given value or other else.

After the tree-building phase, the tree-pruning phase is used to prune the generated tree with test data. Since the tree is built with training data, it may grow to be one that fits the noisy training data. Pruning tree phase removes the overfitting branches of the tree given the estimated error rate.

Decision tree has been used to build predictive models and discover understandable rules. In this paper, decision tree is applied to discover rules.

2.2   Radial Basis Function Method

Radial basis function algorithm is used to learn from examples, usually used for prediction. RBF can be viewed as a feedforward neural network with only one hidden layer. The outputs from the hidden layer are not simply the product of the input data and a weight. All the input data to each neuron in the hidden layer are treated as a measure of distance which can be viewed as how far the data are from a center. The center is the position of the neuron in a spatial system. The transfer functions of the nodes are used to measure the influence that neurons have at the center. These transfer functions are usually radial spline, Guassian or power functions. For example, 2-dimension Gaussian radial basis function centered in t can be written as:

$$G(\|x - t\|^2) = e^{\|x-t\|^2} = e^{(x-t_x)^2}e^{(y-t_y)^2}. \tag{1}$$

This function can be easily extended for dimensions higher than 2 (see [14]).

As a regularization network, RBF is equivalent to generalized splines. The architecture of backpropagation neural network consists of multilayer networks where one hidden layer and a set of adjustable parameters are configured. Their Boolean version divides the input space into hyperspheres, each corresponding to a center. This center, also call it a radial unit, is active if the input vector is within a certain radius of its center and is otherwise inactive. With an arbitrary number of units, each network can approximate the other, since each can approximate continuous functions on a limited interval.

This property, we call it "divide and conquer", can be used to identify the primary factors of the related cancer patients within the questionnaires. With the "divide and conquer", RBF is able to deal with training data, of which the distribution of the training data is extremely severity.

RBF is also effect on solving the problem in which the training data includes noise. Because the transfer function can be viewed as a linear combination of nonlinear basis functions which effectively change the weights of neurons in the hidden layer. In addition, the RBF allows its model to be generated in an efficient way.

2.3 Back Propagation Neural Network

BPN can be used for both neural prediction and neural classification. BPN consists of one layer of input nodes, one layer of output nodes, and one or more hidden layers between the input and output layers. The input data (called vectors) x_i, each multiplied by a weight w_i and adjusted with a threshold θ, is mapped into the set of two binary values $R^n \rightarrow \{0,1\}$. The threshold function is usually a sigmoid function

$$f(sum) = \frac{1}{1 + e^{-sum}} \tag{2}$$

where the sum is the weighted sum of the signals at the unit input. The unit outputs a real value between 0 and 1. For $sum = 0$, the output is 0.5; for large negative values of sum, the output converges to 0; and for large positive value sum, the output converges to 1. The weight adjustment procedure in backpropagation learning is explained as: (1) Determine the layers and the units in each layer of a neural net; (2) Set up initial weights $w1_{ij}$ and $w2_{ij}$; (3) Input a input vector to the input layer; (4) Propagate the input value from the input layer to the hidden layer, where the output value of the jth unit is calculated by the function $h_j = \frac{1}{1 + e^{-\sum_i (w1_{ij} \cdot x_i)}}$. The value is propagated to the output layer, and the output value of the jth unit in this layer is defined by the function: $o_j = \frac{1}{1 + e^{-\sum_i (w2_{ij} \cdot h_i)}}$; (5) Compare the outputs o_j with the given classification y_j, calculate the correction error $\delta 2_j = o_j(1-o_j)(y_j - o_j)$, and adjust the weight $w2_{ij}$ with the function: $w2_{ij}(t+1) = w2_{ij}(t) + \delta 2_j \cdot h_j \cdot \eta$, where $w2_{ij}(t)$ are the respective weights at time t, and η is a constant ($\eta \in (0,1)$); (6) Calculate the correction error for the hidden layer by means of the formula $\delta 1_j = h_j(1-h_j)\sum_i \delta 2_i \cdot w2_{ij}$, and adjust the weights $w1_{ij}(t)$ by: $w1_{ij}(t+1) = w1_{ij}(t) + \delta 1_j \cdot x_j \cdot \eta$; (7) Return to step 3, and repeat the process.

The weight adjustment is also an error adjustment and propagation process, where the errors (in the form of weights) are feedback to the hidden units. These errors are normalized per unit fields in order to have a sum of all as 100%. This process is often considered as a sensitivity analysis process which shows the input field (variable) contributions to the classification for a *class label*. Therefore, omitting the variables that do not contribute will improve the training time and those variables are not included in the classification run. As we know, real data sets often include many irrelevant or redundant input fields. By examining the weight matrix of the trained neural network itself, the significance of inputs can be determined. A comparison is made by sensitivity analysis, where the sensitivity of outputs to input perturbation is used as a measure of the significance of inputs. Practically, in the decision tree classification, by making use of sensitivity analysis and removing the lowest contributed variables, understandable and clear decision trees are easily generated.

3   Application Template Overview

Our task for this study is to uncover the primary factors of cancer incidences and living habits of cancer patients, and further compare these factors and habits with healthy or non-cancer people.

The mining sources are from an investigation organization which collected data via questionnaires. The questionnaire data set consists of 250 attributes and is full of 47,000 records. These attributes are from 14 categories. These categories mainly include: personal information (the date of birth, living area, etc.); records of one's illnesses (apoplexy, high blood pressure, myocardial infarction, tuberculosis, cancer, etc.); the health statute of one's families (parents, brothers and sisters); the health status of one in the recent one year (bowels movement, sleeping, etc.); one's drinking activity (what kind of liquor, how often, how much, etc.); one's smoking records (when begun, how many cigarettes a day, etc.); one's eating habit (regular meal time, what kind of food, what kind of meat and fish, etc.); occupation (teacher, doctor, company staff, etc.), and so on. A questionnaire record may contain missing values of some attributes. For example, a female-oriented question is not answered by males. In other cases, missing data is due to lack of responses. There are several ways to deal with missing-data (see [15]). One effective way is EM (Expectation and Maximization) [16]. This method has been implemented in some analytical tool, such as SPSS. We use SPSS to deal with the missing values before mining operations.

Mining data marts are generated from data sources and used for mining. Several data marts are created, which are used for decision tree, RBF and BPN mining. In fact, decision tree could not directly applied to the whole dataset. The decision tree mining operation is applied to the output from clustering operation, where the distribution for a selected objective variable is almost balanced. For example, to classify the cancer/non-cancer (with value 1/0) people, the variable "cancer flag" is selected as the class variable. For efficiently generating decision trees, removing irrelevant or redundant processes are performed by first applying the BPN sensitivity analysis. In addition, the data marts and mining processes are also repeated with BPN operation, for acquiring a list of significant cancer incidence factors.

When building a data mart for RBF analysis, the analysis object is to predict the probability of the cancer accident. The variable "cancer flag" is mapping to a new variable "probV26" with value of [0,1]. This new variable is used as a dependence variable, whose values (e.g., probability) will be predicted using the other variables (independence variables).

4   Mining Process and Mining Result

IBM INTELLIGENT MINER FOR DATA (IM4D) [17] is used as the mining tool, since the combined mining processes can be performed with IM4D, which includes decision tree, RBF and BPN algorithms as well as clustering. In this application, we clean the data source with SPSS, build data marts for mining, and perform mining operations to acquire useful cancer incidence factors and related rules.

The mining process includes building data marts, creating mining bases, mining with decision trees, RBF and BPN. As we know, not all the questionnaire objects are cancer patients. In fact, only 561 persons were or are cancer patients in the given records. The missing values are allocated as *unknown* (more detail processes see [18]).

4.1   Mining with Decision Tree

Decision tree is performed based on the output data from a clustering model, where the class variable distribution can be well balanced. With carefully selected data, objective-oriented trees are generated. For example, a decision tree can be created for describing the male cancer patients or the female ones. In order to further investigate the cancer factors, decision trees are generated with selected variables from personal information, from illness category, health statute of family category, from drinking, smoking and eating activity, respectively.

The results of the decision tree mining are useful in understanding primary factors of cancer incidences. For instance, with respect to male cancer patients, there are tree rules generated like: (a) the cancer patients were alcohol drinkers, there were smokers in their family, and their smoking period was more than 9 years; (b) They were accepted surgery on the abdomen, 62 age over, suffering from apoplexy, experiencing blood transfusion; (c) They have no work now but are living with stresses, they ever had been teachers, or doing management work in company or government. From another decision tree, for both male and female cancer patients, there is a rule: among 122 cancer patients, 42 of them accepted surgery on the abdomen, contracted gallstone/gallbladder inflammation, and suffered from diabetes. Another rule denotes: among 372 cancer patients, 100 of female cancer patients' menses were stopped by surgery, their initial marriage ages were less than 26, and suffering from both constipation and diabetes.

4.2   Mining with RBF

As shown above, these rules from decision trees are useful for understanding the primary factors of cancers. But there is no information for comparison of cancer patients with non-cancer people.

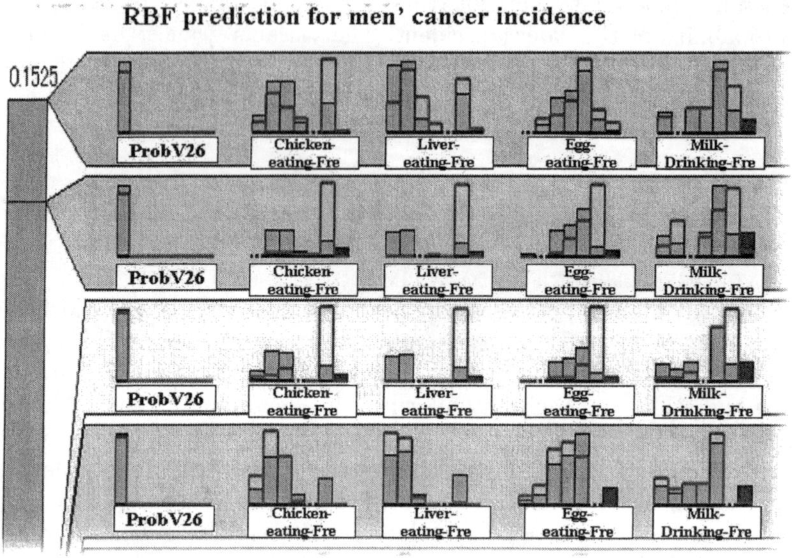

RBF prediction for men' cancer incidence

Fig. 1. The "divide and conquer" of RBF method

With RBF, several predictive models have been generated. First, one predictive model is generated with the dependence variable "probV26" (mentioned before) and all independence variables. More predictive models have been built for male and female cancer patients. Second, in order to further discover the different living habits between the cancer patient group and the non-cancer people, the independent variables of predictive models are selected from only personal information and illness information, from only health statute of families, and from only drinking activity and smoking information respectively. With these data marts, related RBF predictive models are built respectively.

Fig. 1 shows the RBF predictive models which predict probability of cancer incidences, where RBF automatically builds small, local predictive models for different regions of data space. This "divide and conquer" strategy appears well for prediction and factor identifier. This chart indicates eating habits in terms of food-eating frequency. The segment with low probability of cancer incidence segment (at bottom) shows the chicken-eating frequency (the variable located in the second from the left) is higher than that of the segment (at top) with higher probability of cancer incidences. The detailed explanation of distribution is described in Fig. 2, where for a numerical variable, the distributions in the population and in the current segment are indicated. Moreover, the percentage of each distribution can be given if necessary. With RBF predictive ability, the characteristic of every segment can be identified. By means of RBF, the living habits of cancer patients and non-cancer or healthy people are discovered.

Fig. 2 shows an example of distributions of a variable. The histogram chart is for a numerical variable in a segment of RBF models, where the distributions of population and current segment of the variable are described, respectively.

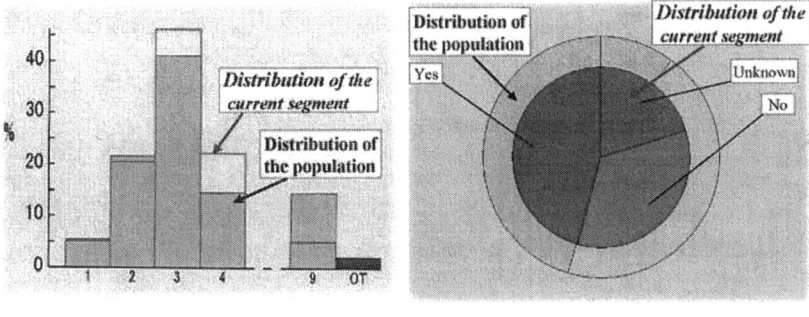

Histogram chart   Pie chart

Fig. 2. Variable distribution in the population and current segment in RBF

Table 1. Comparison among female patients and non-cancer women in suffered illness

Illness	Female cancer patients	non-cancer women
Kidney	6.5%	3.5%
Womb illness	24.6%	14.2%
Blood transfusion	12.7%	7.1%
Diabetes	3.5%	1.2%

For instance, the percentage of partition 4 in the current segment is higher than that of the population (the entire data set). The pie chart is for a categorical variable. The outside ring of the pie chart shows the distribution for the variable over the population. The inside ring shows the distribution for this variable in the current segment. In the pie chart of Fig. 2, the distribution of *No* in the current segment is less than that of the population.

The results of RBF mining are interesting. The results provide comparable information among cancer patients and non-cancer people in suffered illness. Some results from RBF are described in Table 1. In this table, there is a prediction case of cancer incidence of women, 6.5% of a high cancer incidence group has kidney illness, while the percentage for non-cancer people is 3.5%. For womb illness and blood transfusion, the figures for female cancer patients are higher than those of non-cancer women.

The eating habits between the group of female cancer incidences and the group of non-cancer women are compared. The results of RBF (described in Fig. 3) show the characteristics in the segment with highest cancer incidence probability (with 0.15 probability and segment ID 98) and that of lowest probability as well (with 0 probability and segment ID 57). By picking up the variables with obviously different distributions in these two segments, comparable results are obtained. Within eating habits, by comparing regular breakfast habit category, 87% of female cancer patients have regular breakfast habit, which is lower than 93.3% of non-cancer women. With meat-eating and chicken-eating 3-4 times per-week, the percentage figures are 12% and 8% of female cancer patients, 27.7% and

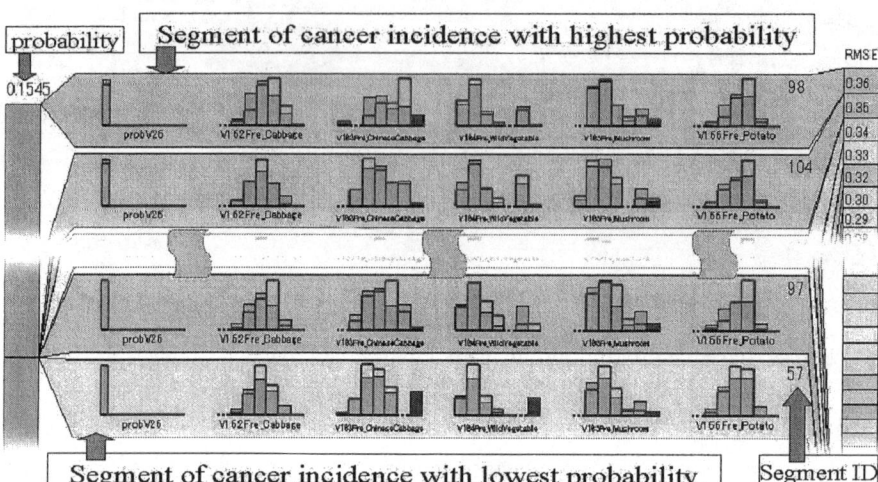

Fig. 3. Comparison of eating habits: female cancer incidences and non-cancer women

18% of non-cancer women, respectively. With one's personal life, 54.5% of female cancer patients are living in a state of stress, far higher than 15% the percentage of non-cancer women. For judgment on matters, 36% of female cancer patients gives out their judgments very quickly. This percentage is also higher than 13%, the percentage figure of non-cancer women.

4.3   Mining with Back Propagation Neural Network

This section describes the mining results with back propagation neural network. When the back propagation method is used for classification, it is also used as sensitivity analysis simultaneously. With sensitivity analysis, the important factors of cancer incidences can be acquired. In this case study, sensitivity analysis has been performed with the data marts built for in decision tree classification. With BPN, mining run on these data sets tries to discover the relationship between the input variables and the class variable *cancer flag*.

Table 2 shows those variables with most contributions to the cancer incidence, which is the BPN mining results with a data mart where both male and female cancer patients' records are included. The important factors are those with high sensitivity. *blood transfusion* (sensitivity 1.4) and *job-category* (sensitivity 1.3) are important factors. For a female patient, *menstruation* (if her menstruation is regular or not) and *lactation type* (which type of lactation was applied for her children) are indicated as important factors. It also shows that *smoking* and *alcohol* are tightly related to cancer incidences, which is similar to the results acquired in the decision tree rules. The fact that if one's biological father/mother

Table 2. Most important factors of cancer incidences

Attribute related cancer	Sensitivity
blood transfusion	1.4
job-category (now)	1.3
menstruation	1.2
surgery experience or not	1.2
volume of meal	1
the longest occupation	0.8
lactation type (of woman)	0.8
site of uterine cancer check	0.8
site of breast cancer check	0.8
somking	0.7
site of stomach cancer check	0.7
biological mother suffered cancer	0.7
volume of alcolhol	0.6
hot favorance	0.6
rich oil favorance	0.6
biological father suffered cancer	0.6

has suffered cancer is also important. The factor *hot favorance* and *rich oil favorance* are also noticed.

As described above, decision tree classification, RBF and BPN mining processes generate useful rules, patterns and cancer incidence factors. By carefully prepared mining data marts and removing irrelevant or redundant input variables, decision tree rules show the primary factors of cancer patients. RBF predictive models reveal more detail information for comparison of cancer patients with non-cancer people. BPN obviously reports the important cancer incidence factors. These results enable us to discover the primary factors and living habits of cancer patients, their different characteristics compared with non-cancer people, further indicating what are the most related factors contributing to cancer incidences.

5   Concluding Remarks

In applying data mining to medical and healthcare area, the special issue in [6] describes more detail of the mining results from variety of mining methods, where common medical databases are presented. This is a very interesting way to identifying the mined results. However, for a specific mining propose, the researchers have not described which algorithm is effective and which result (or part of results) is more useful or accurate compared to that generated with other algorithms.

In applying decision tree to medical data, our earlier work [19] was done with clustering and classification, where comparison between the cancer patient group and the non-cancer people could not be given. In addition, the critical cancer incidence factors were not acquired. The study with RBF has successfully compared the difference between the cancer patient group and non-cancer people. BPN is used to find significant cancer incidence factors. With applying RBF in factor identification, a case study of semiconductor yield forecasting can be found in [20]. The work of [9, 10] are applications of BPN in genome. However, these applications are based on single method for mining. Therefore, the mining results can be improved with multistrategy data mining. The integration of decision tree, RBF and BPN to do mining is an effective way to discover rules, patterns and important factors.

Data mining is a very useful tool in the healthcare and medical area. Ideally, large amounts of data (e.g., the human genome data) are continuously collected. These data are then segmented, classified, and finally reduced suited for generating a predictive model. With an interpretable predictive model, significant factors of a predictive object can be uncovered. This paper has described an integrated mining method that includes multiple algorithms, and mining operations for efficiently obtaining results.

Acknowledgements

This work was supported in part by the Project (No.2004D006) from Hubei Provincial Department of Education, P. R. China.

References

1. S. L. Pomeroy et al. *Prediction of central nervous system embryonal tumour outcome based on gene expression. Nature*, 405:436–442, 2002.
2. Y. Kawamura and X. Zhang and A. Konagaya. *Inference of genetic network in cluster level. 18th AI Symposium of Japanese Society for Artificial Intelligence, SIG-J-A301-12P, 2003.*
3. R. Agrawal, T. Imielinski, and A. Swami. Database mining: A performance perspective. *IEEE Transactions on Knowledge and Data Engineering*, 5:914–925, 1993.
4. M.S. Chen, J. Han, and P.S. Yu. Data mining: An overview from a database perspective. *IEEE Transactions on Knowledge and Data Engineering*, 8:866–883, 1996.
5. Xiaolong Zhang. *Knowledge Acqusition and Revision with First Order Logic Induction.* PhD Thesis, Tokyo Institute of Technology, 1998.
6. Special Issue. Comparison and evaluation of KDD methods with common medical databases. *Journal of Japanese Society for Artificial Intelligence*, 15:750–790, 2000.
7. C. Apte, E. Grossman, E. Pednault, B. Rosen, F. Tipu, and B. White. Probablistic estimation based data mining for discovering insurance risks. Technical Report IBM Research Report RC-21483, T. J. Watson Research Center, IBM Research Division, Yorktown Heights, NY 10598, 1999.
8. Gedeon TD. Data mining of inputs: analysing magnitude and functional measures. *Int. J. Neural Syst*, 8:209–217, 1997.
9. Wu Cathy and S. Shivakumar. Back-propagation and counter-propagation neural networks for phylogenetic classification of ribosomal RNA sequences. *Nucleic Acids Research*, 22:4291–4299, 1994.

10. Wu Cathy, M. Berry, S. Shivakumar, and J. McLarty. Neural networks for full-scale protein sequence classification: Sequence encoding with singular value decomposition. *Machine Learning*, 21:177–193, 1994.
11. L. Breiman, J. Friedman amd R. Olshen, and C. Stone. *Classification and Regression Trees*. Belmont, CA: Wadsworth, 1984.
12. J.R. Quinlan. *C4.5: Programs for Machine Learning*. Morgan Kaufmann, 1993.
13. J.C. Shafer, R. Agrawal, and M. Mehta. SPRINT: A scalable parallel classifier for data mining. In *Proc. of the 22th Int'l Conference on Very Large Databases*, Bombay, India, 1996.
14. T. Poggio and F. Girosi. Networks for approximation and learning. *Proceedings of the IEEE*, 78:1481–1497, 1990.
15. Roderick J. A. Little and Donald B. Rubin. *Statistical analysis with missing data*. John Wiley & Sons, 1987.
16. Dempster A., Laird N., and Rubin D. Maximun likelihood from incomplete data via the EM algorithm. *J. Roy. Statist. Soc. B*, 39:1–38, 1977.
17. IBM Intelligent Miner for Data. *Using the Intelligent Miner for Data*. IBM Corp., Third Edition, 1998.
18. P. Cabena et al. *Discovering data mining*. Prentice Hall PTR, 1998.
19. X. Zhang and T. Narita. Discovering the primary factors of cancer from health and living habit questionaires. In S. Arikawa and K. Furukawa, editors, *Discovery Science: Second International Conference (DS'99)*. LNAI 1721 Springer, 1999.
20. Ashok N. Srivastava. Data mining for semiconductor yield forecasting. *Future Fab International*, 1999.

Author Index

Akutsu, Tatsuya   11

Bachimont, Bruno   34

Dardzińska, Agnieszka   255
Dong, Juzhen   210

Fujie, Hajime   312
Fujishima, Daisuke   152
Fujishima, Satoshi   303
Fujita, Yasuo   210
Fusamoto, Issey   152

Geamsakul, Warodom   126

Hamuro, Yukinobu   152
Hirano, Shoji   268

Ichise, Ryutaro   112
Iida, Akira   74
Ikeda, Takaya   152

Katoh, Naoki   152
Kitaguchi, Shinya   174
Kitamura, Yasuhiko   74

Matsumoto, Yuji   236
Matsumura, Naohiro   312
Morizet-Mahoudeaux, Pierre   34
Motoda, Hiroshi   1, 126
Murata, Hiroshi   59

Narita, Tetsuo   336
Nattee, Cholwich   92
Niitsuma, Hirotaka   287
Nishikoori, Katsumi   303
Numao, Masayuki   1, 92, 112

Ohara, Kouzou   126
Ohsaki, Miho   174
Ohsawa, Yukio   312
Ohshima, Muneaki   210
Okada, Takashi   92, 287
Okazaki, Naoaki   312
Okuno, Tomohiro   210
Onoda, Takashi   59

Park, Keunsik   74

Raś, Zbigniew W.   255

Saiura, Akio   312
Shimbo, Masashi   236
Sinthupinyo, Sukree   92
Suzuki, Einoshin   190

Takabayashi, Katsuhiko   126, 190
Takahashi, Yoshimasa   303
Tsumoto, Shusaku   1, 268

Washio, Takashi   126, 152

Yada, Katsutoshi   152
Yamada, Seiji   59
Yamada, Yuu   190
Yamaguchi, Takahira   1, 174
Yamakawa, Masumi   287
Yamasaki, Takahiro   236
Yokoi, Hideto   126, 174, 190, 210
Yoshida, Tetsuya   126

Zhang, Xiaolong   336
Zhong, Ning   210

Lecture Notes in Artificial Intelligence (LNAI)

Vol. 3518: T.B. Ho, D. Cheung, H. Li (Eds.), Advances in Knowledge Discovery and Data Mining. XXI, 864 pages. 2005.

Vol. 3508: P. Bresciani, P. Giorgini, B. Henderson-Sellers, G. Low, M. Winikoff (Eds.), Agent-Oriented Information Systems II. X, 227 pages. 2005.

Vol. 3505: V. Gorodetsky, J. Liu, V. A. Skormin (Eds.), Autonomous Intelligent Systems: Agents and Data Mining. XIII, 303 pages. 2005.

Vol. 3501: B. Kégl, G. Lapalme (Eds.), Advances in Artificial Intelligence. XV, 458 pages. 2005.

Vol. 3492: P. Blache, E. Stabler, J. Busquets, R. Moot (Eds.), Logical Aspects of Computational Linguistics. X, 363 pages. 2005.

Vol. 3488: M.-S. Hacid, N.V. Murray, Z.W. Raś, S. Tsumoto (Eds.), Foundations of Intelligent Systems. XIII, 700 pages. 2005.

Vol. 3464: S.A. Brueckner, G.D.M. Serugendo, A. Karageorgos, R. Nagpal (Eds.), Engineering Self-Organising Systems. XIII, 299 pages. 2005.

Vol. 3452: F. Baader, A. Voronkov (Eds.), Logic for Programming, Artificial Intelligence, and Reasoning. XI, 562 pages. 2005.

Vol. 3438: H. Christiansen, P.R. Skadhauge, J. Villadsen (Eds.), Constraint Solving and Language Processing. VIII, 205 pages. 2005.

Vol. 3430: S. Tsumoto, T. Yamaguchi, M. Numao, H. Motoda (Eds.), Active Mining. XII, 349 pages. 2005.

Vol. 3419: B. Faltings, A. Petcu, F. Fages, F. Rossi (Eds.), Constraint Satisfaction and Constraint Logic Programming. X, 217 pages. 2005.

Vol. 3416: M. Böhlen, J. Gamper, W. Polasek, M.A. Wimmer (Eds.), E-Government: Towards Electronic Democracy. XIII, 311 pages. 2005.

Vol. 3415: P. Davidsson, B. Logan, K. Takadama (Eds.), Multi-Agent and Multi-Agent-Based Simulation. X, 265 pages. 2005.

Vol. 3403: B. Ganter, R. Godin (Eds.), Formal Concept Analysis. XI, 419 pages. 2005.

Vol. 3398: D.-K. Baik (Ed.), Systems Modeling and Simulation: Theory and Applications. XIV, 733 pages. 2005.

Vol. 3397: T.G. Kim (Ed.), Artificial Intelligence and Simulation. XV, 711 pages. 2005.

Vol. 3396: R.M. van Eijk, M.-P. Huget, F. Dignum (Eds.), Agent Communication. X, 261 pages. 2005.

Vol. 3394: D. Kudenko, D. Kazakov, E. Alonso (Eds.), Adaptive Agents and Multi-Agent Systems II. VIII, 313 pages. 2005.

Vol. 3392: D. Seipel, M. Hanus, U. Geske, O. Bartenstein (Eds.), Applications of Declarative Programming and Knowledge Management. X, 309 pages. 2005.

Vol. 3374: D. Weyns, H.V.D. Parunak, F. Michel (Eds.), Environments for Multi-Agent Systems. X, 279 pages. 2005.

Vol. 3371: M.W. Barley, N. Kasabov (Eds.), Intelligent Agents and Multi-Agent Systems. X, 329 pages. 2005.

Vol. 3369: V.R. Benjamins, P. Casanovas, J. Breuker, A. Gangemi (Eds.), Law and the Semantic Web. XII, 249 pages. 2005.

Vol. 3366: I. Rahwan, P. Moraitis, C. Reed (Eds.), Argumentation in Multi-Agent Systems. XII, 263 pages. 2005.

Vol. 3359: G. Grieser, Y. Tanaka (Eds.), Intuitive Human Interfaces for Organizing and Accessing Intellectual Assets. XIV, 257 pages. 2005.

Vol. 3346: R.H. Bordini, M. Dastani, J. Dix, A.E.F. Seghrouchni (Eds.), Programming Multi-Agent Systems. XIV, 249 pages. 2005.

Vol. 3345: Y. Cai (Ed.), Ambient Intelligence for Scientific Discovery. XII, 311 pages. 2005.

Vol. 3343: C. Freksa, M. Knauff, B. Krieg-Brückner, B. Nebel, T. Barkowsky (Eds.), Spatial Cognition IV. XIII, 519 pages. 2005.

Vol. 3339: G.I. Webb, X. Yu (Eds.), AI 2004: Advances in Artificial Intelligence. XXII, 1272 pages. 2004.

Vol. 3336: D. Karagiannis, U. Reimer (Eds.), Practical Aspects of Knowledge Management. X, 523 pages. 2004.

Vol. 3327: Y. Shi, W. Xu, Z. Chen (Eds.), Data Mining and Knowledge Management. XIII, 263 pages. 2005.

Vol. 3315: C. Lemaître, C.A. Reyes, J.A. González (Eds.), Advances in Artificial Intelligence – IBERAMIA 2004. XX, 987 pages. 2004.

Vol. 3303: J.A. López, E. Benfenati, W. Dubitzky (Eds.), Knowledge Exploration in Life Science Informatics. X, 249 pages. 2004.

Vol. 3301: G. Kern-Isberner, W. Rödder, F. Kulmann (Eds.), Conditionals, Information, and Inference. XII, 219 pages. 2005.

Vol. 3276: D. Nardi, M. Riedmiller, C. Sammut, J. Santos-Victor (Eds.), RoboCup 2004: Robot Soccer World Cup VIII. XVIII, 678 pages. 2005.

Vol. 3275: P. Perner (Ed.), Advances in Data Mining. VIII, 173 pages. 2004.

Vol. 3265: R.E. Frederking, K.B. Taylor (Eds.), Machine Translation: From Real Users to Research. XI, 392 pages. 2004.

Vol. 3264: G. Paliouras, Y. Sakakibara (Eds.), Grammatical Inference: Algorithms and Applications. XI, 291 pages. 2004.

Vol. 3259: J. Dix, J. Leite (Eds.), Computational Logic in Multi-Agent Systems. XII, 251 pages. 2004.

Vol. 3257: E. Motta, N.R. Shadbolt, A. Stutt, N. Gibbins (Eds.), Engineering Knowledge in the Age of the Semantic Web. XVII, 517 pages. 2004.

Vol. 3249: B. Buchberger, J.A. Campbell (Eds.), Artificial Intelligence and Symbolic Computation. X, 285 pages. 2004.

Vol. 3248: K.-Y. Su, J. Tsujii, J.-H. Lee, O.Y. Kwong (Eds.), Natural Language Processing – IJCNLP 2004. XVIII, 817 pages. 2005.

Vol. 3245: E. Suzuki, S. Arikawa (Eds.), Discovery Science. XIV, 430 pages. 2004.

Vol. 3244: S. Ben-David, J. Case, A. Maruoka (Eds.), Algorithmic Learning Theory. XIV, 505 pages. 2004.

Vol. 3238: S. Biundo, T. Frühwirth, G. Palm (Eds.), KI 2004: Advances in Artificial Intelligence. XI, 467 pages. 2004.

Vol. 3230: J.L. Vicedo, P. Martínez-Barco, R. Muñoz, M. Saiz Noeda (Eds.), Advances in Natural Language Processing. XII, 488 pages. 2004.

Vol. 3229: J.J. Alferes, J. Leite (Eds.), Logics in Artificial Intelligence. XIV, 744 pages. 2004.

Vol. 3228: M.G. Hinchey, J.L. Rash, W.F. Truszkowski, C.A. Rouff (Eds.), Formal Approaches to Agent-Based Systems. VIII, 290 pages. 2004.

Vol. 3215: M.G.. Negoita, R.J. Howlett, L.C. Jain (Eds.), Knowledge-Based Intelligent Information and Engineering Systems, Part III. LVII, 906 pages. 2004.

Vol. 3214: M.G.. Negoita, R.J. Howlett, L.C. Jain (Eds.), Knowledge-Based Intelligent Information and Engineering Systems, Part II. LVIII, 1302 pages. 2004.

Vol. 3213: M.G.. Negoita, R.J. Howlett, L.C. Jain (Eds.), Knowledge-Based Intelligent Information and Engineering Systems, Part I. LVIII, 1280 pages. 2004.

Vol. 3209: B. Berendt, A. Hotho, D. Mladenic, M. van Someren, M. Spiliopoulou, G. Stumme (Eds.), Web Mining: From Web to Semantic Web. IX, 201 pages. 2004.

Vol. 3206: P. Sojka, I. Kopecek, K. Pala (Eds.), Text, Speech and Dialogue. XIII, 667 pages. 2004.

Vol. 3202: J.-F. Boulicaut, F. Esposito, F. Giannotti, D. Pedreschi (Eds.), Knowledge Discovery in Databases: PKDD 2004. XIX, 560 pages. 2004.

Vol. 3201: J.-F. Boulicaut, F. Esposito, F. Giannotti, D. Pedreschi (Eds.), Machine Learning: ECML 2004. XVIII, 580 pages. 2004.

Vol. 3194: R. Camacho, R. King, A. Srinivasan (Eds.), Inductive Logic Programming. XI, 361 pages. 2004.

Vol. 3192: C. Bussler, D. Fensel (Eds.), Artificial Intelligence: Methodology, Systems, and Applications. XIII, 522 pages. 2004.

Vol. 3191: M. Klusch, S. Ossowski, V. Kashyap, R. Unland (Eds.), Cooperative Information Agents VIII. XI, 303 pages. 2004.

Vol. 3187: G. Lindemann, J. Denzinger, I.J. Timm, R. Unland (Eds.), Multiagent System Technologies. XIII, 341 pages. 2004.

Vol. 3176: O. Bousquet, U. von Luxburg, G. Rätsch (Eds.), Advanced Lectures on Machine Learning. IX, 241 pages. 2004.

Vol. 3171: A.L.C. Bazzan, S. Labidi (Eds.), Advances in Artificial Intelligence – SBIA 2004. XVII, 548 pages. 2004.

Vol. 3159: U. Visser, Intelligent Information Integration for the Semantic Web. XIV, 150 pages. 2004.

Vol. 3157: C. Zhang, H. W. Guesgen, W.K. Yeap (Eds.), PRICAI 2004: Trends in Artificial Intelligence. XX, 1023 pages. 2004.

Vol. 3155: P. Funk, P.A. González Calero (Eds.), Advances in Case-Based Reasoning. XIII, 822 pages. 2004.

Vol. 3139: F. Iida, R. Pfeifer, L. Steels, Y. Kuniyoshi (Eds.), Embodied Artificial Intelligence. IX, 331 pages. 2004.

Vol. 3131: V. Torra, Y. Narukawa (Eds.), Modeling Decisions for Artificial Intelligence. XI, 327 pages. 2004.

Vol. 3127: K.E. Wolff, H.D. Pfeiffer, H.S. Delugach (Eds.), Conceptual Structures at Work. XI, 403 pages. 2004.

Vol. 3123: A. Belz, R. Evans, P. Piwek (Eds.), Natural Language Generation. X, 219 pages. 2004.

Vol. 3120: J. Shawe-Taylor, Y. Singer (Eds.), Learning Theory. X, 648 pages. 2004.

Vol. 3097: D. Basin, M. Rusinowitch (Eds.), Automated Reasoning. XII, 493 pages. 2004.

Vol. 3071: A. Omicini, P. Petta, J. Pitt (Eds.), Engineering Societies in the Agents World. XIII, 409 pages. 2004.

Vol. 3070: L. Rutkowski, J. Siekmann, R. Tadeusiewicz, L.A. Zadeh (Eds.), Artificial Intelligence and Soft Computing - ICAISC 2004. XXV, 1208 pages. 2004.

Vol. 3068: E. André, L. Dybkjær, W. Minker, P. Heisterkamp (Eds.), Affective Dialogue Systems. XII, 324 pages. 2004.

Vol. 3067: M. Dastani, J. Dix, A. El Fallah-Seghrouchni (Eds.), Programming Multi-Agent Systems. X, 221 pages. 2004.

Vol. 3066: S. Tsumoto, R. Słowiński, J. Komorowski, J.W. Grzymała-Busse (Eds.), Rough Sets and Current Trends in Computing. XX, 853 pages. 2004.

Vol. 3065: A. Lomuscio, D. Nute (Eds.), Deontic Logic in Computer Science. X, 275 pages. 2004.

Vol. 3060: A.Y. Tawfik, S.D. Goodwin (Eds.), Advances in Artificial Intelligence. XIII, 582 pages. 2004.

Vol. 3056: H. Dai, R. Srikant, C. Zhang (Eds.), Advances in Knowledge Discovery and Data Mining. XIX, 713 pages. 2004.

Vol. 3055: H. Christiansen, M.-S. Hacid, T. Andreasen, H.L. Larsen (Eds.), Flexible Query Answering Systems. X, 500 pages. 2004.

Vol. 3048: P. Faratin, D.C. Parkes, J.A. Rodríguez-Aguilar, W.E. Walsh (Eds.), Agent-Mediated Electronic Commerce V. XI, 155 pages. 2004.

Vol. 3040: R. Conejo, M. Urretavizcaya, J.-L. Pérez-de-la-Cruz (Eds.), Current Topics in Artificial Intelligence. XIV, 689 pages. 2004.

Vol. 3035: M.A. Wimmer (Ed.), Knowledge Management in Electronic Government. XII, 326 pages. 2004.